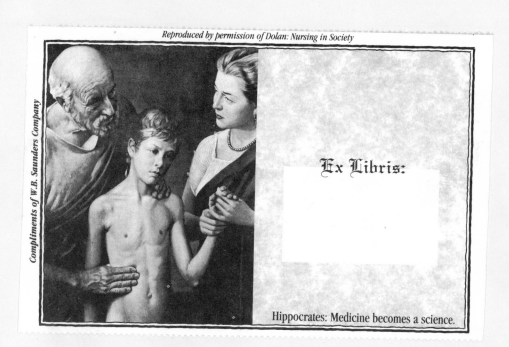

Compliments of W.B. Saunders Company

Ex Libris:

Hippocrates: Medicine becomes a science.

ATLAS OF
HUMAN HISTOLOGY

MARIANO S. H. DI FIORE

*Associate Professor of Histology and Embryology, Faculty of Medical Sciences,
University of Buenos Aires and Head of the Laboratory of the
Juan A. Fernandez Hospital*

FOURTH EDITION

114 ORIGINAL COLOR PLATES
207 FIGURES

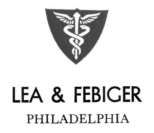

LEA & FEBIGER
PHILADELPHIA

ATLAS DE HISTOLOGIA NORMAL

Libreria "El Ateneo" Editorial

BUENOS AIRES-ARGENTINA

First Edition, 1957
Reprinted 1958, 1959, 1960, 1961, 1962

Second Edition, 1963
Reprinted 1964, 1965

Third Edition, 1967
Reprinted 1968, 1969, 1970, 1971, 1972, 1973

Fourth Edition, 1974
Reprinted 1975, 1976, 1977, 1978, 1979

ISBN 0–8121–0421–8

Library of Congress Catalog Card Number: 72–79345
Printed in the United States of America

FOREWORD TO THE FOURTH EDITION

The medical student is frequently left on his own to pursue his studies. In some schools the instructor purposely employs such a procedure to develop initiative and self-reliance in the student. In other schools the marked growth in medical education has produced a shortage of personnel to meet instructional needs in the basic medical sciences. It is with these thoughts in mind that Dr. di Fiore's ATLAS OF HUMAN HISTOLOGY is presented by the publisher as a right hand to the student receiving initial instruction in histology and to the instructor as an aid in conserving his time.

The illustrations are designed as composite drawings of what may be seen by the student only after a study of several slides. This is done for the pure didactic purpose of reducing the number of illustrations necessary for study, and to curtail the cost of publication. The illustrations are designed to cover the *principles of histology* clearly and concisely. They are not intended to present the student with a bewildering array of every last item known to the professional histologist.

It is felt that Dr. di Fiore's ATLAS offers an admirable reference work for the student. It is not intended to supplant a textbook of histology but rather to stand as a supplementary book.

The earlier editions of Dr. di Fiore's ATLAS met with unusual success. From the many students and faculty members who use the book have come excellent suggestions. This fourth edition has been revised by Dr. Ida G. Schmidt of the Department of Anatomy, University of Alabama Medical Center, Birmingham. She has utilized many of the suggestions in rewriting much of the text and in improving the illustrations. Under her direction the ATLAS has been enhanced by 27 new plates and numerous changes and additions to many of the plates previously used. This fourth edition, therefore, should be even more useful to its audience than heretofore.

THE PUBLISHER

CONTENTS

FOREWORD TO THE FOURTH EDITION   3

INDEX OF PLATES   8

ABBREVIATIONS ON PLATES   13

EPITHELIUM

    Simple Squamous Epithelium   14
    Simple Columnar Epithelium   16
    Stratified Squamous Epithelium   18
    Pseudostratified Columnar Ciliated Epithelium; Transitional
       Epithelium   20
    Simple Branched Tubular Gland (Diagram)   22
    Compound Tubuloalveolar Gland (Diagram)   24
    Compound Alveolar Gland (Diagram)   26

CONNECTIVE TISSUES

    Loose Connective Tissue: Spread   28
    Loose and Dense Irregular Connective Tissue   30
    Dense Regular Connective Tissue   32
    Adipose Tissue; Embryonic Connective Tissue   34
    Cartilage   36
    Bone, Mature   40
       Compact (Dried)   40
       Cancellous   42
    Bone, Developing   42
       Intramembranous Formation   42
       Intracartilaginous Formation   44
       Development of Haversian Systems   48

BLOOD

    Peripheral Blood: Formed Elements   50
    Bone Marrow   54
       Development of Myeloid Elements   56

MUSCLE TISSUE

    Smooth and Skeletal Muscle Fibers   58
    Skeletal, Smooth and Cardiac Muscle   60

NERVOUS TISSUE AND NERVOUS SYSTEM

    Neurons of the Spinal Cord   62
    Neuroglia   66

Nerve Fibers and Peripheral Nerves 68
Dorsal Root Ganglion 72
Sympathetic Trunk Ganglion 72
Spinal Cord: Cervical 74
Spinal Cord: Thoracic 76
Cerebellum 78
Cerebral Cortex 80

CARDIOVASCULAR SYSTEM

Blood and Lymphatic Vessels 82
Blood Vessels, Neurovascular Bundle 84
Heart: Atrium, Ventricle, Mitral Valve 86
Heart: Pulmonary Artery, Semilunar Valve, Ventricle; Purkinje Fibers 88

LYMPHATIC ORGANS

Lymph Node 90
Tonsil 94
Thymus 96
Spleen 98

INTEGUMENT

Skin 100
Scalp; Hair Follicle; Sebaceous Gland 102
Sweat Gland (Diagram) 104

DIGESTIVE SYSTEM

Lip 106
Tongue 108
Tooth, Dried 112
Tooth, Developing 114
Parotid Gland 116
Submandibular Gland 118
Sublingual Gland 120
Esophagus 122
Cardia 128
Stomach, Fundus or Body 130
Stomach, Pyloric 136
Pylorus-Duodenum 138
Small Intestine 140
Large Intestine 146
Appendix 148
Rectum 150
Anal Canal 152
Liver 154
Gall Bladder 160
Pancreas 162

RESPIRATORY SYSTEM

Larynx 164
Trachea 166
Lung 168

Excretory System

    Kidney   172
    Ureter   178
    Bladder   180

Endocrines

    Hypophysis   182
    Thyroid   186
    Thyroid and Parathyroid   188
    Suprarenal   190

Male Reproductive System

    Testis, Rete, Ductuli Efferentes   192
    Testis: Seminiferous Tubules   194
    Ductus Epididymidis   196
    Ductus Deferens   198
    Seminal Vesicle   198
    Prostate   200
    Penis   202

Female Reproductive System

    Ovary   204
    Uterine Tube   212
    Uterus   214
    Placenta   220
    Cervix   222
    Vagina   224
    Vagina: Exfoliate Cytology   226
    Mammary Gland   228

Organs of Special Sense and Associated Structures

    Eyelid   232
    Lacrimal Gland and Cornea   234
    Eye: Panoramic View   236
    Eye: Retina   238
    Ear   241

Index   243

INDEX OF PLATES

TISSUES

EPITHELIAL TISSUE

Plate

1. Fig. 1. Dissociated squamous epithelial cells.
   Fig. 2. Mesothelium of the peritoneum (surface view).
   Fig. 3. Mesothelium of the peritoneum (transverse section).
2. Fig. 1. Simple columnar epithelial tissue.
   Fig. 2. Simple columnar epithelium with striated border.
3. Fig. 1. Stratified squamous epithelium (transverse section).
   Fig. 2. Stratified squamous epithelium (tangential section).
4. Fig. 1. Pseudostratified columnar ciliated epithelium.
   Fig. 2. Transitional epithelium.
5. Simple branched tubular gland (diagram).
6. Compound tubuloalveolar gland (diagram).
7. Compound alveolar gland (diagram).

CONNECTIVE TISSUE

8. Fig. 1. Loose connective tissue: spread.
   Fig. 2. Cells of loose connective tissue in sections.
9. Fig. 1. Loose connective tissue.
   Fig. 2. Dense irregularly arranged connective tissue.
10. Fig. 1. Dense regular connective tissue: tendon (longitudinal section).
    Fig. 2. Dense regular connective tissue: tendon (transverse section).
11. Fig. 1. Dense irregular and loose connective tissue (elastic stain).
    Fig. 2. Adipose tissue.
    Fig. 3. Embryonic connective tissue.
12. Fig. 1. Hyaline cartilage (fresh preparation).
    Fig. 2. Hyaline cartilage (stained).
    Fig. 3. Hyaline cartilage of the trachea.
13. Fig. 1. Fibrous cartilage: intervertebral disc.
    Fig. 2. Elastic cartilage: epiglottic cartilage.
14. Fig. 1. Compact bone, dried: diaphysis of the tibia (transverse section).
    Fig. 2. Compact bone, dried: diaphysis of the tibia (longitudinal section).
15. Fig. 1. Cancellous bone: adult sternum (transverse section).
    Fig. 2. Intramembranous bone formation: mandible of a fetus of five months.
16. Intracartilaginous bone formation: developing metacarpal bone (panoramic view, longitudinal section).
17. Intracartilaginous bone formation (sectional view).
18. Formation of bone: development of Haversian systems (transverse section).
19. Peripheral blood smear.
20. Fig. 1. Supravital stain: blood cells.
    Fig. 2. Pappenheim's and Celani's stains: blood smears.
21. Fig. 1. Hemopoietic bone marrow (section).
    Fig. 2. Bone marrow of a rabbit, India ink preparation.
22. Bone marrow: smear.

Plate

MUSCLE TISSUE

23. Fig. 1. Smooth muscle fibers.
    Fig. 2. Skeletal muscle (dissociated).
24. Fig. 1. Skeletal muscle: muscles of the tongue.
    Fig. 2. Smooth muscle: muscle layer of the intestine.
    Fig. 3. Cardiac muscle: myocardium.
    Fig. 4. Skeletal muscle (longitudinal section).
    Fig. 5. Cardiac muscle (longitudinal section).

NERVOUS TISSUE AND NERVOUS SYSTEM

25. Fig. 1. Gray matter: anterior horn of the spinal cord. Nissl's method.
    Fig. 2. Gray matter: anterior horn of the spinal cord. Cajal's method.
26. Fig. 1. Gray matter: anterior horn of the spinal cord. Golgi's method.
    Fig. 2. Gray matter: anterior horn of the spinal cord. Weigert-Pal's method.
27. Fig. 1. Fibrous astrocytes of the brain.
    Fig. 2. Oligodendrocytes of the brain.
    Fig. 3. Microglia of the brain.
28. Fig. 1. Myelinated nerve fibers (dissociated).
    Fig. 2. Nerve (transverse section).
29. Fig. 1. Nerve (panoramic view, longitudinal section). Hematoxylin-eosin.
    Fig. 2. Nerve, longitudinal section. Hematoxylin-eosin.
    Fig. 3. Nerve, transverse section. Hematoxylin-eosin.
    Fig. 4. Nerve, longitudinal section. Protargol and aniline blue.
    Fig. 5. Nerve, transverse section. Protargol and aniline blue.
    Fig. 6. Nerve, transverse section. Mallory-Azan.
30. Fig. 1. Dorsal root ganglion: panoramic view.
    Fig. 2. Section of a dorsal root ganglion.
    Fig. 3. Section of a sympathetic trunk ganglion.
31. Fig. 1. Spinal cord: cervical region (panoramic view).
    Fig. 2. Spinal cord: anterior (gray) horn and adjacent white matter.
32. Fig. 1. Spinal cord: mid-thoracic region (panoramic view).
    Fig. 2. Nerve cells of some typical regions of the cord.
33. Fig. 1. Cerebellum: sectional view.
    Fig. 2. Cerebellum: cortex.
34. Fig. 1. Cerebral cortex: section.
    Fig. 2. Cerebral cortex: central area of cortex.

ORGANS

35. Fig. 1. Blood and lymphatic vessels.
    Fig. 2. Large vein: portal vein (transverse section).
36. Fig. 1. Neurovascular bundle (transverse section).
    Fig. 2. Large artery: aorta (transverse section).
37. Heart: Left atrium and ventricle (panoramic view, longitudinal section).
38. Fig. 1. Heart: pulmonary artery, pulmonary valve, right ventricle (panoramic view, longitudinal section).
    Fig. 2. Heart: Purkinje fibers (hematoxylin-eosin).
    Fig. 3. Heart: Purkinje fibers (Mallory-Azan).
39. Lymph node (panoramic view).
40. Fig. 1. Lymph node (sectional view).
    Fig. 2. Lymph node (reticular fiber stain).
41. Fig. 1. Lymph node: proliferation of lymphocytes.
    Fig. 2. Palatine tonsil.

Plate

42. Fig. 1. Thymus (panoramic view).
    Fig. 2. Thymus (sectional view).
43. Fig. 1. Spleen (panoramic view).
    Fig. 2. Spleen: red and white pulp.
    Fig. 3. Development of lymphocytes and related cells.
44. Fig. 1. Integument: skin, general body surface (Cajal's trichrome stain).
    Fig. 2. Skin, palm: superficial layers.
45. Fig. 1. Skin: scalp.
    Fig. 2. Skin: a sebaceous gland and adjacent hair follicle.
    Fig. 3. Skin: the bulb of a hair follicle and adjacent sweat glands.
46. Sweat gland (diagram).
47. Lip (longitudinal section).
48. Tongue: apex (panoramic view, longitudinal section).
49. Fig. 1. Tongue: circumvallate papilla (vertical section).
    Fig. 2. Posterior tongue (longitudinal section).
50. Fig. 1. Dried tooth (panoramic view, longitudinal section).
    Fig. 2. Dried tooth: layers of the crown.
    Fig. 3. Dried tooth: layers of the root.
51. Fig. 1. Developing tooth (panoramic view).
    Fig. 2. Developing tooth (sectional view).
52. Salivary gland: parotid.
53. Salivary gland: submandibular.
54. Salivary gland: sublingual.
55. Upper esophagus: wall (transverse section).
56. Upper esophagus: mucosa and submucosa (transverse section).
57. Fig. 1. Upper esophagus (Mallory's stain).
    Fig. 2. Lower esophagus (Van Gieson's trichrome stain).
58. Cardia (longitudinal section).
59. Stomach: fundus or body (transverse section).
60. Stomach: mucosa of the fundus or body (transverse section).
61. Fig. 1. Stomach: superficial region of the mucosa of the fundus or body.
    Fig. 2. Stomach: deep region of the mucosa of the fundus or body.
62. Stomach: mucosa of the pyloric region.
63. Pyloric-duodenal junction (longitudinal section).
64. Small intestine: duodenum (longitudinal section).
65. Fig. 1. Small intestine: jejunum-ileum (transverse section).
    Fig. 2. Intestinal glands with Paneth cells.
    Fig. 3. Intestinal glands with argentaffin cells.
66. Fig. 1. Small intestine: ileum.
    Fig. 2. Small intestine: villi.
67. Large intestine: colon, wall (transverse section).
68. Appendix (panoramic view, transverse section).
69. Rectum (panoramic view, transverse section).
70. Anal canal (longitudinal section).
71. Liver lobule (panoramic view).
72. Fig. 1. Liver lobule (sectional view).
    Fig. 2. Liver: reticuloendothelium.
    Fig. 3. Liver: bile canaliculi.
73. Fig. 1. Mitochondria and fat droplets in liver cells (Altmann's stain).
    Fig. 2. Glycogen in liver cells (Best's carmine stain).
    Fig. 3. Reticular fibers in a hepatic lobule (Del Rio Hortega's stain).
74. Gall bladder.
75. Fig. 1. Pancreas (sectional view).
    Fig. 2. Pancreatic acini (special preparation).
    Fig. 3. Pancreatic islets (special preparation).
76. Larynx (frontal section).

Plate

77. Fig. 1. Trachea (panoramic view, transverse section).
    Fig. 2. Trachea (sectional view).
    Fig. 3. Trachea, elastic stain (sectional view).
78. Lung (panoramic view).
79. Fig. 1. Lung: secondary (lobar) bronchus.
    Fig. 2. Lung: bronchiole.
    Fig. 3. Lung: respiratory bronchiole.
    Fig. 4. Lung: alveolar walls.
80. Kidney: cortex and one pyramid (panoramic view).
81. Kidney: deep cortical area and outer medulla.
82. Fig. 1. Kidney medulla: papilla, transverse section.
    Fig. 2. Kidney medulla: papilla adjacent to a calyx (sectional view).
83. Fig. 1. Ureter (transverse section).
    Fig. 2. Ureter: a sector of the wall.
84. Fig. 1. Urinary bladder: wall.
    Fig. 2. Urinary bladder: mucosa.
85. Fig. 1. Hypophysis (pituitary gland): panoramic view, sagittal section.
    Fig. 2. Hypophysis (pituitary gland): sectional view.
86. Fig. 1. Hypophysis: pars distalis (Azan stain).
    Fig. 2. Hypophysis: cellular groups (Azan stain).
87. Fig. 1. Thyroid gland: lobules (sectional view).
    Fig. 2. Thyroid gland: follicles (sectional view).
88. Fig. 1. Thyroid and parathyroid glands.
    Fig. 2. Parathyroid gland.
89. Suprarenal gland.
90. Fig. 1. Testis.
    Fig. 2. Seminiferous tubules, straight tubules, rete testis and ductuli efferentes.
91. Testis: seminiferous tubules.
92. Fig. 1. Ductuli efferentes and transition to ductus epididymidis.
    Fig. 2. Ductus epididymidis.
93. Fig. 1. Ductus deferens (transverse section).
    Fig. 2. Seminal vesicle.
94. Fig. 1. Prostate gland with prostatic urethra.
    Fig. 2. Prostate gland (sectional view).
95. Penis (transverse section).
96. Ovary (panoramic view).
97. Fig. 1. Ovary: cortex, primary and growing follicles.
    Fig. 2. Ovary: wall of a mature vesicular follicle.
98. Ovary: corpora lutea and atretic follicles.
99. Fig. 1. Corpus luteum (panoramic view).
    Fig. 2. Corpus luteum (peripheral wall).
100. Fig. 1. Uterine tube: ampulla (panoramic view, transverse section).
     Fig. 2. Uterine tube: mucosal folds.
101. Uterus: follicular phase.
102. Uterus: progravid phase.
103. Uterus: menstrual phase.
104. Fig. 1. Placenta: five months' pregnancy.
     Fig. 2. Placenta: chorionic villi (placenta at five months).
     Fig. 3. Placenta: chorionic villi (placenta at term).
105. Cervix (longitudinal section).
106. Fig. 1. Vagina (longitudinal section).
     Fig. 2. Glycogen in human vaginal epithelium.
107. Vagina: exfoliate cytology (vaginal smears).
108. Fig. 1. Mammary gland, inactive.
     Fig. 2. Mammary gland during the first half of pregnancy.

Plate

109. Fig. 1. Mammary gland, seventh month of pregnancy.
     Fig. 2. Mammary gland during lactation.
110. Eyelid (sagittal section).
111. Fig. 1. Lacrimal gland.
     Fig. 2. Cornea (transverse section).
112. Eye (sagittal section).
113. Fig. 1. Retina, choroid and sclera (panoramic view).
     Fig. 2. Layers of the retina and choroid.
114. Fig. 1. Inner ear: cochlea (vertical section).
     Fig. 2. Inner ear: cochlear duct.

ABBREVIATIONS ON PLATES

h.s. — horizontal section
l.s. — longitudinal section
o.s. — oblique section
tg.s. — tangential section
t.s. — transverse section
v.s. — vertical section

PLATE 1 (Fig. 1)

DISSOCIATED SQUAMOUS EPITHELIAL CELLS

Illustrated is a "fresh" preparation of epithelial cells obtained by scraping the superficial layers of the epithelium which lines the oral cavity. These superficial cells are squamous cells. They are seen as isolated cells (1, 6), or as sheets of cells (2). In the sheets, the cells remain firmly attached to each other.

In surface view, the squamous cells have the shape of irregular polygons (1, 6). Their cell membranes (plasma membranes) are distinct (3). Their cytoplasm is finely granular (4). The small rounded or oval nuclei (5) are usually centrally placed, but may be eccentric in position (8). In lateral view (7), the squamous cells are thin and tapered at their ends (spindle-shaped). The nuclei appear thin and rod-like.

PLATE 1 (Fig. 2)

SIMPLE SQUAMOUS EPITHELIUM: MESOTHELIUM OF THE PERITONEUM (SURFACE VIEW)

A piece of rabbit mesentery, treated with silver nitrate solution and exposed to light, has been dehydrated and mounted in balsam. Mesentery is covered with a simple squamous epithelium (mesothelium), seen here in surface view. Outlines of the squamous cells (1) are greatly accentuated and appear dark brown because of reduction of the silver. The thickened areas between some cells are probably desmosomes (4). Nuclei (3) are not stained but they occupy the clear oval or rounded areas within the light brown granular cytoplasm (2).

These squamous cells adhere tightly to each other and form a sheet a single layer in thickness, a simple squamous epithelium, sometimes called pavement epithelium because of its appearance in surface view.

PLATE 1 (Fig. 3)

SIMPLE SQUAMOUS EPITHELIUM: MESOTHELIUM OF THE PERITONEUM (TRANSVERSE SECTION)

Illustrated is a simple squamous epithelium, mesothelium, seen in transverse section as it covers the wall of the jejunum. The cells are spindle-shaped with prominent, oval nuclei (1). Cell boundaries are not seen distinctly but are indicated in the depressed areas (2) where the cells taper and join each other. A fine basement membrane is recognizable in places (3). In surface view, these cells look like those in Fig. 2.

Mesothelium and the layer of underlying loose connective tissue (4) form the serosa (peritoneum), the outermost layer of the wall of the jejunum; this is attached to the muscularis externa (6). In the connective tissue layer may be seen small blood vessels, which are lined by a simple squamous endothelium (5).

PLATE 1

EPITHELIAL TISSUE

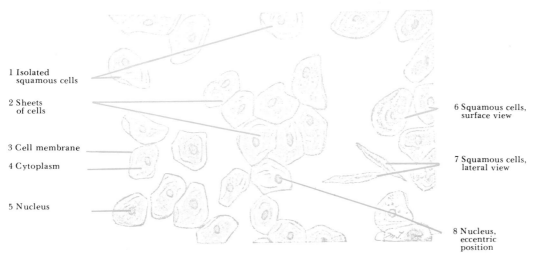

1 Isolated
squamous cells

2 Sheets
of cells

3 Cell membrane

4 Cytoplasm

5 Nucleus

6 Squamous cells,
surface view

7 Squamous cells,
lateral view

8 Nucleus,
eccentric
position

FIG. 1. *Dissociated squamous epithelial cells.*

Observed in the fresh state. 110×.

2 Cytoplasm

3 Nuclei

4 Desmosomes

1 Cell membranes

FIG. 2. *Mesothelium of the peritoneum.*

Stain: silver nitrate. 230×.

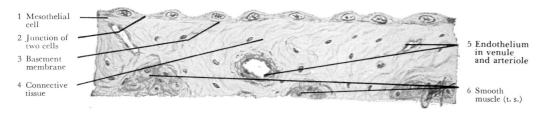

1 Mesothelial
cell

2 Junction of
two cells

3 Basement
membrane

4 Connective
tissue

5 Endothelium
in venule
and arteriole

6 Smooth
muscle (t. s.)

FIG. 3. *Simple squamous epithelium (transverse section).*

Stain: hematoxylin-eosin. 500×.

PLATE 2 (Fig. 1)

SIMPLE COLUMNAR EPITHELIAL TISSUE

A simple columnar epithelium which lines the stomach is illustrated.

Tall columnar cells (2) are arranged in a single row. The ovoid nuclei (7), oriented perpendicularly in the cells, are in the basal region. A thin basement membrane (3), scarcely visible in this preparation, separates the epithelium from the underlying zone of connective tissue (4, 10) which is the lamina propria of the gastric mucosa. Small blood vessels (5) lined with endothelium are seen in the connective tissue.

In some areas the epithelium has been sectioned transversely or obliquely. Where this occurs close to the free surface, the cut ends of the apices of the cells are seen and have the appearance of a mosaic of enucleated polygonal cells (1). Where the plane of section passes through the basal ends of the cells, the nuclei are cut transversely (6), resembling somewhat a stratified epithelium.

These columnar cells are mucus-secreting columnar cells. The light appearance of the cytoplasm is due to solution of mucigen droplets in section preparation. Mucigen droplets had filled the supranuclear or apical portions of the cells (9). The more granular cytoplasm has been displaced basally (8) and stains more deeply with eosin (acidophilic).

Examples of other columnar epithelia may be seen as the lining of the gall bladder (Plate 74: 14); in some of the ducts of salivary glands (Plate 52: 6, 14, IV; Plate 53: 1, 7, III); in bile ducts of the liver (Plate 72, Fig. 1: 6, 13); and in interlobular ducts of the pancreas (Plate 75, Fig. 1: 19, III).

A simple cuboidal epithelium is illustrated in the smallest ducts of the pancreas (Plate 75, Fig. 1: 1, 5, 20) and in the thyroid gland (Plate 87, Fig. 1: 6, and Fig. 2: 2).

PLATE 2 (Fig. 2)

SIMPLE COLUMNAR EPITHELIUM: CELLS WITH STRIATED BORDERS AND GOBLET CELLS

Free ends of intestinal villi (1) illustrate simple columnar epithelium with two types of cells: columnar cells with a striated border (2, 14) and goblet cells (8, 12). The striated border (13) is seen as a bright red membrane with faint vertical striations (microvilli) on the free margin of the columnar cells. In an area of contiguous cells, the striated border appears continuous. Cytoplasm of these cells is finely granular; the oval nuclei are in the basal portions of the cells.

Goblet cells (8, 12) are interspersed among the striated-bordered cells. In section preparation, mucigen was removed, thus the goblet appears clear or only faintly stained (12). The goblet occupies the apical or supranuclear portion of the cell (8); nucleus and cytoplasm are displaced basally (8).

The epithelium at the tip of the villus in the lower center of the figure has been sectioned obliquely. The apical parts of the columnar cells appear as a mosaic (7) of enucleated cells, and the basal parts, where the section passes through nuclei, appear stratified (7).

The basement membrane (5) is slightly more visible than in Fig. 1. In the connective tissue (10) underlying the epithelium may be seen a lymphatic vessel (3) and capillaries (9) lined with endothelium, and smooth muscle fibers (4, 11) as single fibers or in small groups.

Other examples of cells with striated borders and goblet cells may be seen in a section of jejunum-ileum (Plate 65, Fig. 2: 1, 2 and unlabeled in Fig. 3, and at a low magnification in Fig 1: 11).

—16—

PLATE 2

EPITHELIAL TISSUE

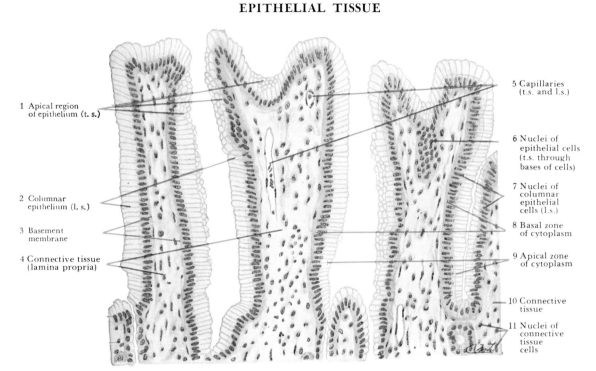

1 Apical region of epithelium (t. s.)

2 Columnar epithelium (l. s.)

3 Basement membrane

4 Connective tissue (lamina propria)

5 Capillaries (t.s. and l.s.)

6 Nuclei of epithelial cells (t.s. through bases of cells)

7 Nuclei of columnar epithelial cells (l.s.)

8 Basal zone of cytoplasm

9 Apical zone of cytoplasm

10 Connective tissue

11 Nuclei of connective tissue cells

FIG. 1. *Simple columnar epithelial tissue.*
Stain: hematoxylin-eosin. 250×.

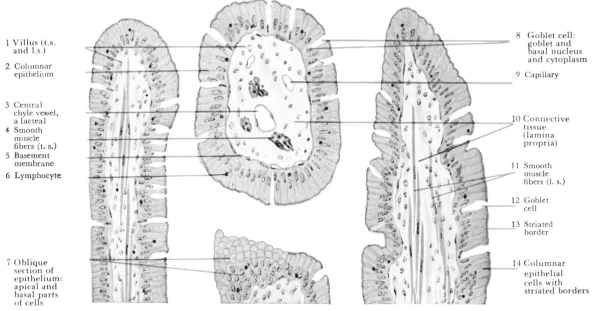

1 Villus (t.s. and l.s.)

2 Columnar epithelium

3 Central chyle vessel, a lacteal

4 Smooth muscle fibers (t. s.)

5 Basement membrane

6 Lymphocyte

7 Oblique section of epithelium: apical and basal parts of cells

8 Goblet cell: goblet and basal nucleus and cytoplasm

9 Capillary

10 Connective tissue (lamina propria)

11 Smooth muscle fibers (l. s.)

12 Goblet cell

13 Striated border

14 Columnar epithelial cells with striated borders

FIG. 2. *Simple columnar epithelial tissue.*
Stain: hematoxylin-eosin. 250×.

PLATE 3 (Fig. 1)

STRATIFIED SQUAMOUS EPITHELIUM (TRANSVERSE SECTION)

Stratified squamous epithelium is composed of numerous superimposed layers of cells having a characteristic structure and arrangement. The thickness of the epithelium varies in its different locations, and some resultant modifications may occur.

The epithelium illustrated (1) is an example of a moist epithelium such as lines the esophagus. The cells in the basal or deepest layer are columnar or cylindrical (5) with finely granular cytoplasm and an oval nucleus, rich in chromatin, which occupies most of the cell.

Cells of the intermediate layers are polyhedral (4) with rounded or oval nuclei. Cell membranes become more visible. Mitosis (7) occurs in the deeper layers as well as in the basal columnar cells.

Above the polyhedral cells are several rows of squamous cells (3). Cells and nuclei become progressively flatter toward the free surface, and outlines of cells are more distinct.

A fine basement membrane (8), hardly visible, separates the epithelium (1) from the underlying connective tissue (2), the lamina propria. Papillae of connective tissue (12) indent the lower surface of the epithelium, giving it a characteristic wavy appearance. In the connective tissue are collagenous fibers (11), connective tissue cells, the fibroblasts (10) and small blood vessels (6, 9, 13, 14).

Other examples of moist stratified squamous epithelium may be seen on Plates 49, 55, 56, 105, and 106.

When stratified squamous epithelium is exposed to drying or much wear and tear, the stratum corneum becomes very thick and consists of many layers of non-nucleated cornified (keratinized) cells, as in the epidermis on Plate 44, Fig. 2.

An example of a thin, non-papillated stratified squamous epithelium may be seen in the cornea of the eye, Plate 111, Fig. 2. The lower surface is smooth, not indented by connective tissue papillae. This epithelium is only a few cell layers in thickness but shows the characteristic arrangement of basal columnar cells, polyhedral cells, and squamous cells.

PLATE 3 (Fig. 2)

STRATIFIED SQUAMOUS EPITHELIUM (TANGENTIAL SECTION)

A section has been made parallel to the surface of the epithelium, at the level of line a-a in Fig. 1. It passes through several epithelial downgrowths and their surrounding connective tissue papillae, both of which are therefore seen sectioned transversely.

In the connective tissue papillae (1, 5, 8) are seen fibers, fibroblasts (3), and capillaries (2, 4). Basal columnar cells of the epithelium (6) surround the papillae. Polyhedral cells (7) of the intermediate layers occupy the remaining area.

EPITHELIAL TISSUE

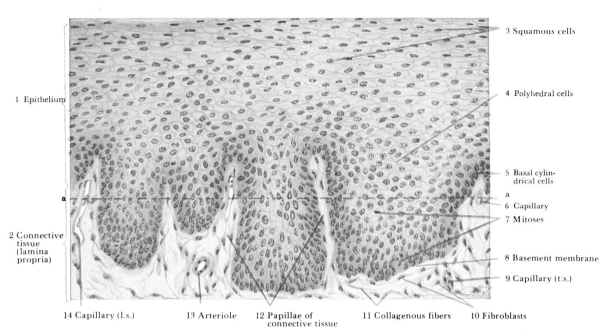

1 Epithelium

2 Connective
tissue
(lamina
propria)

a

3 Squamous cells

4 Polyhedral cells

5 Basal cylin-
drical cells

a

6 Capillary

7 Mitoses

8 Basement membrane

9 Capillary (t.s.)

14 Capillary (l.s.)   13 Arteriole   12 Papillae of   11 Collagenous fibers   10 Fibroblasts
connective tissue

F<small>IG</small>. 1. *Stratified squamous epithelium, taken from a transverse section of the esophagus.*
Stain: hematoxylin-eosin. 215×.

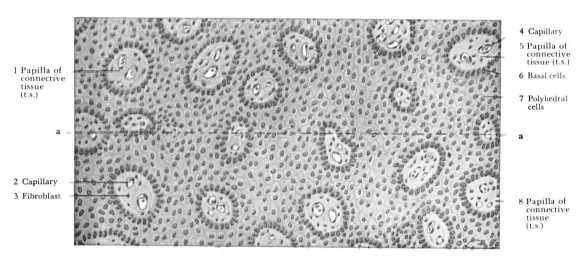

1 Papilla of
connective
tissue
(t.s.)

a

2 Capillary
3 Fibroblast

4 Capillary
5 Papilla of
connective
tissue (t.s.)

6 Basal cells

7 Polyhedral
cells

a

8 Papilla of
connective
tissue
(t.s.)

F<small>IG</small>. 2. *Stratified squamous epithelium, a tangential section from the esophagus.*
Stain: hematoxylin-eosin. 215×.

PLATE 4 (Fig. 1)

PSEUDOSTRATIFIED COLUMNAR CILIATED EPITHELIUM

The epithelium illustrated is from the upper respiratory passages. In this type of epithelium, the cells appear to be in several layers because their nuclei are situated at different levels. Serial sections show that all cells are in contact with the basement membrane, but the cells are of different shapes and heights and all do not reach the free surface. The epithelium is therefore not stratified but pseudostratified.

The more deeply placed nuclei are those belonging to short basal cells (7) and intermediate cells. The more superficial, more oval nuclei are those of columnar ciliated cells (5). Interspersed goblet cells (6) are also present. The small, round, heavily stained nuclei, without any visible surrounding cytoplasm, are those of lymphocytes (9) migrating from the connective tissue through the epithelium.

The short, motile cilia (3) are numerous and close together. Each cilium arises from a basal body (centriole) (4), located just beneath the surface membrane of the columnar cell. The basal bodies are lined up adjacent to each other and often give the appearance of a continuous membrane.

The basement membrane (8) is clearly seen, separating the epithelium (1) from the underlying connective tissue of the lamina propria (2, 11). It is thick and prominent, in contrast to the very thin basement membrane seen under other epithelia.

In the connective tissue (11) are seen its fibers and cells (fibroblasts), scattered lymphocytes and small blood vessels (10). Deeper down is glandular epithelium in the form of serous alveoli (12) and mucous alveoli (13).

Other examples of pseudostratified columnar ciliated epithelium are seen on Plate 76: 14, and Plate 77, Fig. 1: 13 and Fig. 2: 5, 6.

PLATE 4 (Fig. 2)

TRANSITIONAL EPITHELIUM

Transitional epithelium (1), found in the excretory passages, is a stratified epithelium composed of several layers of generally similar cells (4, 5, 6) which are more or less rounded, with rounded nuclei. This similarity of cells differentiates this epithelium from stratified squamous epithelium (which it may resemble somewhat at times) in which the cells of the various layers have different shapes.

This epithelium (1) has the ability to rearrange the number of cell layers according to whether it is in expanded or contracted condition. When contracted, the cells are generally rounded or may be somewhat cuboidal or columnar (4, 5, 6). When distended, the number of cell layers is reduced. The cells of the outer layers are then more elongated or flattened, but not so much that they appear typically squamous. (Compare this transitional epithelium with stratified squamous epithelium of the cornea, Plate 111, Fig. 2.)

The epithelium (1) rests on connective tissue (2, 7). A basement membrane is not distinct. The base of the epithelium is not indented by connective tissue papillae, thus it presents an even contour. Small blood vessels (8, 9, 10) are present in the connective tissue. Deeper, groups of smooth muscle fibers (11) indicate the beginning of a layer of smooth muscle.

Other examples of transitional epithelium are seen in both figures on Plates 83 and 84.

PLATE 4

EPITHELIAL TISSUE

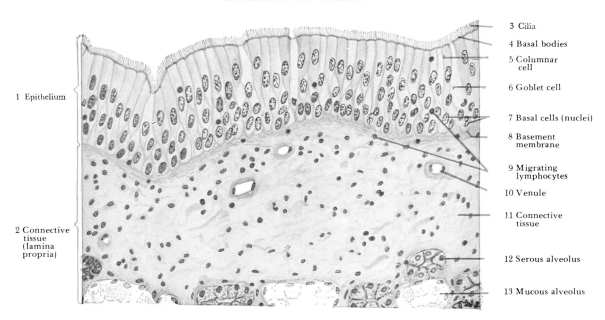

1 Epithelium

2 Connective
tissue
(lamina
propria)

3 Cilia

4 Basal bodies

5 Columnar
cell

6 Goblet cell

7 Basal cells (nuclei)

8 Basement
membrane

9 Migrating
lymphocytes

10 Venule

11 Connective
tissue

12 Serous alveolus

13 Mucous alveolus

Fig. 1. *Pseudostratified columnar ciliated epithelium.*
Stain: hematoxylin-eosin. 330×.

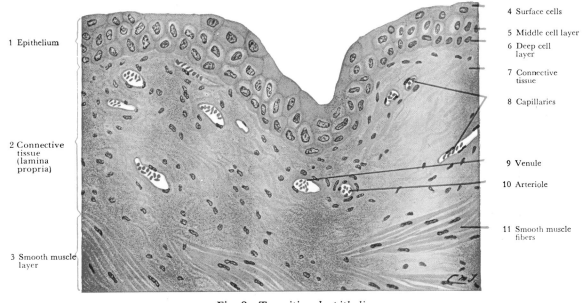

1 Epithelium

2 Connective
tissue
(lamina
propria)

3 Smooth muscle
layer

4 Surface cells

5 Middle cell layer

6 Deep cell
layer

7 Connective
tissue

8 Capillaries

9 Venule

10 Arteriole

11 Smooth muscle
fibers

Fig. 2. *Transitional epithelium.*
Stain: hematoxylin-eosin. 300×.

PLATE 5

SIMPLE BRANCHED TUBULAR GLAND (DIAGRAM)

In the center of the plate is a diagram of a simple branched tubular gland consisting of a long duct (2) and a branched terminal secreting portion of four tubules (3) arising from the basal portion of the duct. The diagram illustrates the general structure of a gland of this type, but there are variations in different glands.

The duct (2) is lined with simple low columnar epithelium whose oval nuclei are oriented vertically in the lower parts of the cells. The duct opens onto an epithelial surface of similar cells (1). Duct epithelium decreases in height, becoming lower columnar, toward the secreting part of the gland. The glandular epithelium (3) is low columnar or cuboidal. Nuclei are flattened at the bases of the cells, indicating that the cells are filled with secretion.

The diagram in the center also illustrates the appearance of sections resulting from cuts passing at different angles through various parts of the gland.

At A is a section taken at the level of the blue line a-a', which passes through the nuclear region of the surface epithelial cells in a plane parallel to the surface. In the center of the section is the orifice or opening of the gland with its wall of low columnar cells (A-1). Surrounding this are transverse sections of the surface epithelial cells (A-2).

B represents a sagittal section of the same gland along the vertical red line b-b', which extends through the entire length of the gland. At B-1, the cut passes through the surface epithelium and tangentially through the wall of the duct so that the lumen is not seen; the wall appears as a solid column of stratified epithelium. The cut next passes through the lumen of the duct (B-2) and then through the lumen of one of the secretory tubules (B-3). At the bottom, the cut passes transversely through the curved basal portion of the adjacent secretory tubule (B-4) so that it is seen as a circular structure with a central lumen surrounded by pyramid-shaped cells.

C represents an oblique section through the duct along the blue line c-c'. The lumen has an elliptical shape (C-1). At both ends of the section, the epithelium appears as a mosaic of cells (C-2) because the oblique cut has passed across different parts of duct cells, through both nucleated and non-nucleated parts.

D represents a sagittal section through the wall of one of the secretory tubules along the blue line d-d'. The section thus appears as a solid mass of cells.

E represents an oblique section (E-1) and a transverse section (E-2) through the lumen and wall of a secretory tubule along the blue line e-e'.

F illustrates transverse sections through three secretory tubules along the red line f-f'. Each shows the small central lumen and cuboidal or pyramidal cells forming the wall.

G represents part of a secretory tubule sectioned longitudinally along the blue line g-g'. It passes through the lumen of the tubule except at the upper part where the wall has been sectioned obliquely.

EXAMPLES

There are probably no tubular glands in the human that have the exact structure represented in this general diagram but tubular glands with variations occur in several locations.

Unbranched simple tubular glands without ducts are represented by the intestinal glands (crypts of Lieberkühn) of the large intestine (Plate 67: 20) and rectum (Plate 70: 7). These are lined with goblet cells and columnar cells with thin striated borders.

Similar shorter intestinal glands are found in the small intestine (Plate 65, Fig. 1:3). These are also lined with goblet cells and striated-bordered cells, and in addition, cells in the deep part of the gland (Paneth cells) are specialized for enzymatic secretion (Plate 65, Fig. 2).

The simple or slightly branched tubular gastric glands, without ducts, are lined with modified columnar cells highly specialized for secreting enzymes and the precursor of HCl (Plate 60: 4, 15–17). Pyloric glands, in contrast, are coiled tubular glands whose columnar cells secrete mucus; cells are therefore lightly stained (Plate 62: 5, 14).

A coiled tubular gland with a long duct is the sweat gland (Plate 46).

Highly branched tubular glands, lined with mucus-secreting columnar cells, are the glands of the cervix (Plate 105: 2). A narrow constricted portion serves as a duct.

PLATE 5

TUBULAR GLAND (DIAGRAM)

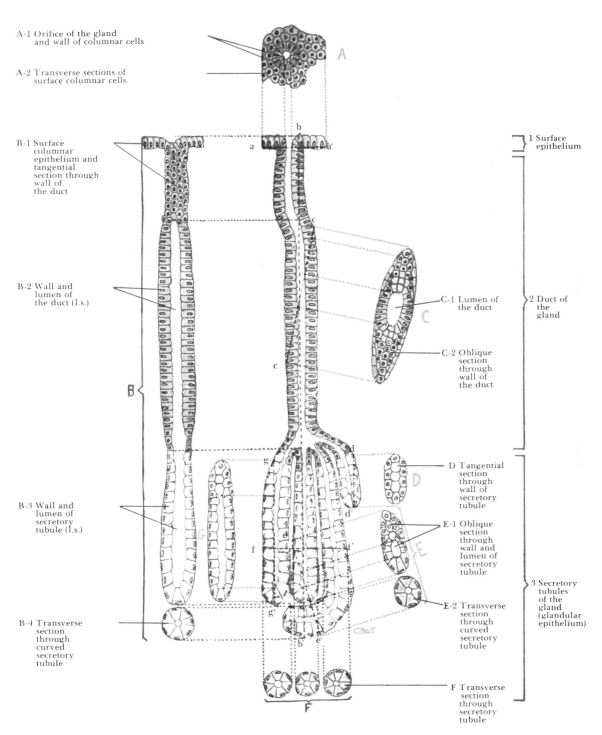

A-1 Orifice of the gland
and wall of columnar cells

A-2 Transverse sections of
surface columnar cells

B-1 Surface
columnar
epithelium and
tangential
section through
wall of
the duct

1 Surface
epithelium

B-2 Wall and
lumen of
the duct (l.s.)

C-1 Lumen of
the duct

2 Duct of
the
gland

C-2 Oblique
section
through
wall of
the duct

D Tangential
section
through
wall of
secretory
tubule

B-3 Wall and
lumen of
secretory
tubule (l.s.)

E-1 Oblique
section
through
wall and
lumen of
secretory
tubule

3 Secretory
tubules
of the
gland
(glandular
epithelium)

E-2 Transverse
section
through
curved
secretory
tubule

B-4 Transverse
section
through
curved
secretory
tubule

F Transverse
section
through
secretory
tubule

PLATE 6

COMPOUND TUBULOALVEOLAR GLAND (DIAGRAM)

This diagram represents, in general, the type of gland associated with the oral cavity and some other parts of the digestive system, and with the respiratory system. A large excretory duct (A-1) opens onto an epithelial surface (not indicated in the diagram). This divides or gives off successively smaller ducts (A-5, A-6). At the terminal ends of these are the rounded or elongated secretory units (alveoli) with small lumens surrounded by pyramidal or columnar cells.

Illustrated is the general structure of ducts and secretory units, and the appearance of these when sectioned in various planes.

A illustrates the appearance of sections resulting when red line a-a' passes obliquely (A-2) through a large duct (A-1), transversely through two small ducts (A-3) and transversely through two alveoli (A-4).

At B are seen sections of small ducts (B-1, B-3) and alveoli (B-2, B-4) when the red line b-b' passes through these in transverse or oblique planes.

At C-1 are seen sections when the blue line c-c' passes through different parts of two alveoli. Since these are rounded units, both sections appear generally similar. At C-2, the same blue line c-c' has passed longitudinally through two small ducts and through the lumen of the alveolus which opens into the smallest duct.

EXAMPLES

The major salivary glands are glands of this type (Plates 52, 53, 54), being composed of masses of alveoli and ducts of various sizes. These illustrate two major types of secretory alveoli, serous alveoli and mucous alveoli. Serous alveoli are described on page 116, and are present in the glands on Plates 52, 53, and 54. Mucous alveoli are described and are compared with serous alveoli on page 118. They are seen on Plates 53 and 54. Ducts are distinct structures, lined with cuboidal, columnar or stratified epithelium, and are named according to their location in the gland.

A less complex tubuloalveolar gland, consisting of mucous alveoli and ducts, is illustrated on Plate 55:11, 12 (esophageal glands). Similar glands, with mucous and serous alveoli and ducts, are the tracheal glands (Plate 77).

PLATE 6

COMPOUND TUBULOALVEOLAR GLAND (DIAGRAM)

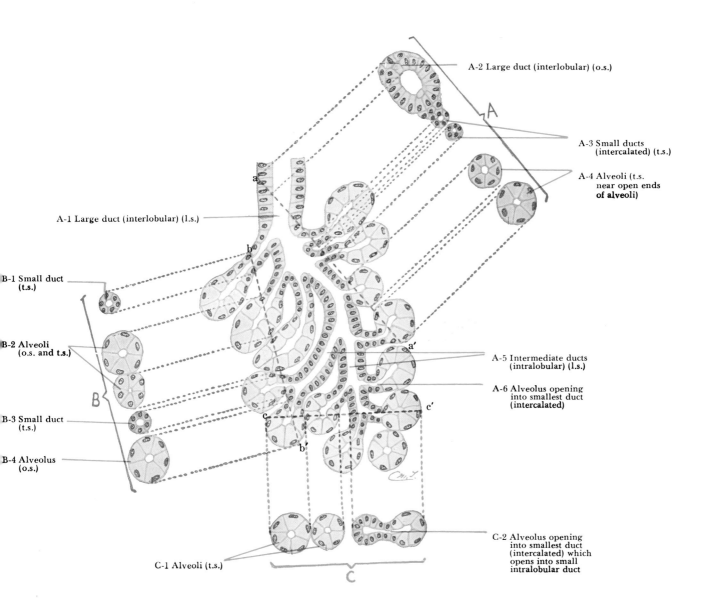

A-2 Large duct (interlobular) (o.s.)

A-3 Small ducts (intercalated) (t.s.)

A-4 Alveoli (t.s. near open ends of alveoli)

A-1 Large duct (interlobular) (l.s.)

B-1 Small duct (t.s.)

B-2 Alveoli (o.s. and t.s.)

A-5 Intermediate ducts (intralobular) (l.s.)

A-6 Alveolus opening into smallest duct (intercalated)

B-3 Small duct (t.s.)

B-4 Alveolus (o.s.)

C-2 Alveolus opening into smallest duct (intercalated) which opens into small intralobular duct

C-1 Alveoli (t.s.)

Plate 7

COMPOUND ALVEOLAR GLAND (DIAGRAM)

This is representative, in general, of a gland like the mammary gland. The terminal secreting units are also alveoli but are large rounded sacs with a large central lumen, and a thin wall of glandular cuboidal or low columnar epithelium (4, 6, 7). The alveoli may branch (6).

As previously, these alveoli open into small ducts (2, 3) lined with low columnar cells, which then pass into successively larger ducts (1, 5, 8). The final excretory duct is not indicated in the diagram.

The blue line a-a' and the red line b-b' pass through alveoli and ducts at different angles. The resulting sections are shown at A and B respectively.

EXAMPLES

The mammary gland is the outstanding example of this type of gland (Plates 108, 109). The large lumened secretory alveoli are seen in inactive and active states, and several ducts are illustrated.

PLATE 7

COMPOUND ALVEOLAR GLAND (DIAGRAM)

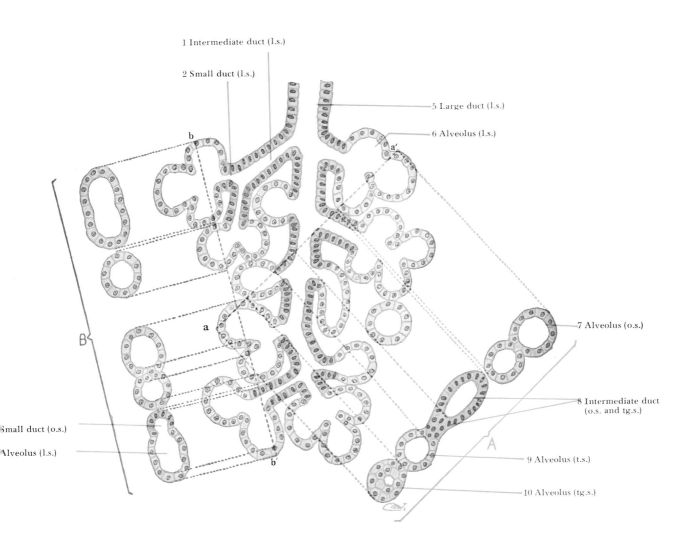

1 Intermediate duct (l.s.)

2 Small duct (l.s.)

5 Large duct (l.s.)

6 Alveolus (l.s.)

7 Alveolus (o.s.)

8 Intermediate duct (o.s. and tg.s.)

9 Alveolus (t.s.)

10 Alveolus (tg.s.)

Small duct (o.s.)

Alveolus (l.s.)

PLATE 8 (Fig. 1)

LOOSE (IRREGULARLY ARRANGED) CONNECTIVE TISSUE: SPREAD, STAINED WITH NEUTRAL RED

The plate illustrates subcutaneous connective tissue from a white rat, stained by injection of a dilute solution of neutral red in normal saline. This solution permits the tissue elements to remain in their natural state for some time, but it separates them so that they are much farther apart than normally, or when seen in prepared sections. Fibers and cells may be identified.

Collagenous fibers, unstained, are the most numerous and the largest of the fibers (2, 9). They course in all directions. They are thick, somewhat wavy, and faint longitudinal striations (their component fibrils) may be seen. No cut ends are visible.

Elastic fibers are fine, single fibers (1, 10) which are straight, but may be wavy after cutting when tension has been released. They form branching and anastomosing networks. Although unstained, they are highly refringent, in contrast to the dull appearance of collagenous fibers. Fine reticular fibers are not apparent.

The fixed permanent cells of this and other connective tissues proper are fibroblasts (8, I). In this preparation, they are seen as flattened, branching cells with an oval nucleus in which chromatin is sparse (8), but one or two nucleoli may be present (I:14, 15). Fixed macrophages or histiocytes (4, 11, II) are always present in varying numbers. When inactive, they appear much like fibroblasts, although their processes may be more irregular and their nuclei smaller. Phagocytic inclusions, however, give varied appearances to their cytoplasm. Here, cytoplasmic vacuoles are filled with neutral red (small vacuoles in 4, large ones in 11 and II:17).

Mast cells (7, III) are a usual component of loose connective tissue, seen singly or often grouped along small blood vessels (7). They are usually ovoid cells with a small, pale, centrally placed nucleus (18) and cytoplasm filled with large, closely packed granules which are stained a deep brick-red with neutral red (7, 19).

Present also are groups of adipose cells (fat cells) (3). Each cell is a spherical, colorless globule. The minute, eccentric nucleus is not visible.

Other blood and tissue cells may be seen in small numbers. These are not stained with neutral red, but it may be possible to identify eosinophils (5) by the lobulated nucleus and coarse granules in the cytoplasm, and small round lymphocytes (6) in which the nucleus occupies most of the cell.

The faint background stain is ground substance which has been infiltrated with the injected fluid.

PLATE 8 (Fig. 2)

CELLS OF LOOSE CONNECTIVE TISSUE IN SECTIONS

In this figure are shown some cells of loose connective tissue as they appear in histological preparations after fixation and staining with hematoxylin-eosin.

Free macrophages (1) usually appear rounded, but the cell outline may be slightly irregular. Their appearance varies; this one has a small nucleus rich in chromatin, and slightly acidophilic cytoplasm. The fibroblast (2) is elongated with some projections, the nucleus is ovoid with sparse chromatin and has one or two nucleoli. The fibrocyte (3), a more mature cell, is smaller, without cytoplasmic projections; the nucleus is similar but smaller.

The large lymphocyte (4) and the small lymphocyte (5) are rounded cells which differ principally in the larger amount of cytoplasm in the former. Their darkly-staining nuclei have condensed chromatin clumps but no nucleoli.

Plasma cells (6) are distinguished from lymphocytes by their smaller eccentrically placed nucleus whose condensed chromatin is in peripheral clumps and one central mass, and by a clear halo in the cytoplasm adjacent to the nucleus. The cytoplasm takes a grayish stain.

Eosinophils (7) of the circulating blood are readily distinguished by their large size, a bilobed nucleus, and large granules in the cytoplasm which stain intensely with eosin.

Occasional pigment cells (8) may be seen. Adipose cells (9) are seen as clear cells with a narrow rim of cytoplasm and a small eccentrically placed nucleus. The large globule of fat of the living cell has been dissolved by reagents used in section preparation.

PLATE 8

LOOSE (IRREGULARLY ARRANGED) CONNECTIVE TISSUE

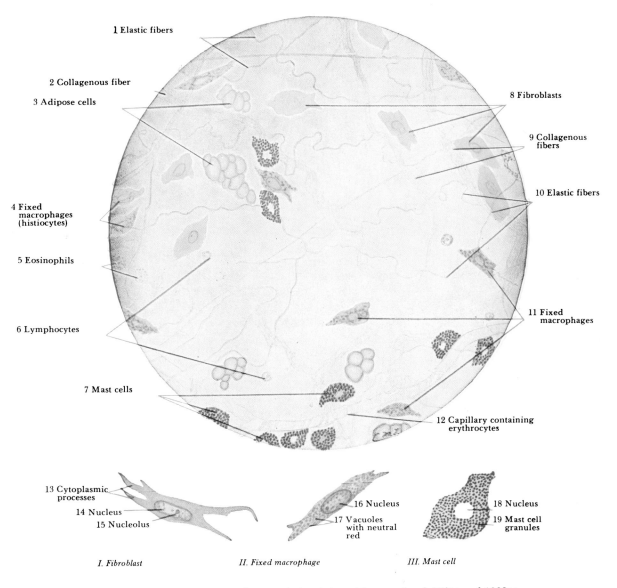

1 Elastic fibers

2 Collagenous fiber

3 Adipose cells

8 Fibroblasts

9 Collagenous fibers

4 Fixed macrophages (histiocytes)

10 Elastic fibers

5 Eosinophils

6 Lymphocytes

11 Fixed macrophages

7 Mast cells

12 Capillary containing erythrocytes

13 Cytoplasmic processes

16 Nucleus

18 Nucleus

14 Nucleus

17 Vacuoles with neutral red

19 Mast cell granules

15 Nucleolus

I. Fibroblast   *II. Fixed macrophage*   *III. Mast cell*

FIG. 1. *Connective tissue spread:* supravital staining with neutral red. 320× and 1200×.

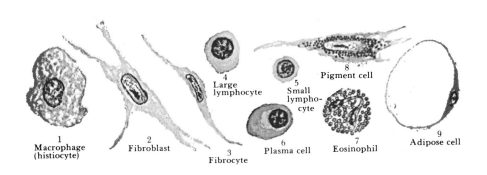

1 Macrophage (histiocyte)

2 Fibroblast

3 Fibrocyte

4 Large lymphocyte

5 Small lymphocyte

6 Plasma cell

7 Eosinophil

8 Pigment cell

9 Adipose cell

FIG. 2. *Cells of loose connective tissue.* Stain: hematoxylin-eosin. 1200×.

PLATE 9 (Fig. 1)

LOOSE (IRREGULARLY ARRANGED) CONNECTIVE TISSUE

The field reproduced represents a portion of the submucosa of the esophagus.

Collagenous fibers (1, 9) are the predominant components of loose connective tissue. They course in different directions, forming a loosely arranged meshwork. They are sectioned in various planes, and cut ends may be seen. The fibers are of different diameters (1, 9). They may appear longitudinally striated because of their fibrillar structure (1). They are acidophilic, staining pink with eosin. Thin elastic fibers are present but not easily distinguishable with this stain and magnification.

Fibroblasts (2, 3, 4) are the most numerous cells. They, too, may be sectioned in various planes, so that only parts of cells might be seen. Cytoplasm may shrink during section preparation. A typical fibroblast in surface view (4) shows an oval nucleus with sparse chromatin and lightly acidophilic cytoplasm with a few short processes. A fibroblast may be seen in profile (upper 3), in surface view but without much cytoplasm (lower 3), and in transverse section (2) in which the nucleus appears rounded.

Also seen are occasional neutrophils (5, 11) with lobulated nuclei, and small lymphocytes (6, 12) with large, round nuclei. Fat cells or adipose cells are characteristically empty with a thin rim of cytoplasm (7) and peripheral nuclei (8). Capillaries (10) lined with endothelium are seen.

Examples of loose connective tissue in organs may be seen on Plate 24, Fig. 1 (10) and on Plate 83, Fig. 2 (5).

PLATE 9 (Fig. 2)

DENSE IRREGULARLY ARRANGED CONNECTIVE TISSUE
(DENSE FIBROELASTIC CONNECTIVE TISSUE)

This figure illustrates dense irregular connective tissue from the dermis of the skin. Fibers, cells and arrangement of fibers are like those in loose connective tissue but are modified to conform to areas where a more firm support is required.

Collagenous fibers are large, typically in thick bundles (1, 2) and are sectioned in different planes since they course in various directions. Arrangement is very compact. Thin, wavy elastic fibers (10) form fine networks.

Fibroblasts (5) are often compressed among the fibers. Also seen are an undifferentiated mesenchymal cell (6) along a small blood vessel, and a few cells of the circulating blood: neutrophils with lobulated nuclei (3) and lymphocytes (9) with large rounded nuclei and no visible cytoplasm. Small blood vessels are seen (4, 8).

Dense irregular connective tissue in the dermis of the skin is illustrated on Plate 44, Fig. 1 (3).

PLATE 9

CONNECTIVE TISSUE

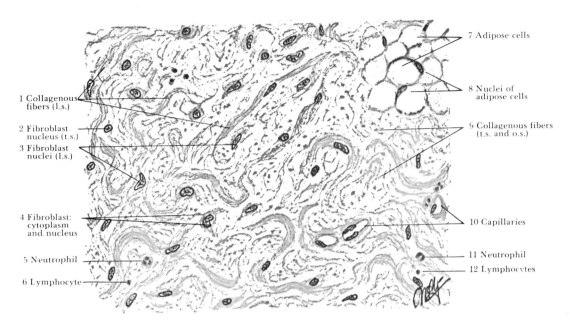

1 Collagenous fibers (l.s.)

2 Fibroblast nucleus (t.s.)

3 Fibroblast nuclei (l.s.)

4 Fibroblast: cytoplasm and nucleus

5 Neutrophil

6 Lymphocyte

7 Adipose cells

8 Nuclei of adipose cells

9 Collagenous fibers (t.s. and o.s.)

10 Capillaries

11 Neutrophil

12 Lymphocytes

FIG. 1. *Loose connective tissue.* Stain: hematoxylin-eosin. 300×.

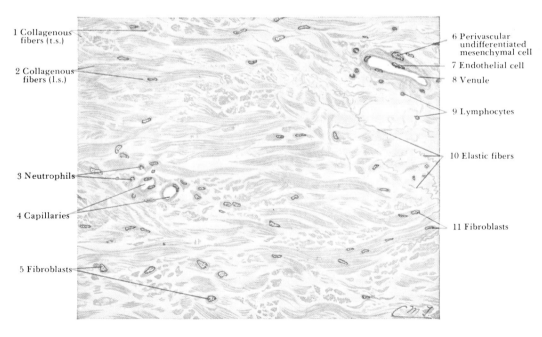

1 Collagenous fibers (t.s.)

2 Collagenous fibers (l.s.)

3 Neutrophils

4 Capillaries

5 Fibroblasts

6 Perivascular undifferentiated mesenchymal cell

7 Endothelial cell

8 Venule

9 Lymphocytes

10 Elastic fibers

11 Fibroblasts

FIG. 2. *Dense irregularly arranged connective tissue.*
Stain: hematoxylin-eosin. 300×.

PLATE 10 (Fig. 1)

DENSE REGULAR CONNECTIVE TISSUE: TENDON
(LONGITUDINAL SECTION)

Dense regular collagenous connective tissue (dense fibrous tissue) occurs where great tensile strength is required, principally in ligaments and tendons. Tendon represents the highest development of this structure. A portion of tendon is shown here at a high magnification.

Collagenous fibers are arranged in compact, parallel bundles (2, 3). Between the bundles are thin partitions of looser connective tissue in which are rows of modified fibroblasts, the tendon cells (1, 4, 5). They are thick cells with short processes (not visible here) and nuclei which are ovoid (4) when seen in surface view, or rod-like in lateral view (5).

Dense regular connective tissue in a less highly specialized form (compact collagenous fibers with interspersed flattened fibroblasts) also forms fibrous membranes or capsules which surround specific structures or organs. Examples are the perichondrium around the tracheal cartilage (Plate 77, Fig. 1:2), the dura mater around the spinal cord (Plate 32, Fig. 1:13), and the tunica albuginea around the testis (Plate 90, Fig. 1:1).

PLATE 10 (Fig. 2)

DENSE REGULAR CONNECTIVE TISSUE: TENDON
(TRANSVERSE SECTION)

A tendon in transverse section is seen at a much lower magnification than that in Fig. 1. Within each large bundle of tendon fibers (1) are seen tendon cells (nuclei) in transverse section (2). These lie between small bundles of tendon fibers whose cut ends are not distinguishable at this magnification but may be seen in the insert (10).

Between the large bundles are thin partitions of connective tissue (3). Bundles are grouped into fasciculi between which course larger partitions (septa or trabeculae) of interfascicular connective tissue (4, 8). In these may be seen blood vessels (5), nerves, and occasionally lamellar (Pacinian) corpuscles (6) which are pressure receptors.

At a higher magnification, the small bundles of collagenous fibers (10) are distinguishable with the fibers sectioned transversely, and the branched or wing-shaped structure of the tendon cells (9) may be seen.

Also present is a small section of skeletal muscle (7) in transverse section. It is adjacent to the tendon but separated from it by connective tissue.

—32—

PLATE 10

CONNECTIVE TISSUE

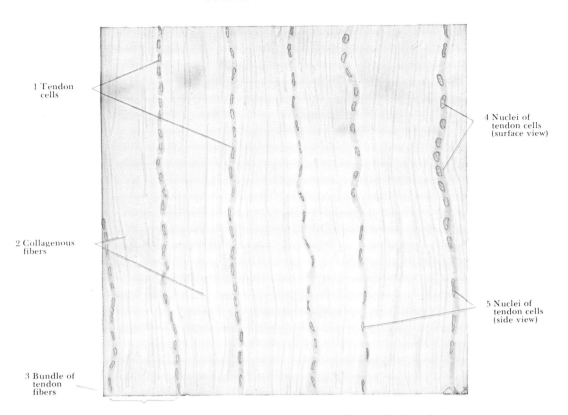

1 Tendon cells

4 Nuclei of tendon cells (surface view)

2 Collagenous fibers

5 Nuclei of tendon cells (side view)

3 Bundle of tendon fibers

FIG. 1. *Dense regular connective tissue: tendon (longitudinal section).*
Stain: hematoxylin-eosin. 250×.

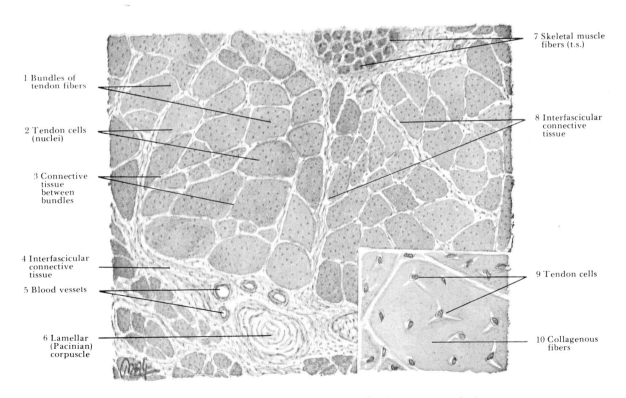

7 Skeletal muscle fibers (t.s.)

1 Bundles of tendon fibers

2 Tendon cells (nuclei)

8 Interfascicular connective tissue

3 Connective tissue between bundles

4 Interfascicular connective tissue

5 Blood vessels

9 Tendon cells

6 Lamellar (Pacinian) corpuscle

10 Collagenous fibers

FIG. 2. *Dense regular connective tissue: tendon (transverse section).*
Stain: hematoxylin-eosin. 80× and 300×.

PLATE 11 (Fig. 1)

DENSE IRREGULAR AND LOOSE CONNECTIVE TISSUE
(ELASTIC STAIN)

Illustrated is a field with dense irregular connective tissue at the left side, a transition zone and loose connective tissue on the right.

Using Verhoeff's method, elastic fibers are selectively stained a deep blue color (1, 4). Using Van Gieson's as a counterstain, acid fuchsin gives a red color to collagenous fibers (2, 5). Cellular detail of fibroblasts is not revealed, but the nuclei stain deep blue (3, 6).

The characteristics of dense irregular and loose connective tissues are readily apparent with this technique. Collagenous fibers are of larger size, more numerous and more concentrated in the dense irregular connective tissue (2). Elastic fibers likewise are somewhat larger and more numerous (1). In the loose connective tissue, both fiber types are smaller (4, 5) and more loosely arranged. Fine elastic networks are seen in both tissues.

PLATE 11 (Fig. 2)

ADIPOSE TISSUE

Illustrated is a section of mesentery in which adipose cells (fat cells) are present in large accumulations, organized into adipose tissue.

Here the connective tissue of the peritoneum (6) serves as a capsule around the masses of adipose cells.

Adipose cells (2) are close together, separated by small amounts of connective tissue in which the fibroblasts (7) are compressed. Lobules of adipose tissue are marked off by trabeculae (septa) of connective tissue (3) in which course blood vessels (1, 4) and nerves; capillaries (5) are distributed to the intercellular connective tissue.

Individual adipose cells show their characteristic structure, empty cells (2) due to solution of fat during section preparation, with nuclei compressed in the peripheral rim of cytoplasm (8). It is not always easy to distinguish between fibroblast nuclei (7) and nuclei of adipose cells (8) in sections.

PLATE 11 (Fig. 3)

EMBRYONIC CONNECTIVE TISSUE

Illustrated is a representative field of embryonic connective tissue, which, structurally, could be mesenchyme or mucous connective tissue. The difference in ground substance (semi-fluid or more viscid and jelly-like respectively) is not apparent in sections.

Fibroblasts (2) are numerous. Fine collagenous fibrils (3) course everywhere between them; some of these are in close contact with fibroblasts. The tissue is vascular (1, 4).

At a higher magnification, a primitive fibroblast (5) is seen as a large, branching cell with abundant cytoplasm and prominent cytoplasmic processes, and an oval nucleus with fine chromatin and one or more nucleoli. The widely separated collagenous fibrils (6) are more apparent.

PLATE 11

CONNECTIVE TISSUE

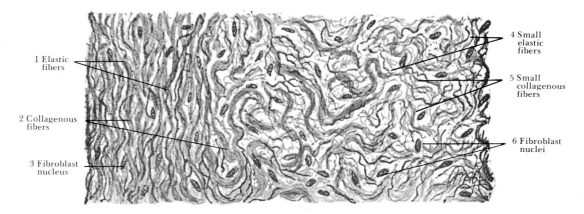

1 Elastic
fibers

2 Collagenous
fibers

3 Fibroblast
nucleus

4 Small
elastic
fibers

5 Small
collagenous
fibers

6 Fibroblast
nuclei

FIG. 1. *Dense irregular and loose connective tissue.*
Stain: Verhoeff's elastin stain and Van Gieson's. 240×.

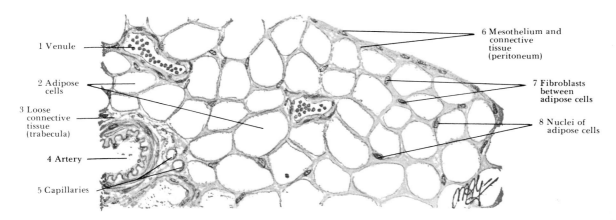

1 Venule

2 Adipose
cells

3 Loose
connective
tissue
(trabecula)

4 Artery

5 Capillaries

6 Mesothelium and
connective
tissue
(peritoneum)

7 Fibroblasts
between
adipose cells

8 Nuclei of
adipose cells

FIG. 2. *Adipose tissue.* Stain: hematoxylin-eosin. 240×.

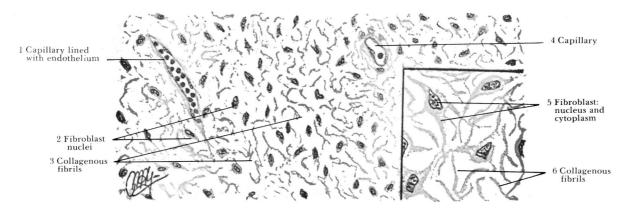

1 Capillary lined
with endothelium

2 Fibroblast
nuclei

3 Collagenous
fibrils

4 Capillary

5 Fibroblast:
nucleus and
cytoplasm

6 Collagenous
fibrils

Embryonic connective tissue. Stain: hematoxylin-eosin. 240× and 900×.

PLATE 12 (Fig. 1)

HYALINE CARTILAGE (FRESH PREPARATION)

This section represents an area in the interior or central portion of a plate of hyaline cartilage. Distributed throughout a homogeneous substance, the matrix (5), are numerous lacunae which contain the cartilage cells or chondrocytes (1).

In normal intact cartilage, the chondrocytes fill the lacunae. Each cell has granular cytoplasm and a nucleus (2) which is seen as a small vesicle more highly refringent than the cytoplasm. In removed cartilage, the chondrocytes may contract slightly and the lacunae can then be seen as clear spaces (3).

The intercellular matrix (interterritorial matrix) (5) appears homogeneous but is actually composed of ground substance and collagenous fibrils. It is modified around each lacuna to form the cartilage capsule (6), and around groups of lacunae to form the territorial matrix.

PLATE 12 (Fig. 2)

HYALINE CARTILAGE (STAINED)

A section of hyaline cartilage, similar to that in Fig. 1, is shown as it appears after fixation and staining. Chondrocytes (1) shrink somewhat during section preparation, thus more of the lacunar space is visible. Nuclei (2) are smaller than in a fresh preparation. The matrix (5) again appears homogeneous; it takes a faint basophilic stain. Basophilia is intensified around groups of lacunae, and this region is termed the territorial matrix (4). The cartilage capsules (3) appear as thin, darkened boundaries around each lacuna.

PLATE 12 (Fig. 3)

HYALINE CARTILAGE (STAINED)

In this stained preparation of a plate of hyaline cartilage from the trachea, lacunae with their contained chondrocytes may be seen singly (12) or as isogenous groups (13). The chondrocytes appear to fill their lacunae, thus only the margins of lacunae are visible (16). Lacunae and chondrocytes in the interior of the plate are large, rounded or ovoid (12, 13), but toward the periphery they are progressively flattened (11); these are younger forms.

The interterritorial (intercellular) matrix stains lightly (14), and the territorial matrix stains more deeply (15).

A perichondrium of dense connective tissue (4, 9, 18) surrounds the entire cartilage plate. Its inner layer is the chondrogenic area (10). Here chondrocytes are being formed (17) by differentiation of fibroblasts of the perichondrium (18) (appositional growth).

Other examples of hyaline cartilage may be seen on Plates 76 and 77.

PLATE 12

CARTILAGE

1 Cartilage cell
(chondrocyte)

2 Nuclei of
cartilage cells

3 Lacuna

4 Lacuna with
two cells

5 Hyaline matrix
(interterritorial
matrix)

6 Cartilage
capsules

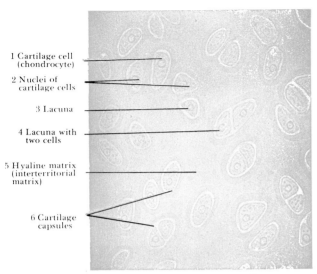

FIG. 1. *Hyaline cartilage.*
Fresh preparation. 320×.

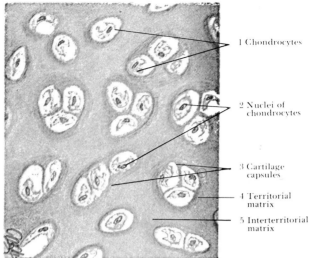

1 Chondrocytes

2 Nuclei of
chondrocytes

3 Cartilage
capsules

4 Territorial
matrix

5 Interterritorial
matrix

FIG. 2. *Hyaline cartilage.*
Stain: hematoxylin-eosin. 320×.

1 Tracheal
glands

3 Mucous
alveoli

2 Serous
alveoli

4 Perichondrium

5 Surrounding
connective
tissue

6 Glandular duct

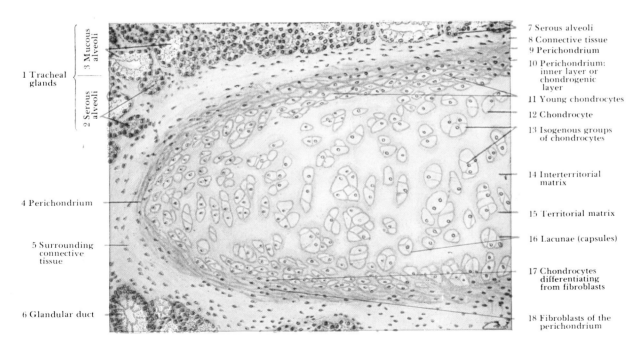

7 Serous alveoli

8 Connective tissue

9 Perichondrium

10 Perichondrium:
inner layer or
chondrogenic
layer

11 Young chondrocytes

12 Chondrocyte

13 Isogenous groups
of chondrocytes

14 Interterritorial
matrix

15 Territorial matrix

16 Lacunae (capsules)

17 Chondrocytes
differentiating
from fibroblasts

18 Fibroblasts of the
perichondrium

FIG. 3. *Hyaline cartilage of the trachea (stained)*
Stain: hematoxylin-eosin. 120×.

PLATE 13 (Fig. 1)

FIBROUS CARTILAGE: INTERVERTEBRAL DISC

In fibrous cartilage, the matrix (6) is permeated with many small collagenous fibers (5), which are frequently in parallel arrangement as in a tendon.

Small chondrocytes in lacunae (1, 2, 4) usually lie in rows (3) within this fibrous matrix, not in random arrangement or in isogenous groups as in hyaline or elastic cartilage. All chondrocytes and lacunae are about the same size; there is not the gradation from larger central ones to smaller and more flattened peripheral ones.

A perichondrium is absent, since fibrous cartilage usually forms a transition area between hyaline cartilage and tendon or ligament.

The proportion of fibers to matrix, the number of chondrocytes and their arrangement may vary. Fibers may be so dense that matrix is virtually invisible; chondrocytes and lacunae would then be flattened. Fibers within a bundle may be parallel but different bundles may course at various angles.

PLATE 13 (Fig. 2)

ELASTIC CARTILAGE: EPIGLOTTIC CARTILAGE

Elastic cartilage differs from hyaline cartilage principally by the presence of elastic fibers in its matrix (1). These are well demonstrated, as deep purple fibers, by staining with orcein (3). They enter the cartilaginous matrix from the perichondrium (4), usually as small fibers, and distribute in the interior as branching and anastomosing fibers of varying sizes (3); some of these are of considerable thickness (3, middle leader). The density of fibers in the matrix varies in different elastic cartilages, as well as in the same one under different conditions.

As in hyaline cartilage, large chondrocytes in lacunae are seen in the interior of the plate and smaller ones toward the periphery (2, 5), finally making a transition to fibroblasts of the perichondrium.

—38—

PLATE 13

CARTILAGE

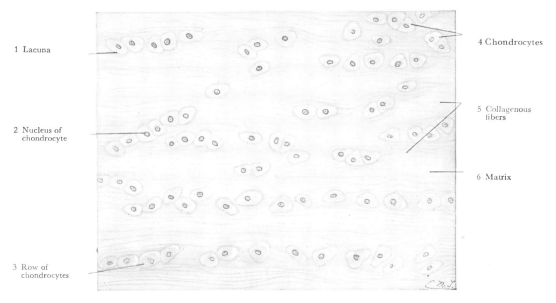

1 Lacuna

2 Nucleus of
chondrocyte

3 Row of
chondrocytes

4 Chondrocytes

5 Collagenous
fibers

6 Matrix

FIG. 1 *Fibrous cartilage: intervertebral disc.*
Stain: hematoxylin-eosin. 320×.

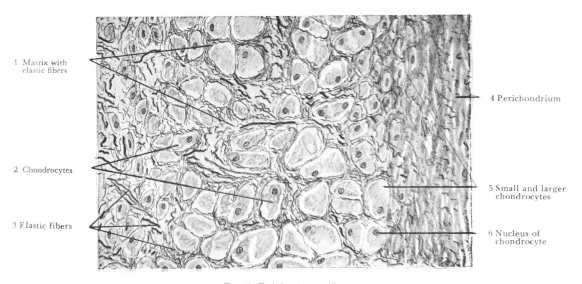

1 Matrix with
elastic fibers

2 Chondrocytes

3 Elastic fibers

4 Perichondrium

5 Small and larger
chondrocytes

6 Nucleus of
chondrocyte

FIG. 2 *Epiglottic cartilage.*
Stain: hematoxylin-orcein. 320×.

PLATE 14 (Fig. 1)

COMPACT BONE, DRIED: DIAPHYSIS OF THE TIBIA
(TRANSVERSE SECTION)

The units of structure of bone are lamellae, which are thin plates of bony tissue containing osteocytes or bone cells in almond-shaped lacunae (11, 15), from which radiate minute canals, the canaliculi (12). These anastomose with canaliculi from other lacunae, and some open into central or Haversian canals and marrow cavities of bones. Lamellae may be flattened, curved, tubular or irregular in shape.

The outer portion of a compact bone (beneath the periosteum) is formed of external circumferential lamellae (10) which are parallel to each other and to the long axis of the bone. Comparably, the inner wall (along the marrow cavity) is composed of internal circumferential lamellae (6). Between these external and internal circumferential lamellae are many osteons or Haversian systems (4, 8), which are seen here in transverse or oblique sections. The small irregular areas of bone between osteons or Haversian systems are interstitial or intercalated lamellae (7, 9).

Each osteon or Haversian system (4, 8) consists of a number of concentric (tubular) lamellae (3) surrounding a central or Haversian canal (2, 14) which in the living state contains reticular connective tissue and blood vessels (a miniature marrow cavity). The boundary of each osteon or Haversian system is a thin, homogeneous layer of modified matrix, the cementing line (5). Cross-connections or anastomoses between central or Haversian canals are seen (13).

PLATE 14 (Fig. 2)

COMPACT BONE, DRIED: DIAPHYSIS OF THE TIBIA
(LONGITUDINAL SECTION)

This figure represents a small area of a longitudinal section of the diaphysis of a compact bone.

Since the central or Haversian canals course longitudinally in the bone, each canal (3) is seen as a tube sectioned parallel to the long axis of the bone. It is surrounded by numerous lamellae (1) within or between which are lacunae (4) with their canaliculi (6). Lamellae, lacunae, and the boundaries of osteons or Haversian systems (cementing lines) (2) are, in general, parallel to the corresponding central or Haversian canals.

—40—

PLATE 14

COMPACT BONE, DRIED

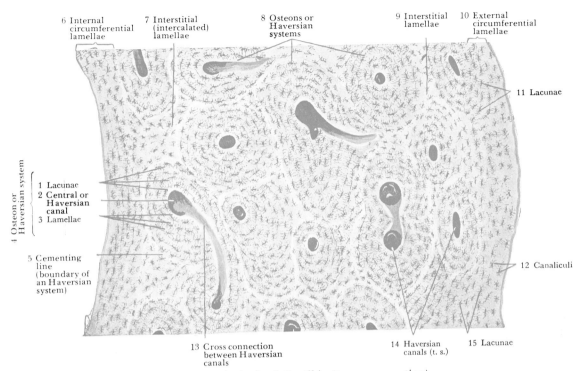

6 Internal circumferential lamellae   7 Interstitial (intercalated) lamellae   8 Osteons or Haversian systems   9 Interstitial lamellae   10 External circumferential lamellae

11 Lacunae

4 Osteon or Haversian system

1 Lacunae
2 Central or Haversian canal
3 Lamellae

5 Cementing line (boundary of an Haversian system)

12 Canaliculi

13 Cross connection between Haversian canals   14 Haversian canals (t. s.)   15 Lacunae

FIG. 1. *Diaphysis of the tibia (transverse section).*
Stain: aniline blue. 80×

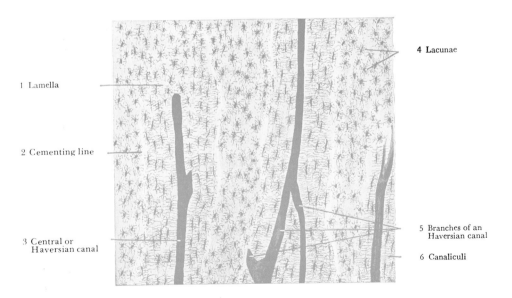

4 Lacunae

1 Lamella

2 Cementing line

5 Branches of an Haversian canal

3 Central or Haversian canal

6 Canaliculi

FIG. 2. *Diaphysis of the tibia (longitudinal section).*
Stain: aniline blue. 80×.

PLATE 15 (Fig. 1)

CANCELLOUS BONE: ADULT STERNUM
(TRANSVERSE SECTION, DECALCIFIED)

Cancellous bone consists primarily of slender, bony trabeculae which ramify and anastomose (6), and enclose irregular marrow cavities of various sizes (5). Peripherally, these trabeculae merge with a thin shell of compact bone (3) in which may be observed scattered osteons or Haversian systems (4, 7). The surrounding periosteum (2) may dip into the bone at intervals. It merges with adjacent loose connective tissue (1) which is rich in blood vessels.

Except for concentric lamellae in the osteons or Haversian systems (7), the peripheral rim of bone and the trabeculae are composed of parallel lamellae, which (in this figure) are more apparent on the margins of the bony areas (8). Lacunae with osteocytes (9) are present throughout the bone.

The framework of reticular connective tissue of the marrow cavities is obscured by adipose cells (10) and groups of hemopoietic cells (11). Arteries may be seen, but sinusoids are not distinguishable in this illustration. Marrow fills the cavities, but a thin endosteum of condensed stroma becomes visible when marrow is mechanically separated from the bone (12).

PLATE 15 (Fig. 2)

INTRAMEMBRANOUS BONE FORMATION
(MANDIBLE OF A FETUS OF FIVE MONTHS, DECALCIFIED)

The upper part of the section shows the gum covering the developing mandible. The mucosa of the gum consists of stratified squamous epithelium (1) and a wide lamina propria (2) with blood vessels and nerves.

Below the lamina propria is seen the bony tissue in the process of development. The periosteum (3) is differentiated, and numerous anastomosing trabeculae constitute the bone. These trabeculae surround primitive marrow cavities of various sizes (14). The primitive marrow consists of embryonic connective tissue with blood vessels and nerves (16). At the periphery of the bone, collagenous fibers of the inner periosteum are in continuity with the fibrils of the embryonic connective tissue of adjacent marrow cavities (6) and with collagenous fibers within the bony trabeculae (10).

In close contact with some of the developing trabeculae are seen osteoblasts (7, 15) in linear arrangement, associated with bone deposition, and osteoclasts (5, 8), which are multinucleated giant cells related to the process of bone resorption.

Within the bony trabeculae are osteocytes in their lacunae (4, 9). Although collagenous fibers embedded in the bony matrix are obscured, the continuity with fibers of the embryonic connective tissue in the marrow cavities may be seen at the margins of many trabeculae (13).

It should be noted that formation of new bone is not constantly in progress. Many inactive areas are present, where bone deposition has ceased temporarily: neither osteoid nor osteoblasts are present. In some of the primitive marrow cavities, fibroblasts are enlarging preparatory to differentiating to osteoblasts (12). Elsewhere, osteoid may be seen on the margins of the bony trabeculae (11,17); osteoblasts may (11) or may not be present (17). Definitive myeloid tissue is not yet present in the marrow cavities.

PLATE 15

FIG. 1. CANCELLOUS BONE: ADULT STERNUM
(TRANSVERSE SECTION, DECALCIFIED)

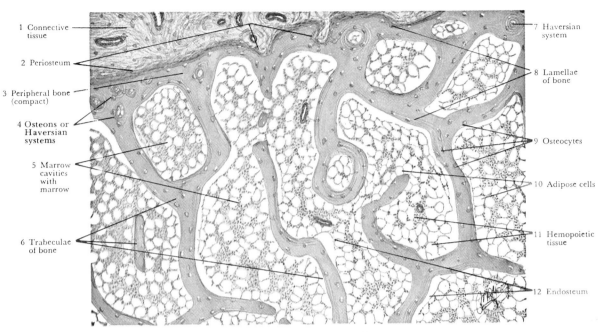

1 Connective tissue

2 Periosteum

3 Peripheral bone (compact)

4 Osteons or Haversian systems

5 Marrow cavities with marrow

6 Trabeculae of bone

7 Haversian system

8 Lamellae of bone

9 Osteocytes

10 Adipose cells

11 Hemopoietic tissue

12 Endosteum

Stain: hematoxylin-eosin. 35×.

FIG. 2. INTRAMEMBRANOUS BONE FORMATION: MANDIBLE OF A FETUS OF
FIVE MONTHS (TRANSVERSE SECTION, DECALCIFIED)

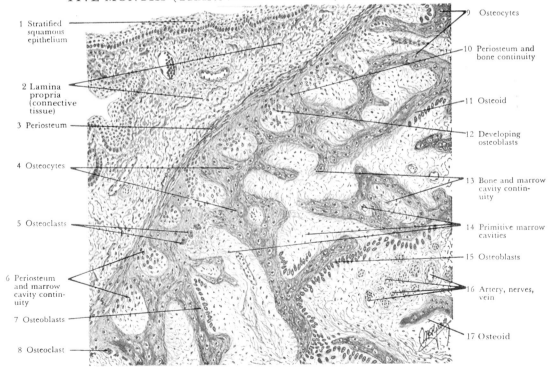

1 Stratified squamous epithelium

2 Lamina propria (connective tissue)

3 Periosteum

4 Osteocytes

5 Osteoclasts

6 Periosteum and marrow cavity continuity

7 Osteoblasts

8 Osteoclast

9 Osteocytes

10 Periosteum and bone continuity

11 Osteoid

12 Developing osteoblasts

13 Bone and marrow cavity continuity

14 Primitive marrow cavities

15 Osteoblasts

16 Artery, nerves, vein

17 Osteoid

Stain: Mallory-Azan. 50×.

— 43 —

PLATE 16

INTRACARTILAGINOUS BONE FORMATION: DEVELOPING METACARPAL BONE (PANORAMIC VIEW, LONGITUDINAL SECTION)

This illustration shows endochondral or intracartilaginous bone formation, in which the future bone is first formed as a plate of embryonic hyaline cartilage. The cartilage is then gradually destroyed and replaced by bone. In the center of the shaft of the bone illustrated, this has already occurred, and in addition, most of the original spongy bone so formed has been destroyed and resorbed to form the central marrow cavity, thus leaving only scattered, thin spicules of bone of endochondral origin (11, 30). Red marrow (13) fills the cavity. The stroma of reticular connective tissue is obscured by masses of developing erythrocytes and granulocytes, mature forms of these, megakaryocytes (14) and numerous venous sinusoids (12) and capillaries, as well as other blood vessels.

The process of continued endochondral bone formation can be followed from the upper part of the illustration downward toward the central marrow cavity. Uppermost is seen the zone of reserve normal hyaline cartilage (17) in which the chondrocytes in their lacunae are distributed singly or in small groups (2). Chondrocytes then multiply rapidly and become arranged in columns of cells (3, 18); cells and lacunae increase in size toward the lower area of this zone of proliferating cartilage (19). These chondrocytes then hypertrophy by swelling of nucleus and cytoplasm, lacunae enlarge (4), the cells then degenerate and the thin partitions of intervening matrix calcify (20). The calcified cartilage stains a deep purple.

Tufts of vascular marrow penetrate into this area (5, 21), erode the lacunar walls and calcified cartilage (5, 21), thus forming new, small marrow spaces. Osteoblasts are differentiated, osteoid and bone are deposited around remaining spicules of calcified cartilage (6). This is the zone of ossification (21).

The lower, lateral two-thirds of the illustration shows the development of periosteal bone. Osteoblasts become differentiated from embryonic fibroblasts in the inner layer of the periosteum (9) and a bone collar is formed (10) by the intramembranous method. Formation of new periosteal bone keeps pace with formation of new endochondral bone (22). The bone collar increases in thickness and compactness as development of the bone proceeds, the greatest thickness at any time being in the central part of the diaphysis at the initial site of formation of periosteal bone (29) around the primary ossification center.

Surrounding the shaft of the developing bone are soft tissues: muscle (7), subcutaneous layer and dermis of the skin (15, 25) with hair follicles (26), sebaceous glands (28) and sweat glands (16), and the epidermis (24).

PLATE 16

INTRACARTILAGINOUS BONE FORMATION: DEVELOPING
METACARPAL BONE (PANORAMIC VIEW,
LONGITUDINAL SECTION)

1 Perichondrium

2 Chondrocytes
in lacunae

3 Column of
chondrocytes

4 Hypertrophied
chondrocytes
and calcified
matrix

5 Vascular tufts
of osteogenic
marrow

6 Osteoid and
bone tissue
around a
spicule of
calcified cartilage

7 Muscle

8 Periosteum
(outer
layer)

9 Periosteum
(inner layer
with
osteoblasts)

10 Periosteal
bone
(bone collar)

11 Spicules of
bone of
endochondral
origin

12 Venous sinusoid

13 Red bone
marrow with
myeloid elements

14 Megakaryocytes

15 Subcutaneous
connective tissue
and dermis

16 Sweat
gland

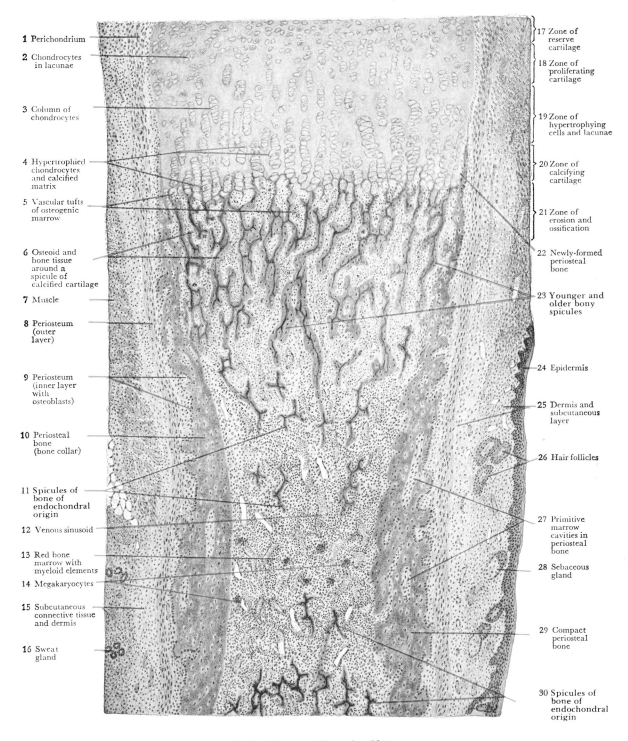

17 Zone of
reserve
cartilage

18 Zone of
proliferating
cartilage

19 Zone of
hypertrophying
cells and lacunae

20 Zone of
calcifying
cartilage

21 Zone of
erosion and
ossification

22 Newly-formed
periosteal
bone

23 Younger and
older bony
spicules

24 Epidermis

25 Dermis and
subcutaneous
layer

26 Hair follicles

27 Primitive
marrow
cavities in
periosteal
bone

28 Sebaceous
gland

29 Compact
periosteal
bone

30 Spicules of
bone of
endochondral
origin

Stain: hematoxylin-eosin. 60✕.

PLATE 17

INTRACARTILAGINOUS BONE FORMATION
(SECTIONAL VIEW)

This preparation shows, in more detail, the processes involved in endochondral bone formation at the zone of ossification and adjacent areas, corresponding approximately to 3 through 6 in Plate 16.

Proliferating chondroblasts are arranged in columns (2, 10). The cells in the lower part of this zone hypertrophy because of accumulation of glycogen in their cytoplasm and swelling of their nuclei, and lacunae hypertrophy simultaneously. Cytoplasm then becomes vacuolated, nuclei become pyknotic (3), the thin partitions of cartilaginous matrix become calcified (4, 11).

Sprouts of vascular marrow invading this area (5) produce the zone of erosion. Osteoblasts are formed, line up along remaining spicules of calcified cartilage (14) and lay down osteoid (15) and bone. Osteoblasts entrapped in the osteoid or bone become osteocytes (7).

In the marrow (17) are seen cells belonging to the erythrocytic (18) and granulocytic (19) series, and megakaryocytes (8). Multinucleated osteoclasts (16) are shown adjacent to bone tissue which is being resorbed. They lie in depressions or lacunae of erosion (Howship's lacunae).

On the right side of the illustration is an area of periosteal cancellous bone (13) with osteocytes and primitive marrow cavities. New bone is being added peripherally by osteoblasts derived from primitive fibroblasts of the inner periosteum (12). The outer layer of the periosteum continues upward as the perichondrium (9).

PLATE 17

INTRACARTILAGINOUS BONE FORMATION (SECTIONAL VIEW)

1 Basophilic matrix

2 Columns of cartilage cells

3 Hypertrophied cartilage cells (vacuolized cytoplasm, pyknotic nuclei)

4 Degenerating cartilage cells surrounded by calcified matrix

5 Invading capillaries and embryonic bone marrow in zone of erosion

6 Spicule of calcified cartilage surrounded by osteoid

7 Newly-formed osteocytes

8 Megakaryocytes

9 Perichondrium

10 Columns of cartilage cells

11 Calcified cartilage

12 Periosteum, outer layer, and inner layer with osteoblasts

13 Periosteal bone with osteocytes

14 Osteoblasts

15 Osteoid

16 Osteoclasts in lacunae of erosion (Howship's lacunae)

17 Hematogenous bone marrow (red marrow)

18 Nests of erythroblasts

19 Group of myelocytes

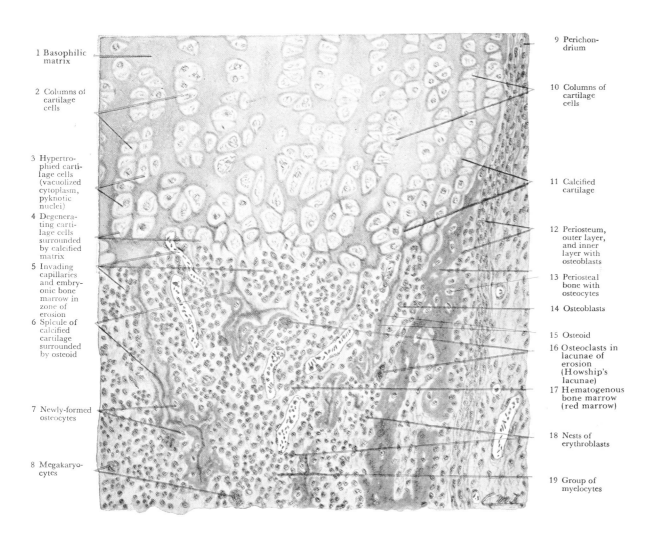

Stain: hematoxylin-eosin. 200×.

PLATE 18

FORMATION OF BONE: DEVELOPMENT OF OSTEONS OR HAVERSIAN SYSTEMS (DECALCIFIED, TRANSVERSE SECTION)

This represents a late stage in the development of a future compact bone. Primitive osteons or Haversian systems have already formed and others are in the process of developing. In a metacarpal bone, such as seen in Plate 16, or in a long bone, the first compact bone will have formed by subperiosteal deposition (Plate 16: 29). Vascular sprouts of connective tissue from the periosteum or endosteum will have eroded this bone to form primitive osteons or Haversian systems, as seen in this illustration. Reconstruction will continue by breakdown of these first and later Haversian systems and formation of new ones.

In this plate is seen a thick wall of immature compact bone; the matrix (11) is stained deeply with eosin. Primitive osteons or Haversian systems are seen in transverse sections, with large central canals or Haversian canals (8) surrounded by a few concentric lamellae of bone (3) and their contained osteocytes (1). The central or Haversian canals contain primitive connective tissue and blood vessels (6, 8). Deposition of bone is continuing in some of these, as indicated by the presence of osteoblasts at the periphery of the Haversian canal (9) along the margin of the innermost lamella of bone. Osteoclasts (2) indicate resorption of bone in some of these primitive Haversian systems, preparatory to reconstruction.

A longitudinal channel of osteogenic connective tissue (10) passes through the bone. From it arise tufts of vascular connective tissue which are central or Haversian canals in the process of formation (4). Osteoblasts are already lined up on the periphery.

In the lower part of the figure is the large central marrow cavity of the bone filled with bone marrow (14) in which hematopoiesis is in progress, thus this is red marrow. Developing erythrocytes and granulocytes are present, also megakaryocytes (16), blood vessels (7), a spicule of bone (15), and osteoclasts (13) in their lacunae of erosion along the wall of the bone.

PLATE 18

FORMATION OF BONE: DEVELOPMENT OF HAVERSIAN SYSTEMS (DECALCIFIED, TRANSVERSE SECTION)

1 Osteocytes

2 Osteoclast

3 Concentric lamellae

4 Central canals or Haversian canals in process of formation from tufts of vascular connective tissue

5 Inactive area

6 Haversian blood vessel

7 Venous sinusoids in the bone marrow

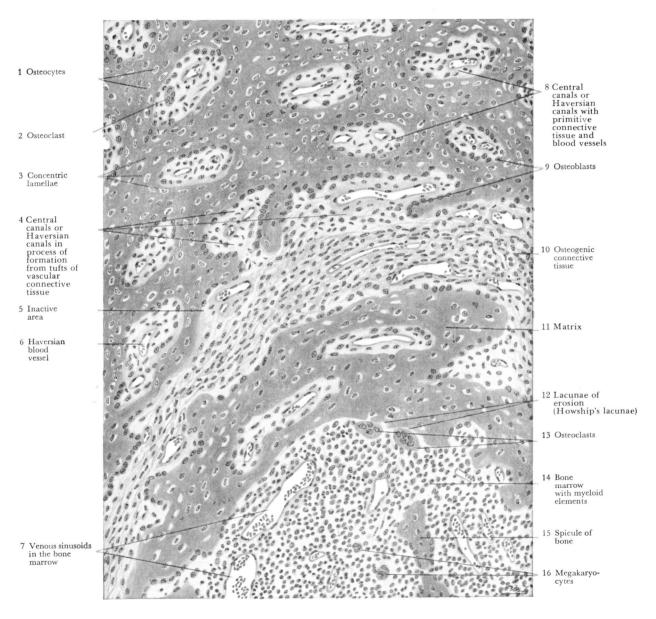

8 Central canals or Haversian canals with primitive connective tissue and blood vessels

9 Osteoblasts

10 Osteogenic connective tissue

11 Matrix

12 Lacunae of erosion (Howship's lacunae)

13 Osteoclasts

14 Bone marrow with myeloid elements

15 Spicule of bone

16 Megakaryo-cytes

Stain: hematoxylin-eosin. 140×.

PLATE 19

PERIPHERAL BLOOD SMEAR

The central circular area presents an idealized blood smear, stained with May-Grünwald-Giemsa stain. Erythrocytes, leukocytes and blood platelets are shown.

The erythrocytes (6) are enucleated cells which stain pink with eosin. They are uniform in size, about 7.6 μ, and can be used as a size reference for other cell types.

The blood platelets (7) are the smallest of the formed elements. These are small irregular masses of basophilic cytoplasm containing azurophilic granules. They tend to form clumps in smears.

The leukocytes are subdivided into types according to the character of the nucleus, the absence or presence of granules in the cytoplasm, and the types of granules.

Those leukocytes with numerous granules and a lobulated nucleus are polymorphonuclear granulocytes. Of these, neutrophils (3) are most numerous. Their cytoplasm contains fine violet or pinkish granules. The nucleus has several lobes connected by chromatin strands. Fewer lobes indicate less mature cells.

Eosinophils (1) have large, bright pink granules which fill the cytoplasm. The nucleus is typically bilobed but a small, third lobe may be present. In basophils (2), the granules are not as numerous as in eosinophils, they vary in size, and stain dark blue or brown. The nucleus is not markedly lobulated, and takes a pale, basophilic stain.

Agranular leukocytes have few or no granules in their cytoplasm and round to horseshoe-shaped nuclei. Lymphocytes show more variations in size than any other leukocytes, ranging from cells smaller than red blood corpuscles to almost twice as large (4). The nucleus occupies a large portion of the cell. It stains heavily, the chromatin being in dense blocks intermingled with less dense areas. The narrow rim of basophilic cytoplasm is agranular but often contains a few non-specific azurophilic granules.

In monocytes (5), the largest of the leukocytes, the nucleus varies from round, oval or indented to horseshoe-shaped, and stains more lightly than in lymphocytes. The chromatin is arranged in skein-like fashion. The abundant cytoplasm is lightly basophilic, and usually has many fine azurophilic granules.

PLATE 19

PERIPHERAL BLOOD SMEAR

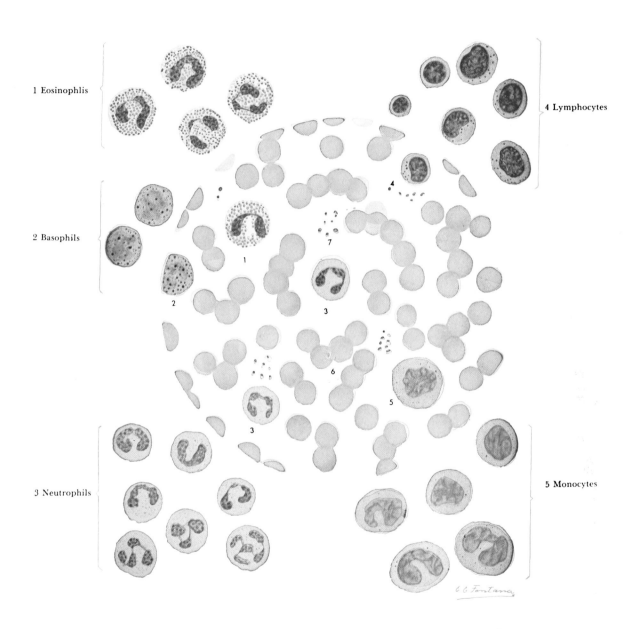

1 Eosinophlis

2 Basophils

3 Neutrophils

4 Lymphocytes

5 Monocytes

Stain: May-Grünwald-Giemsa. 1100×.

PLATE 20 (Fig. 1)

BLOOD CELLS: SUPRAVITAL STAINS

The formation of phagocytic vacuoles within leukocytes is easily demonstrated. A dilute solution of neutral red is placed on a slide, a drop of blood is added, and a cover slip placed over this. In 15 to 50 minutes vacuoles of different sizes appear in the cytoplasm (1, 2, 3:a). The smallest and slowest to appear are in small lymphocytes (2:a).

Mitochondria are demonstrated by using the same technique employing Janus green. Mitochondria stain a bluish green (1, 2, 3:b).

In reticulated erythrocytes, the youngest erythrocytes after extrusion of the nucleus, a reticulum can be demonstrated by placing a drop of blood on a slide on which a solution of cresyl blue has previously been allowed to dry. The reticulum is seen as filamentous networks of darkly staining granular material (4:c).

PLATE 20 (Fig. 2)

BLOOD SMEARS: PAPPENHEIM'S AND CELANI'S STAINS

The various types of blood cells are clearly differentiated by staining a blood film with May-Grünwald's stain, followed by Giemsa's stain. Nuclear structures, the more or less intense basophilic nature of the cytoplasm, and the various types of granules are well demonstrated (a) by this method.

Benzidine is oxidized by hydrogen peroxide activated by the peroxides in the blood cells. Granules which have oxidases stain blue. Polymorphs and monocytes in circulating blood have peroxidases (b); lymphocytes do not have them.

PLATE 20

BLOOD CELLS: SUPRAVITAL STAIN

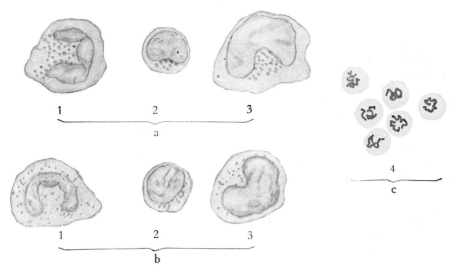

FIG. 1. *Supravital stain: blood cells.*

1. Neutrophilic granulocyte; 2. lymphocyte; 3. monocyte; 4. erythrocytes

   a) Vacuoles stained with neutral red.
   b) Mitochondria stained with Janus green.
   c) Reticulum stained with cresyl blue.

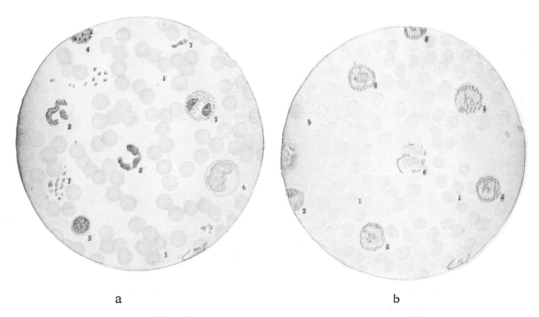

FIG. 2. *Pappenheim's and Celani's stains: blood smears.*

a) Pappenheim's method (May-Grünwald and Giemsa stains). Nuclei: reddish violet; basophilic cytoplasm: blue of varying intensity according to degree of basophilia; acidophilic cytoplasm: more or less deep red; neutrophilic granules: violet; eosinophilic granules: orange red; basophilic granules: dark violet; azurophilic granules: brilliant purple.

b) Peroxidase reaction. Celani's technique. Nuclei: light red; cytoplasm of leukocytes: pale pink; erythrocytes: yellow; granules with peroxidases: blue.

1. erythrocytes; 2. neutrophilic granulocyte; 3. eosinophil granulocyte; 4. basophil granulocyte; 5. lymphocyte; 6. monocyte; 7. platelets.

—53—

PLATE 21 (Fig. 1)

HEMOPOIETIC BONE MARROW (SECTION)

In a section of red bone marrow, it is usually difficult to distinguish all the types of developing blood cells. The cells are densely packed and different types are intermingled, although some of the erythrocytic forms often occur in groups or "nests" (6, 20). Details of structure are not as apparent as in a smear because of cell shrinkage during section preparation. Only parts of cells, rather than entire cells, may be present.

This section is stained with hematoxylin-eosin. At low magnification, little differentiation of cytoplasm is visible, except for brightly staining eosinophilic granules (4). For comparison, the individual cells below are from a marrow smear, where detailed structure can be seen.

The reticular connective tissue stroma of the marrow is largely obscured by hemopoietic cells, but may be seen in less dense areas (8), or, elongated reticular cells are often recognizable (24). Blood vessels of different kinds are seen (9, 10, 19, 25).

Conspicuous in marrow are large adipose cells (14), having a large vacuole (due to removal of fatty substances during section preparation) and a small amount of peripheral cytoplasm surrounding the nucleus (2).

Other cells easily identified are the huge megakaryocytes (5, 23) whose nuclei show varied lobulations.

Erythrocytes are abundant (12). The most easily recognizable of the earlier erythrocytic cells are normoblasts (20) with small, darkly staining nuclei (as in f). Many are in mitosis (18). Polychromatophilic erythroblasts may also occur in groups or "nests" (22) and are larger than normoblasts, with a larger nucleus having a more evident checkerboard appearance (as in e). Basophilic erythroblasts (3) are still larger cells with large, less dense nuclei and basophilic cytoplasm (as in d).

In the granulocytic series, the most easily recognizable are the polymorphonuclear heterophils (16) (corresponding to neutrophils in man) and eosinophils. Their earlier forms, metamyelocytes (21), have bean-shaped or horseshoe-shaped nuclei (as in c). Myelocytes (1, 4, b) have larger, round or ovoid nuclei.

Less easily recognizable in a section are the pale-staining primitive reticular cells (11) and hemocytoblasts (13, 17, a). Nuclei of the latter contain one or two nuclei.

An alternate terminology for the developing erythrocytic forms, in wide use clinically, is as follows:

Proerythroblast = rubriblast
Basophilic erythroblast = prorubricyte
Polychromatophilic erythroblast = rubricyte
Normoblast = metarubricyte

PLATE 21 (Fig. 2)

BONE MARROW OF A RABBIT, INDIA INK PREPARATION (SECTION)

Hemopoietic bone marrow is illustrated in which some of the primitive reticular cells of the stroma (1, 8) and some of the reticuloendothelial cells (2) lining the venous sinusoids (3) are filled with carbon granules which they have ingested following injection of India ink. Carbon granules may be so dense that the nucleus of the cell is obscured (1, 8). These cells are the fixed macrophages, which have the ability to phagocytize foreign matter while they are part of the stroma or the reticuloendothelium.

Other primitive reticular or reticuloendothelial cells do not exhibit such phagocytosis (12).

Various cells of the erythrocytic and granulocytic series are shown (4, 6, 7, 11, 13) as well as a megakaryocyte (10).

PLATE 21
BONE MARROW (SECTION)

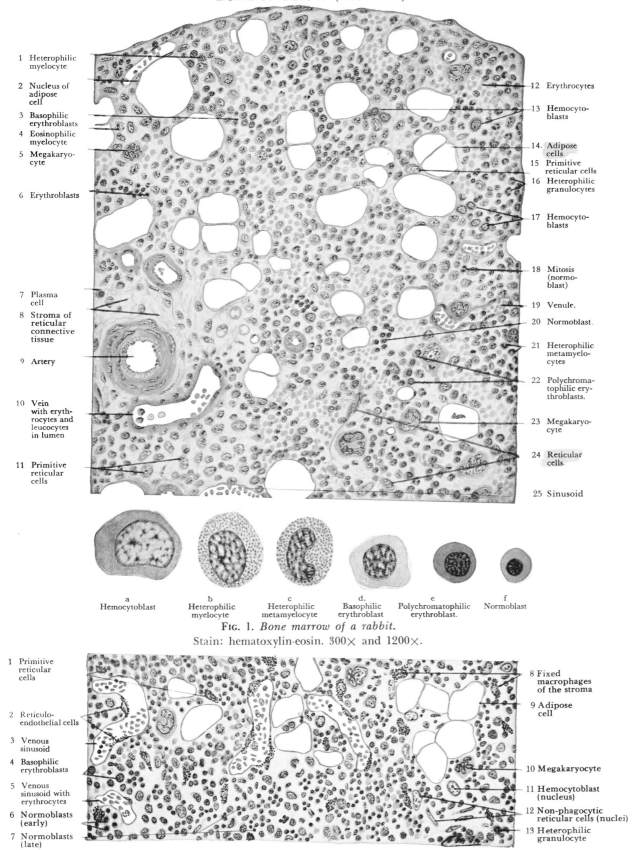

1 Heterophilic myelocyte
2 Nucleus of adipose cell
3 Basophilic erythroblasts
4 Eosinophilic myelocyte
5 Megakaryocyte
6 Erythroblasts
7 Plasma cell
8 Stroma of reticular connective tissue
9 Artery
10 Vein with erythrocytes and leucocytes in lumen
11 Primitive reticular cells

12 Erythrocytes
13 Hemocytoblasts
14. Adipose cells.
15 Primitive reticular cells
16 Heterophilic granulocytes
17 Hemocytoblasts
18 Mitosis (normoblast)
19 Venule.
20 Normoblast.
21 Heterophilic metamyelocytes
22 Polychromatophilic erythroblasts.
23 Megakaryocyte
24 Reticular cells.
25 Sinusoid

a Hemocytoblast
b Heterophilic myelocyte
c Heterophilic metamyelocyte
d. Basophilic erythroblast
e Polychromatophilic erythroblast.
f Normoblast

FIG. 1. *Bone marrow of a rabbit.*
Stain: hematoxylin-eosin. 300× and 1200×.

1 Primitive reticular cells
2 Reticulo-endothelial cells
3 Venous sinusoid
4 Basophilic erythroblasts
5 Venous sinusoid with erythrocytes
6 Normoblasts (early)
7 Normoblasts (late)

8 Fixed macrophages of the stroma
9 Adipose cell
10 Megakaryocyte
11 Hemocytoblast (nucleus)
12 Non-phagocytic reticular cells (nuclei)
13 Heterophilic granulocyte

FIG. 2. *Bone marrow of a rabbit, India ink preparation (section)*
Stain: hematoxylin-eosin. 250x.

PLATE 22

BONE MARROW: SMEAR

In the center of the plate is represented a microscopic field of human bone marrow smear obtained by sternal puncture. Around this are typical cells showing their detailed structure. Formed elements, as seen in the peripheral blood, are easily recognizable: erythrocytes (18, 31), granulocytes (eosinophil 32; neutrophil 33), and platelets (24).

At (1) is an early hemocytoblast differentiating from a reticular cell to become the stem cell of all myeloid elements. It is a large cell with lightly basophilic cytoplasm, sometimes containing azurophilic granules, and a large nucleus with a delicate chromatin network and one or two large pale nucleoli. This cell rounds up, retaining the same characteristics. Cytoplasm becomes more basophilic as numerous mitotic divisions take place. Some workers recognize a myeloblast (2, 25), slightly different from the hemocytoblast, as the parent cell of the granulocytes. It is a large cell (15–18 μ) with deeply basophilic cytoplasm which sometimes contains azurophilic granules. The large nucleus occupies the greater part of the cell; it contains two or three pale nucleoli.

In the erythrocytic series, the parent cell is the proerythroblast* (3, 8), 20–30 μ in diameter, with intensely basophilic cytoplasm. (Azurophilic granules are absent in all cells of this series.) The huge round or oval nucleus occupies most of the cell. Its fine chromatin filaments have a dotted line appearance. One or two large nucleoli may be present. By some authors, this cell is considered as the earliest basophilic erythroblast.

Basophilic erythroblasts (4, 7) are smaller (15–20 μ), cytoplasm is less intensely basophilic, but sufficiently so to obscure the small amount of hemoglobin present. The nucleus has decreased in size, the chromatin is in coarser strands and is beginning to assume the characteristic "checker-board" appearance. Nucleoli are inconspicuous or absent. There follows a series of polychromatophilic erythroblasts (5, 13, 14) of smaller size (12 to 15 μ), whose cytoplasm becomes progressively less basophilic and more acidophilic as more hemoglobin is acquired. Nuclei decrease rapidly in size, chromatin has the coarse "checker-board" arrangement.

When the cells acquire an acidophilic cytoplasm, they are normoblasts of 8–10 μ (6, 11). At first the nucleus has concentrated "checker-board" chromatin (6, 11), cell division continues. The nucleus then decreases rapidly in size, becomes pyknotic, and is extruded. The resulting flattened cell is the reticulocyte or young erythrocyte, with a bluish-pink cytoplasm (9, 16, 17). With special supravital staining, a delicate reticulum is demonstrated (see Plate 20, Fig. 1, 4c). Mature erythrocytes are smaller and have a homogeneous acidophilic cytoplasm (18, 31).

In the granulocytic series, the specific parent is the promyelocyte, 18–20 μ (19, early; 23, later). Cytoplasm is basophilic with variable numbers of azurophilic granules that take a reddish-purple stain. Chromatin in the rounded or oval nucleus is condensing to heavier strands. Nucleoli are less prominent. In the later promyelocytes, the nucleus becomes smaller, nucleoli disappear, azurophilic granules are fewer, and specific granules appear at one side of the nucleus (23, neutrophilic promyelocyte).

Myelocytes are smaller, with a smaller oval, eccentric nucleus with denser chromatin. Cytoplasm is less basophilic with few or no azurophilic granules and more specific granules (neutrophilic early myelocyte, 26; basophilic early myelocyte, 20). More mature myelocytes have abundant specific granules, slightly acidophilic cytoplasm, and a smaller nucleus (12, 21, 22, 27, 29, 34, 35). Cell division ceases with this stage.

In the metamyelocytes, the configuration of the nucleus changes from the oval, eccentric nucleus to that of the mature cells, the greatest change taking place in the neutrophilic forms (in succession: 30 and 36, 28, the two cells in line with erythrocyte 31, 33). Changes in eosinophils and basophils can be followed: (27 lower leader, 27 upper leader, 32; 20, 12).

Megakaryoblasts (37) are 40–60 μ in diameter, have basophilic cytoplasm and a voluminous, unevenly rounded nucleus with chromatin in a screen or sieve arrangement, and poorly defined nucleoli. Megakaryocytes, 80–100 μ, have a larger volume of slightly acidophilic cytoplasm filled with fine azurophilic granules (15, 38). The cell surface forms pseudopodial extensions which apparently form platelets (39). The nucleus is lobulated in various ways; it has a condensed chromatin net, nucleoli are absent.

* For alternate terminology, see page 54, Fig. 1, paragraph 9.

PLATE 22

BONE MARROW: SMEAR

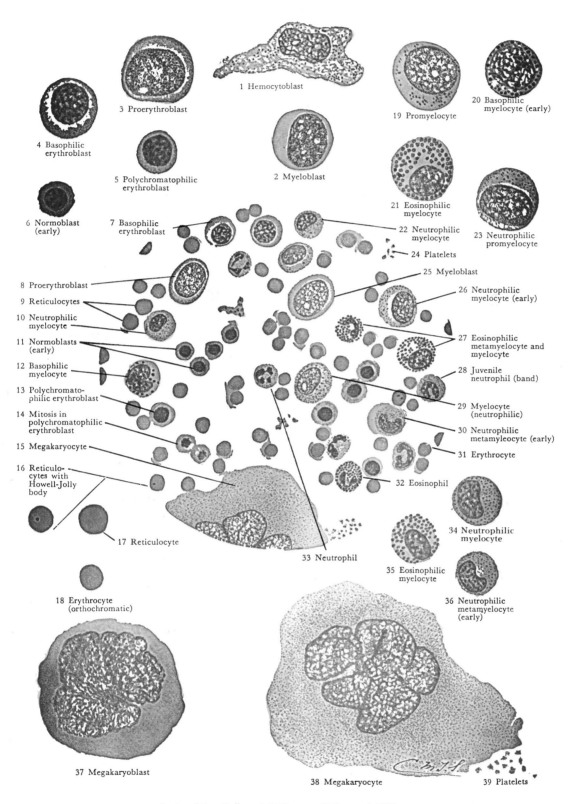

1 Hemocytoblast

3 Proerythroblast

4 Basophilic
erythroblast

5 Polychromatophilic
erythroblast

2 Myeloblast

6 Normoblast
(early)

7 Basophilic
erythroblast

19 Promyelocyte

20 Basophilic
myelocyte (early)

21 Eosinophilic
myelocyte

22 Neutrophilic
myelocyte

23 Neutrophilic
promyelocyte

24 Platelets

25 Myeloblast

26 Neutrophilic
myelocyte (early)

27 Eosinophilic
metamyelocyte and
myelocyte

28 Juvenile
neutrophil (band)

29 Myelocyte
(neutrophilic)

30 Neutrophilic
metamyelocyte (early)

31 Erythrocyte

32 Eosinophil

8 Proerythroblast

9 Reticulocytes

10 Neutrophilic
myelocyte

11 Normoblasts
(early)

12 Basophilic
myelocyte

13 Polychromato-
philic erythroblast

14 Mitosis in
polychromatophilic
erythroblast

15 Megakaryocyte

16 Reticulo-
cytes with
Howell-Jolly
body

17 Reticulocyte

18 Erythrocyte
(orthochromatic)

33 Neutrophil

34 Neutrophilic
myelocyte

35 Eosinophilic
myelocyte

36 Neutrophilic
metamyelocyte
(early)

37 Megakaryoblast

38 Megakaryocyte

39 Platelets

Stain: May-Grünwald-Giemsa. 800× and 1200×.

PLATE 23 (Fig. 1)

SMOOTH MUSCLE FIBERS

In this illustration, from the wall of the distended bladder of the toad, smooth muscle is present in small bundles of different sizes (2, 5). Individual muscle fibers can be distinguished in some of the very small bundles (2). Each one is a spindle-shaped cell, thick in the middle, tapered at the ends, with deeply stained cytoplasm (called sarcoplasm in muscle) and an elongated or ovoid nucleus (3) centrally placed.

In the loose connective tissue between bundles of muscle fibers are seen fibroblasts with clearly defined processes (1, 6), and a capillary containing erythrocytes (4).

Single and small groups of smooth muscle fibers are also illustrated on Plate 2, Fig. 2 (4, 11).

PLATE 23 (Fig. 2)

SKELETAL (STRIATED) MUSCLE FIBERS (DISSOCIATED)

Muscle fibers from the leg of a toad are shown here, teased to separate them, and stained with hematoxylin-eosin. Fibers (1) are much longer and much greater in diameter than are smooth muscle fibers. Each fiber shows distinct cross-striations, which are seen as alternating dark or A bands or discs (4) and light or I bands or discs (5). With higher magnifications, further details are visible, as in Plate 24, Fig. 4. Each fiber is multinucleated. The nuclei lie immediately under the sarcolemma, as is shown in those seen on the sides of the fibers (6). (Sarcolemma is not indicated in the figure.)

A fiber which has been torn by teasing shows its myofibrils joined together in thin bundles (2). Each myofibril has the characteristic cross-striations. These are aligned side by side in adjacent fibrils, thus giving the appearance of continuous cross-striations across a muscle fiber.

Numerous capillaries are present in the connective tissue (endomysium) between muscle fibers. One is shown in close proximity to a fiber (3).

PLATE 23

MUSCLE TISSUE

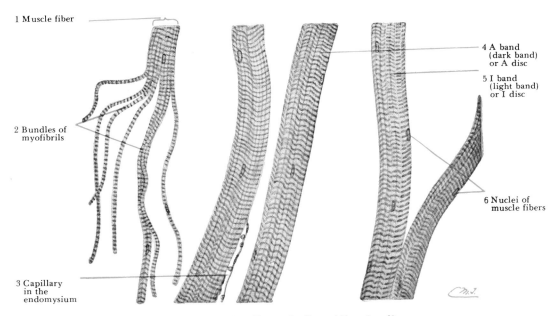

1 Fibroblasts

2 Bundle of smooth muscle fibers

3 Nucleus of a smooth muscle fiber (cell)

4 Capillary with erythrocytes

5 Bundle of smooth muscle fibers

6 Fibroblasts

FIG. 1. *Smooth muscle fibers.*
Stain: hematoxylin-eosin. 360×.

1 Muscle fiber

2 Bundles of myofibrils

3 Capillary in the endomysium

4 A band (dark band) or A disc

5 I band (light band) or I disc

6 Nuclei of muscle fibers

FIG. 2. *Skeletal (striated) muscle fibers (dissociated)*
Stain: hematoxylin-eosin. 250×.

PLATE 24 (Fig. 1)

SKELETAL MUSCLE (MUSCLES OF THE TONGUE)

A section from the central part of the tongue is illustrated, in which many skeletal muscle fibers have been cut longitudinally (3, 6) or transversally (5, 8). The fibers are aggregated into fasciculi (3, 5) which are held together by interfascicular connective tissue (10). Some of this connective tissue forms a compact sheath, the perimysium (2), around each fasciculus of muscle. From the perimysium, thin partitions of connective tissue, the endomysium (1), penetrate into the fasciculus to surround and separate the individual muscle fibers. Small blood vessels are present throughout the connective tissue (7).

Those muscle fibers which have been sectioned longitudinally show their cross-striations (6); those sectioned transversally show bundles of myofibrils cut in cross-section (Cohnheim's fields) (4). Nuclei of muscle fibers are located peripherally (9, 11); this is well demonstrated in transverse sections of fibers (9).

PLATE 24 (Fig. 2)

SMOOTH MUSCLE (MUSCLE LAYERS OF THE INTESTINE)

In one layer, fibers have been sectioned longitudinally (1). The spindle shape of individual fibers can be distinguished. The nucleus (2) is placed in the widest part of each fiber. The muscle fibers in this compact layer are arranged so that the thick parts of fibers are adjacent to the thinner ends of others.

In the second layer, fibers have been sectioned transversally (5). The cross sections are of different diameters, depending on whether the section passed through the central part or through the tapering ends. The largest sections contain the nucleus, also seen in transverse section (5, upper leader).

Small amounts of fine connective tissue envelop the muscle fibers. Larger amounts occur between the two layers of muscle (3) and around blood vessels (4).

PLATE 24 (Fig. 3)

CARDIAC MUSCLE (MYOCARDIUM)

Although resembling skeletal muscle fibers, cardiac muscle fibers branch without much change in diameter. Cross-striations are clearly seen in those fibers sectioned longitudinally (1). Additional transverse striations, the intercalated discs (2), are seen at intervals. They are irregular, are broader than the cross-striations, and represent the interdigitating ends of cardiac muscle cells.

Nuclei of cardiac muscle fibers are centrally placed within the fibers (5, 8). This is clearly visible in those fibers sectioned transversally (8). A clear zone of perinuclear sarcoplasm, free of myofibrils (9), may be seen in some of the sections.

Numerous small blood vessels (6, 7) lie in the interfascicular connective tissue and capillaries are abundant in the endomysium.

PLATE 24 (Fig. 4)

SKELETAL MUSCLE (LONGITUDINAL SECTION)

Several muscle fibers are illustrated as seen at a high magnification and stained with iron hematoxylin, which demonstrates cross-striations well. The A bands or discs or anisotropic discs (2) are the prominent darkly stained bands; the lighter middle region, or H band, is not visible. The I bands or discs or isotropic discs are equally prominent lightly stained acidophilic bands. Crossing the central portion of the I discs are the distinct narrow lines, the Z lines (3).

The closely arranged parallel myofibrils give a faint longitudinally striated appearance to the muscle fibers. Where the myofibrils are exposed because of rupture of the sarcolemma (6), the A and I bands or discs and Z lines are seen on the myofibrils, aligned next to each other on adjacent myofibrils.

Slender ovoid or elongated nuclei (4) of muscle fibers are seen at the periphery of the fibers. In the endomysium (1) between muscle fibers are seen fibroblasts (5) and a capillary (7).

PLATE 24 (Fig. 5)

CARDIAC MUSCLE (LONGITUDINAL SECTION)

Comparison of cardiac with skeletal muscle at the same high magnification and with similar staining illustrates the similarities and differences.

Branching of cardiac fibers (3) is in contrast to individual skeletal fibers. Cross-striations are similar in both but less prominent in cardiac muscle (2, 5). The thicker, more irregular cross-striations seen at intervals are the intercalated discs (7), characteristic of cardiac muscle.

Large, oval nuclei (1) in the center of the cardiac fibers occupy much of the width of the fibers, in contrast to the many elongated nuclei of skeletal fibers located peripherally. Distinctive is the mass of perinuclear sarcoplasm (6). Endomysium (4) fills the spaces between fibers.

PLATE 24

MUSCLE

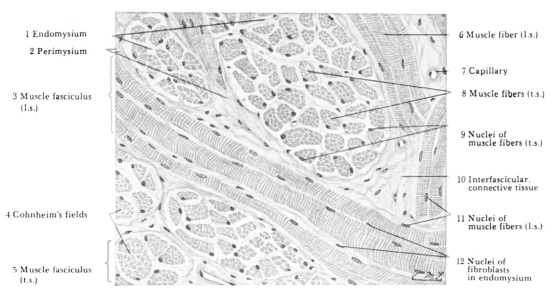

1 Endomysium
2 Perimysium
3 Muscle fasciculus (l.s.)
4 Cohnheim's fields
5 Muscle fasciculus (t.s.)
6 Muscle fiber (l.s.)
7 Capillary
8 Muscle fibers (t.s.)
9 Nuclei of muscle fibers (t.s.)
10 Interfascicular. connective tissue
11 Nuclei of muscle fibers (l.s.)
12 Nuclei of fibroblasts in endomysium

FIG. 1. *Skeletal muscle:* Muscles of the tongue.   Stain: hematoxylin-eosin. 320×.

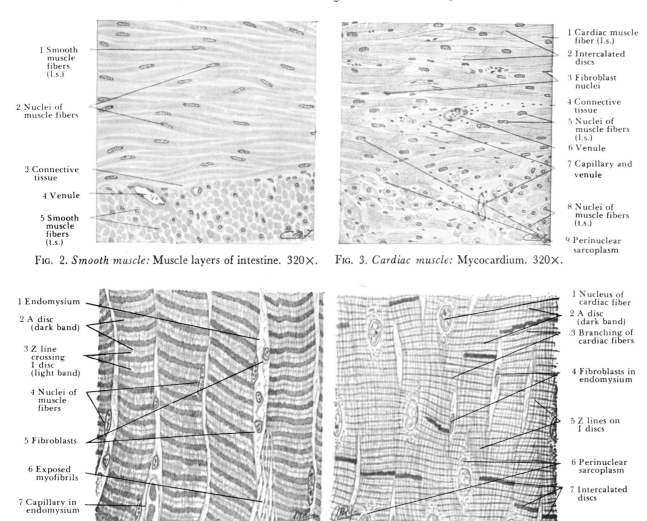

1 Smooth muscle fibers (l.s.)
2 Nuclei of muscle fibers
3 Connective tissue
4 Venule
5 Smooth muscle fibers (t.s.)

1 Cardiac muscle fiber (l.s.)
2 Intercalated discs
3 Fibroblast nuclei
4 Connective tissue
5 Nuclei of muscle fibers (l.s.)
6 Venule
7 Capillary and venule
8 Nuclei of muscle fibers (t.s.)
9 Perinuclear sarcoplasm

FIG. 2. *Smooth muscle:* Muscle layers of intestine. 320×.   FIG. 3. *Cardiac muscle:* Mycocardium. 320×.

1 Endomysium
2 A disc (dark band)
3 Z line crossing I disc (light band)
4 Nuclei of muscle fibers
5 Fibroblasts
6 Exposed myofibrils
7 Capillary in endomysium

1 Nucleus of cardiac fiber
2 A disc (dark band)
3 Branching of cardiac fibers
4 Fibroblasts in endomysium
5 Z lines on I discs
6 Perinuclear sarcoplasm
7 Intercalated discs

FIG. 4. *Skeletal muscle (longitudinal section).* 1000×.   FIG. 5. *Cardiac muscle. (longitudinal section).* 1000×.
Stain: Iron hematoxylin-eosin.

—61—

PLATE 25 (Fig. 1)

GRAY MATTER (ANTERIOR HORN OF THE SPINAL CORD)

The large multipolar anterior horn cells or motor cells (2) of the ventral gray matter of the spinal cord have a proportionally large central nucleus (7, 14) with a prominent nucleolus (6, 13), several cell processes, the dendrites (8, 9), and a single axon (1) which arises from a clear area, the axon hillock (5).

The cytoplasm or neuroplasm of the nerve cell body (perikaryon) contains numerous clumps of coarsely granular chromophilic substance (basophilic substance), the Nissl bodies (12), which stain a deep blue with basic aniline of Nissl's method. The Nissl bodies extend into the dendrites (8, 9) but not into the axon hillock (5) or into the axon (1). The nucleus (7, 14) is distinctly outlined. It stains lightly since the chromatin is dispersed in fine networks (a vesicular nucleus). The nucleolus (6, 13) is large, dense, and stains deeply.

Nuclei of neuroglia cells are stained; the small amount of cytoplasm is not stained. Protoplasmic astrocytes (3, 17) have rounded nuclei with a somewhat loose chromatin network. Nuclei of oligodendrocytes (16) are smaller, also rounded, and stain more deeply. Microglia (11) have elongated dark nuclei.

PLATE 25 (Fig. 2)

GRAY MATTER (ANTERIOR HORN OF THE SPINAL CORD)

This section was prepared by silver impregnation (Cajal's method) which demonstrates neurofibrils. In the large anterior horn cells or motor cells, neurofibrils in their typical arrangement are seen in the nerve cell bodies (3, 6, 11, 13) and in their dendrites (7, 12). Axons are not illustrated but neurofibrils would be seen in parallel arrangement.

Other details of cell structure are not revealed with silver impregnation. The nucleus of the neuron cell body is seen as a lightly stained or almost clear space (14, and in nerve cells 3 and 11). The nucleolus may stain slightly (as in nerve cell 11), but sometimes it is deeply stained (15).

In the intercellular areas are seen many fibrillar processes, some of which are processes of the anterior horn cells and other nerve cells. Some may be processes of neuroglia cells.

Nuclei of neuroglia cells are stained (1, 4, 5, 8, 9, 10) showing characteristics as described in Fig. 1.

PLATE 25

NERVOUS TISSUE

1 Axon of a motor
 neuron (anterior
 horn cell)

2 Cell body (perikaryon)
 of a motor neuron

3 Nuclei of
 protoplasmic
 astrocytes

4 Nerve cell
 sectioned near
 its surface

5 Axon hillock

6 Nucleolus

7 Nucleus of
 a nerve cell

8 Dendrites
 with
 chromophilic
 substance
 (Nissl bodies)

9 Dendrite

10 Capillary

11 Nuclei of
 microglial cells

12 Neuroplasm (cytoplasm)
 with Nissl bodies

13 Nucleolus

14 Nucleus showing
 the chromatin reticulum

15 Capillary

16 Nuclei of
 oligodendrocytes

17 Nuclei of
 protoplasmic astrocytes

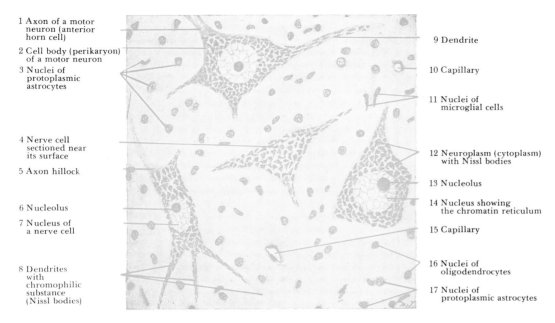

FIG. 1. *Gray matter (anterior horn of the spinal cord).*
Nissl's method. 350×.

1 Protoplasmic astrocytes
 (nuclei)

2 Neurofibrils

3 Cell body
 (perikaryon) of
 a motor neuron

4 Obligodendrocytes
 (nuclei)

5 Protoplasmic astrocytes
 (nuclei)

6 Nerve cell body
 sectioned
 near its surface

7 Dendrites with neurofibrils

8 Microglia (nuclei)

9 Oligodendrocytes
 (nuclei)

10 Protoplasmic astrocytes
 (nuclei)

11 Cell body of
 a motor neuron

12 Dendrite with
 neurofibrils

13 Neurofibrils in
 the cell body

14 Nucleus
15 Nucleolus

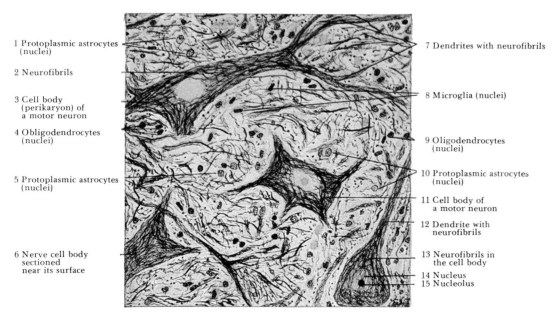

FIG. 2. *Gray matter (anterior horn of the spinal cord).*
Cajal's method. 350×.

PLATE 26 (Fig. 1)

GRAY MATTER (ANTERIOR HORN OF THE SPINAL CORD)

With Golgi's method of silver impregnation, nerve cell bodies and their processes are stained a homogeneous dark brown (4, 2). Their processes can be traced to their finest branches (2). Structural details, as seen in Plate 25, are not demonstrated with this method.

Protoplasmic astrocytes are also stained (1, 3). The small cell body and numerous short, thick branching processes are seen distinctly.

PLATE 26 (Fig. 2)

GRAY MATTER (ANTERIOR HORN OF THE SPINAL CORD)

This staining method, using mordanted sections and hematoxylin, demonstrates nerve fibers. The cytoplasm of the neuron cell bodies is greatly shrunken and retracted and takes only a pale yellowish background stain (1, 4). The nucleus (3) is outlined but also greatly shrunken. No structural details of either cytoplasm or nucleus are visible.

Nerve fibers of varying sizes (2, 5) and fine processes of neuroglia cells fill the intercellular areas. The nerve fibers course in various directions.

PLATE 26

NERVOUS TISSUE

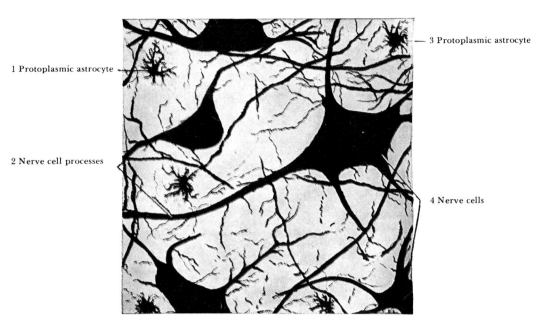

1 Protoplasmic astrocyte

3 Protoplasmic astrocyte

2 Nerve cell processes

4 Nerve cells

Fig. 1. *Gray matter (anterior horn of the spinal cord).*
Golgi's method. 350×.

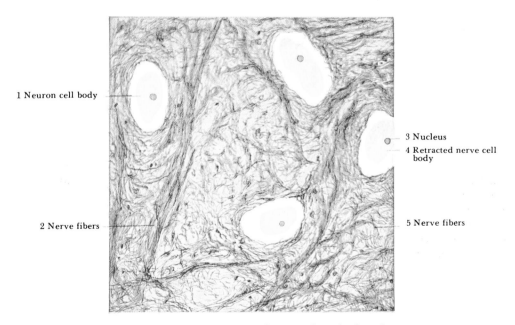

1 Neuron cell body

3 Nucleus

4 Retracted nerve cell body

2 Nerve fibers

5 Nerve fibers

Fig. 2. *Gray matter (anterior horn of the spinal cord).*
Modified Weigert-Pal method. 350×.

PLATE 27 (Fig. 1)

FIBROUS ASTROCYTES OF THE BRAIN

The section has been stained by Del Rio Hortega's method for astrocytes (i.e., macroglia), which demonstrates cell outlines, processes and glial fibers.

In the center of the figure is a fibrous astrocyte with a small cell body and a large nucleus (5), and numerous long, comparatively smooth processes (6), only slightly branched, extending out in all directions. The presence of neuroglia fibers in cell body and processes is indicated. One of these processes terminates on a blood vessel (4) as a vascular pedicle (perivascular foot, foot plate).

In the upper left of the figure, the processes of another fibrous astrocyte are seen in close relationship to a blood vessel (1), and one pedicle is indicated (2, lower leader).

PLATE 27 (Fig. 2)

OLIGODENDROCYTES OF THE BRAIN

The section has been stained with Del Rio Hortega's modification of Golgi's method.

A protoplasmic astrocyte (4) shows its small cell body with a large nucleus, and numerous short, thick, greatly branched processes.

Oligodendrocytes (2, 5) have smaller rounded or oval cell bodies and nuclei than do astrocytes, and only a few thin processes without much branching. Processes may be extremely thin (5, type I oligodendrocyte) or somewhat thicker (2, type II oligodendrocyte).

Oligodendrocytes are found in both gray and white matter. In the white matter, their processes surround nerve fibers (6).

The neuron (1) provides a size contrast.

PLATE 27 (Fig. 3)

MICROGLIA OF THE BRAIN

Del Rio Hortega's method for demonstrating microglia has been used. Cell bodies are very small, variable and often irregular in contour (1, 4). The small nucleus almost fills the cell, and stains deeply. Processes are short, slender but very tortuous, and are covered with minute "spines" (5).

Microglia are found throughout the central nervous system. They are of mesodermal origin, and become macrophages on demand.

The neuron cell body (3) provides a size contrast.

PLATE 27

NEUROGLIA

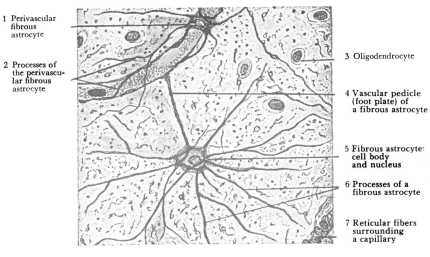

1 Perivascular fibrous astrocyte

2 Processes of the perivascular fibrous astrocyte

3 Oligodendrocyte

4 Vascular pedicle (foot plate) of a fibrous astrocyte

5 Fibrous astrocyte: cell body and nucleus

6 Processes of a fibrous astrocyte

7 Reticular fibers surrounding a capillary

FIG. 1. *Fibrous astrocytes of the brain.*
Del Rio Hortega's method.

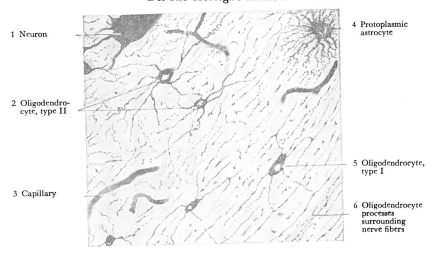

1 Neuron

2 Oligodendrocyte, type II

3 Capillary

4 Protoplasmic astrocyte

5 Oligodendrocyte, type I

6 Oligodendrocyte processes surrounding nerve fibers

FIG. 2. *Oligodendrocytes of the brain.*

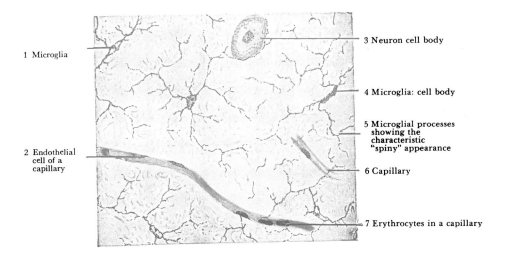

1 Microglia

2 Endothelial cell of a capillary

3 Neuron cell body

4 Microglia: cell body

5 Microglial processes showing the characteristic "spiny" appearance

6 Capillary

7 Erythrocytes in a capillary

FIG. 3. *Microglia of the brain.*
Del Rio Hortega's method.

PLATE 28 (Fig. 1)

MYELINATED NERVE FIBERS (DISSOCIATED)

A portion of the sciatic nerve of a toad has been treated with osmic acid and teased apart. Its constituent fibers appear as fine filaments, stained black by reduction of osmic acid where myelin is present. The myelin sheath is seen as a thick dark band on the periphery of the fibers (4); at intervals it is discontinued, forming the nodes (of Ranvier) (1, 6). At the nodes the fiber consists only of the unstained axon (2, 5, 7) surrounded by the the neurolemma or Schwann's sheath. The neurolemma envelops the full length of the fiber but is not demonstrated by the staining method used. The myelin sheath in the internodal segments shows many oblique unstained lines, the incisures of myelin (Schmidt-Lantermann clefts) (3, 8).

PLATE 28 (Fig. 2)

NERVE (TRANSVERSE SECTION)

Several bundles (fasciculi) of nerve fibers have been sectioned obliquely (8) or transversally (1). They are clearly separated from the neighboring connective tissue by the perineurium (2) which surrounds them. Delicate lamellae of connective tissue arise in the perineurium and penetrate between the fibers of each fasciculus; these fibers are known as the endoneurium (5). Among the nerve fibers there are many nuclei belonging to cells forming the neurolemma (Schwann's sheath) (3) or to fibroblasts of the endoneurium (5).

In the connective tissue (17) between the fasciculi an artery is seen, with its muscular coat (12), inner elastic membrane (14), endothelium (15) and the adventitia with nutritional vessels (13). There are also arteries of smaller diameter sectioned transversally or obliquely (6, 10), venules (16), capillaries (18), and adipose cells (7, 19).

PLATE 28

NERVOUS TISSUE

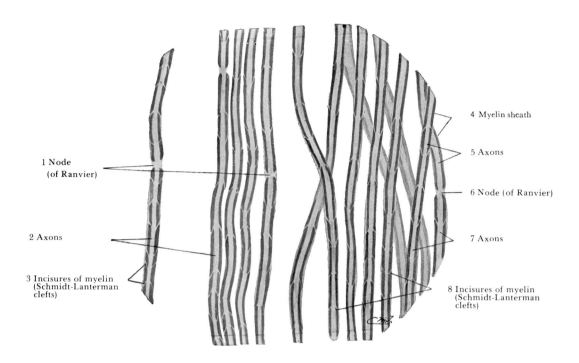

1 Node
(of Ranvier)

2 Axons

3 Incisures of myelin
(Schmidt-Lanterman
clefts)

4 Myelin sheath

5 Axons

6 Node (of Ranvier)

7 Axons

8 Incisures of myelin
(Schmidt-Lanterman
clefts)

FIG. 1. *Myelinated nerve fibers (dissociated).*
Stain: osmic acid. 220×.

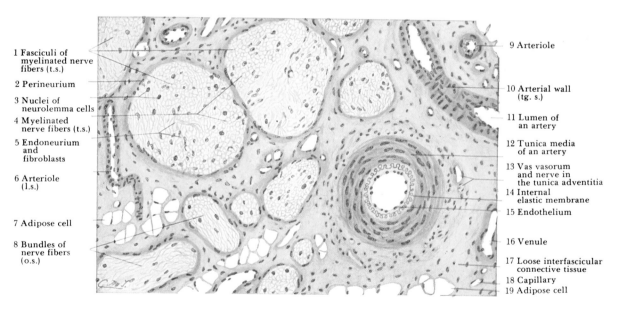

1 Fasciculi of
myelinated nerve
fibers (t.s.)

2 Perineurium

3 Nuclei of
neurolemma cells

4 Myelinated
nerve fibers (t.s.)

5 Endoneurium
and
fibroblasts

6 Arteriole
(l.s.)

7 Adipose cell

8 Bundles of
nerve fibers
(o.s.)

9 Arteriole

10 Arterial wall
(tg. s.)

11 Lumen of
an artery

12 Tunica media
of an artery

13 Vas vasorum
and nerve in
the tunica adventitia

14 Internal
elastic membrane

15 Endothelium

16 Venule

17 Loose interfascicular
connective tissue

18 Capillary

19 Adipose cell

FIG. 2. *Nerve (transverse section).*
Stain: hematoxylin-eosin. 250×.

PLATE 29

NERVOUS TISSUE: NERVES AND NERVE FIBERS

This plate illustrates the appearance of nerves and their fibers after various staining procedures.

FIG. 1 *Nerve (panoramic view, longitudinal section)*

A portion of sciatic nerve is seen at a low magnification, as it appears in a routine preparation stained with hematoxylin-eosin. The outer part of the epineurium, of dense connective tissue, is not shown; the deeper part contains much adipose tissue (2) with many blood vessels (1). Extensions of the epineurium (3) pass between large fasciculi of nerve fibers (5). Perineurium (4) forms a dense sheath around each fasciculus. Many nuclei lined up along nerve fibers are neurolemma nuclei (Schwann cell nuclei) or nuclei of fibroblasts in the endoneurium. It is not possible to differentiate between them at this magnification.

FIG. 2 *Nerve (longitudinal section)*

A small portion of the nerve in Fig. 1 is shown at a high magnification. The axons are seen as slender threads stained lightly with hematoxylin (1). The surrounding myelin sheath has been dissolved, leaving a distinct neurokeratin network (3). The neurolemma is not always distinguishable from surrounding connective tissue, but may be seen in places as a thin, peripheral boundary (4) and at a node (of Ranvier) (2) as it dips in toward the axon. Two neurolemma nuclei (Schwann cell nuclei) are seen (5). Endoneurium (sheath of Henle) (7) surrounds each fiber. It is now possible to distinguish between fibroblasts of the endoneurium (6) and neurolemma nuclei (5).

FIG. 3. *Nerve (transverse section)*

In this transverse section of sciatic nerve, at 800 × as in Fig. 2., one sees centrally placed axons (2), the neurokeratin network (3) as radial lines which do not reach the shrunken axon, and the peripheral neurolemma (4). A neurolemma nucleus (Schwann cell nucleus) appears to encircle the nerve fiber (1).

Collagenous fibers of the endoneurium are faintly distinguishable; fibroblasts, however, are clearly seen (5). Perineurium (6) surrounds fasciculi of nerve fibers. A small blood vessel (7) is present.

FIG. 4 *Nerve (longitudinal section)*

This section is stained with Protargol and aniline blue. Axons (1) are prominent because of silver impregnation of the neurofibrils. The scattered black spots probably represent remnants of neurofibrils remaining after shrinkage of the axon. The neurokeratin network is not stained. Other structures are stained with aniline blue.

FIG. 5. *Nerve (transverse section)*

As in Fig. 4, Protargol stains the axon (1), seen in cross section; the surrounding grayish area and small black droplets probably give an indication of the original diameter of the axon. Endoneurium is well demonstrated by aniline blue staining of the collagenous fibers (4, 6).

FIG. 6. *Nerve (transverse section)*

This figure illustrates still another staining method, and also shows myelinated nerve fibers of varying sizes in a branch of the vagus nerve in the cortex of the thymus. Nuclei, axons and neurokeratin network stain red with azocarmine (1, 3, 4, 6). Endoneurium is again demonstrated clearly, especially in areas where nerve fibers are close together (7) and within groups of small nerve fibers (8).

PLATE 29
NERVOUS TISSUE: NERVES AND NERVE FIBERS

1 Blood vessels

2 Adipose tissue
in epineurium

3 Extensions of
epineurium

4 Perineurium

5 Fasciculi of
nerve fibers

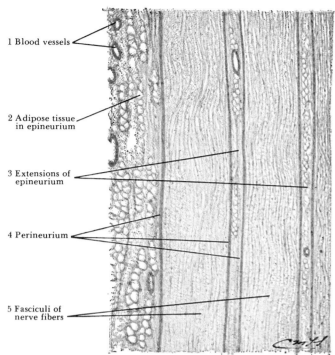

FIG. 1. *Nerve (sciatic), panoramic view, longitudinal section.*
Stain: hematoxylin-eosin. 50×.

1 Axons

2 Node (of Ranvier)

3 Neurokeratin
network

4 Neurolemma
(Schwann's sheath)

5 Neurolemma nucleus
(Schwann cell nucleus)

6 Fibroblast (nucleus)

7 Endoneurium

1 Neurolemma nucleus

2 Axon

3 Neurokeratin
network

4 Neurolemma

5 Fibroblast and
endoneurium

6 Perineurium

7 Venule

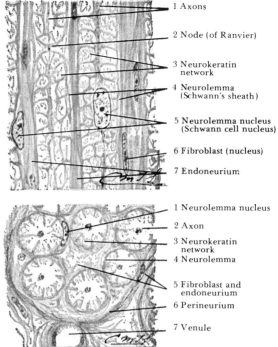

FIG. 2. (above) *Nerve (sciatic), longitudinal section.*
FIG. 3. (below) *Same, transverse section.*
Stain: hematoxylin-eosin. 800×.

1 Axons

2 Myelin sheath

3 Neurolemma

4 Neurolemma
at a node
(of Ranvier)

5 Fibroblasts
nuclei

6 Endoneurium

7 Neurolemma
nuclei

8 Node (of
Ranvier)

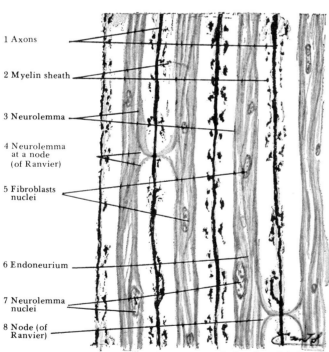

FIG. 4. *Nerve (sciatic), longitudinal section.*
Stain: Protargol and aniline blue. 800×.

1 Axon

2 Myelin sheath

3 Neurolemma

4 Endoneurium

5 Fibroblasts (nuclei)

6 Endoneurium

1 Fibroblast (nucleus)

2 Endoneurium

3 Axon

4 Neurokeratin network

5 Neurolemma

6 Neurolemma nucleus

7 Endoneurium

8 Small myelinated
nerve fibers

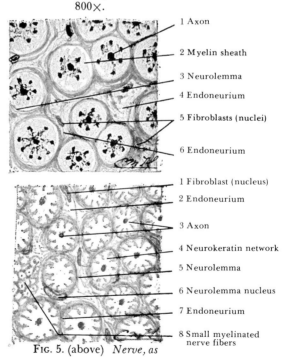

FIG. 5. (above) *Nerve, as in Fig. 4, transverse section.*
FIG. 6. (below) *Nerve (branch of the vagus), transverse section.*
Stain: Mallory-Azan. 800×.

PLATE 30

FIG. 1. DORSAL ROOT GANGLION: PANORAMIC VIEW (LONGITUDINAL SECTION)

A layer of connective tissue, rich in adipose cells and containing many blood vessels, surrounds the mass of nervous tissue (1, 6, 14). It merges with the external capsule of the ganglion, the epineurium (2), which is continuous with the epineurium of the dorsal root (3) and with that of the spinal nerve (11). Larger perineurial septa may be seen (4) but neither perineurium nor endoneurium are distinguishable at this magnification.

Large numbers of rounded unipolar ganglion cells make up the bulk of the ganglion (9), and are conspicuous because of their size and staining capacity. Their vesicular nuclei with nucleoli are visible but will be seen better at a higher magnification (Fig. 2). Bundles of nerve fibers may be seen between groups of ganglion cells. The larger bundles tend to run in a longitudinal direction (10) and will either enter the dorsal root (5) or the spinal nerve (12). These nerve fibers represent, respectively, the central processes and peripheral processes formed by the bifurcation of the single axonal process which emerges from each ganglion cell.

The ventral root (8) joins the nerve fibers emerging from the ganglion (13) to form the spinal nerve.

FIG. 2. SECTION OF A DORSAL ROOT GANGLION

At a higher magnification, one sees ganglion cells of various sizes. The characteristic vesicular nucleus with its prominent nucleolus (2) is conspicuous. The cytoplasm is filled with fine Nissl bodies (3). Some cells display a small clump of lipochrome pigment (5). Each cell has an axon hillock (not illustrated).

Within the perineuronal space, in intimate relationship with the ganglion cells, are satellite cells with rounded or oval nuclei, of neuroectodermal origin, forming a loose inner layer of the capsule (6). An outer capsule of more flattened fibroblasts and fibers (7) is continuous with the endoneurium. In sections, these two layers are not always clearly distinguishable; often the two cell types appear to be intermingled, as around the cell with the lipochrome pigment (5).

Between ganglion cells are seen many fibroblasts (4), randomly arranged in the connective tissue framework, or in rows in the endoneurium between nerve fibers (1, 8). With hematoxylin-eosin, small nerve fibers and connective tissue are not differentiated. Larger myelinated fibers are recognizable when sectioned longitudinally (1).

FIG. 3. SECTION OF A SYMPATHETIC TRUNK GANGLION

Like the dorsal root ganglion cells, sympathetic trunk ganglion cells have the characteristic nucleus and nucleolus (sometimes more than one nucleolus) and small Nissl bodies throughout the cytoplasm.

They are small multipolar cells, therefore cell outlines are often irregular and stumps of processes may be present (6). Nuclei are often eccentrically placed (6); binucleated cells are common. Most cells contain lipochrome pigment.

Satellite cells (2, 5) are usually less numerous than in dorsal root ganglion cells. The connective tissue capsule may or may not be well defined (3).

In the intercellular areas (4) are fibroblasts, supporting connective tissue, blood vessels, unmyelinated and thinly-myelinated fibers. Nerve fibers aggregate into bundles (1, 7) which course through the sympathetic trunk; they represent preganglionic fibers, postganglionic visceral efferent fibers and visceral afferent fibers.

PLATE 30

NERVOUS TISSUE: GANGLIA

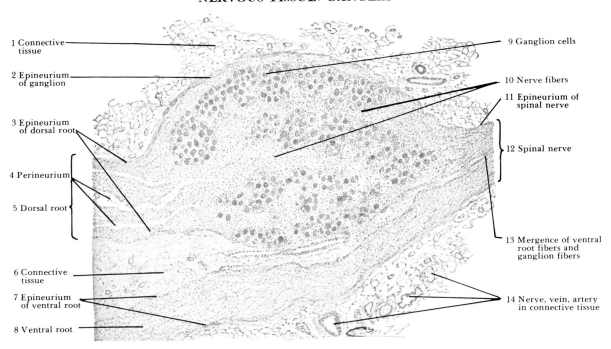

1 Connective tissue

2 Epineurium of ganglion

3 Epineurium of dorsal root

4 Perineurium

5 Dorsal root

6 Connective tissue

7 Epineurium of ventral root

8 Ventral root

9 Ganglion cells

10 Nerve fibers

11 Epineurium of spinal nerve

12 Spinal nerve

13 Mergence of ventral root fibers and ganglion fibers

14 Nerve, vein, artery in connective tissue

FIG. 1. *Dorsal root ganglion: panoramic view (longitudinal section).*
Stain: hematoxylin-eosin. 25×.

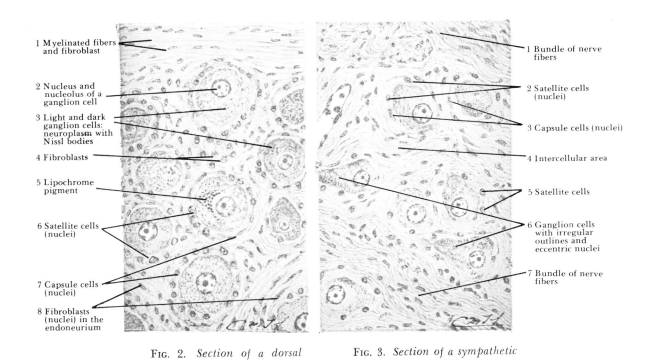

1 Myelinated fibers and fibroblast

2 Nucleus and nucleolus of a ganglion cell

3 Light and dark ganglion cells: neuroplasm with Nissl bodies

4 Fibroblasts

5 Lipochrome pigment

6 Satellite cells (nuclei)

7 Capsule cells (nuclei)

8 Fibroblasts (nuclei) in the endoneurium

1 Bundle of nerve fibers

2 Satellite cells (nuclei)

3 Capsule cells (nuclei)

4 Intercellular area

5 Satellite cells

6 Ganglion cells with irregular outlines and eccentric nuclei

7 Bundle of nerve fibers

FIG. 2. *Section of a dorsal root ganglion.*
Stain: hematoxylin-eosin. 400×.

FIG. 3. *Section of a sympathetic trunk ganglion.*
Stain: hematoxylin-eosin. 400×.

PLATE 31 (Fig. 1)

SPINAL CORD: CERVICAL
REGION (PANORAMIC VIEW,
TRANSVERSE SECTION)

In a transverse section through fresh tissue of a spinal cord, the substance of the cord is seen to be divided into outer white matter and inner gray matter. In stained material, the two areas are readily seen but lose the significance of the terms "white" and "gray." Cajal's silver impregnation method demonstrates neurofibrils.

The inner gray matter has the shape of an H. The crossbar is known as the gray commissure (16). The anterior (ventral) horn or column (17) is thicker and shorter than the posterior (dorsal) horn or column (14). In the anterior (ventral) horn lie two groups of nerve cell bodies: motor cells of the anteromedial column (8) and motor cells of the anterolateral column (7). Unmyelinated fibers (17) are clearly seen in this area. Certain of these fibers (9) penetrate the white matter to the periphery of the cord, at which point they will emerge obliquely as components of the anterior (ventral) roots (20). The posterior (dorsal) horn has isolated large nerve cell bodies (5) and groups of small ones.

The spinal cord on the posterior (dorsal) surface bears a longitudinal shallow groove in the midline, the posterior median sulcus (10). A neuroglial membrane, the posterior (dorsal) median septum (13), extends inward from the sulcus dividing the white matter in the posterior area into right and left halves. Each half in turn is divided by a less conspicuous postero-intermediate septum (12) into a postero-medial column, the fasciculus gracilis (Goll's column) (11) and a postero-lateral column, the fasciculus cuneatus (Burdach's column) (1).

A transverse section of the ependymal canal is seen in the middle of the gray commissure (15). Above and below the canal, the gray matter is referred to as the dorsal and ventral gray commissure (16) respectively. A ventral white commissure is usually seen below the ventral gray one.

The most peripheral part of the spinal cord is the marginal (superficial) glial membrane (4), an area free of nerve fibers. Pia mater is indicated by a yellow zone around the cord; it is seen best in the anterior ventral fissure (19).

PLATE 31 (Fig. 2)

SPINAL CORD: ANTERIOR (VENTRAL) HORN AND VENTRAL
WHITE MATTER (SECTIONAL VIEW)

In the anterior or ventral gray matter are seen multipolar anterior horn cells or motor cells (10) and their dendrites (2) at a higher magnification, showing typical characteristics as described previously. In the nerve cell bodies (8, 10), neurofibrils are in a network arrangement; in the dendrites (2), their arrangement is more parallel. The large, round distinct nucleus shows its prominent nucleolus (7). Other very small cell bodies are neuroglia cells (6).

In the intercellular areas of the ventral gray are seen nerve fibers (9) of different sizes and sectioned in various planes.

Axons of anterior horn cells aggregate into groups and enter the ventral white matter (1). They become myelinated (4) as they pass through the white matter, and leave the cord to become ventral root fibers.

The white matter is composed primarily of myelinated nerve fibers, closely packed, seen here in transverse sections (5). Their darkly stained shrunken axons (3) are surrounded by a clear space which had been occupied by myelin in the living tissue. These fibers compose the ascending and descending tracts that course longitudinally in the spinal cord.

PLATE 31

SPINAL CORD: CERVICAL REGION
(TRANSVERSE SECTION)

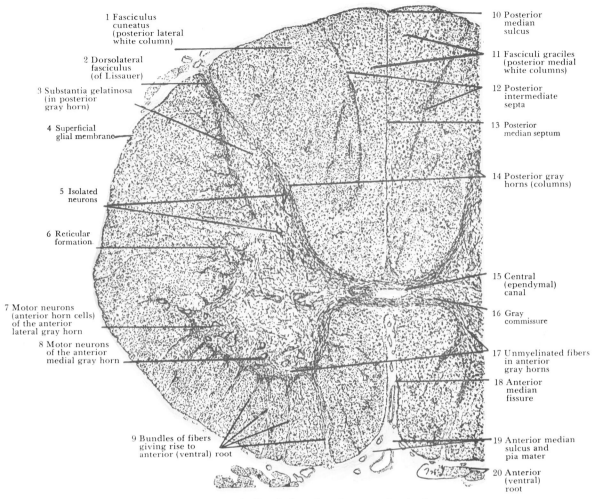

1 Fasciculus cuneatus (posterior lateral white column)

2 Dorsolateral fasciculus (of Lissauer)

3 Substantia gelatinosa (in posterior gray horn)

4 Superficial glial membrane

5 Isolated neurons

6 Reticular formation

7 Motor neurons (anterior horn cells) of the anterior lateral gray horn

8 Motor neurons of the anterior medial gray horn

9 Bundles of fibers giving rise to anterior (ventral) root

10 Posterior median sulcus

11 Fasciculi graciles (posterior medial white columns)

12 Posterior intermediate septa

13 Posterior median septum

14 Posterior gray horns (columns)

15 Central (ependymal) canal

16 Gray commissure

17 Unmyelinated fibers in anterior gray horns

18 Anterior median fissure

19 Anterior median sulcus and pia mater

20 Anterior (ventral) root

FIG. 1. *Cervical region (panoramic view).*
Silver impregnation: Cajal's method. 18×.

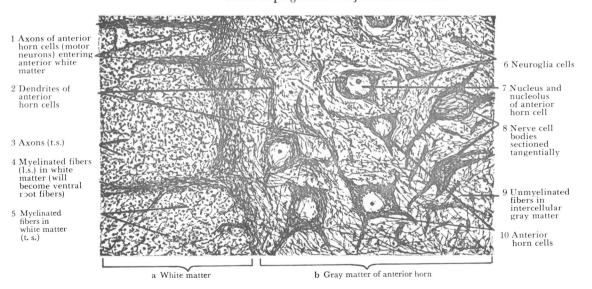

1 Axons of anterior horn cells (motor neurons) entering anterior white matter

2 Dendrites of anterior horn cells

3 Axons (t.s.)

4 Myelinated fibers (l.s.) in white matter (will become ventral root fibers)

5 Myelinated fibers in white matter (t. s.)

6 Neuroglia cells

7 Nucleus and nucleolus of anterior horn cell

8 Nerve cell bodies sectioned tangentially

9 Unmyelinated fibers in intercellular gray matter

10 Anterior horn cells

a White matter

b Gray matter of anterior horn

FIG. 2. *Anterior gray horn and adjacent anterior white matter.*
Silver impregnation: Cajal's method. 160×.

PLATE 32 (Fig. 1)

SPINAL CORD: MID-THORACIC REGION
(TRANSVERSE SECTION, PANORAMIC VIEW)

This illustration represents a transverse section of mid-thoracic cord, as seen in a routine hematoxylin-eosin preparation. It differs in several ways from the section of cervical cord represented in Plate 31. The dorsal gray columns (posterior or dorsal horns) are slender (5). At their ventromedial basal portion one sees the nucleus dorsalis (column of Clarke), a prominent structure because of the number and size of its neuron cell bodies (22). The lateral gray columns are well developed, and contain the small-celled lateral sympathetic nucleus (23). The ventral gray columns (anterior horns) are small; the number of motor cells is reduced to only a few cells in both the medial and lateral motor nuclei (24).

Other structures in this section of mid-thoracic cord are seen in corresponding areas of the cervical cord in Plate 31, differing only in appearance because of the stain used.

Shown here, in addition, are the meninges of the spinal cord. The fibrous pia mater (9), innermost layer of the meninges, adheres closely to the superficial (marginal) glial membrane of the cord, which is seen here indistinctly. In the pia mater are small blood vessels, as well as larger ones (1, 15), which supply the cord. Fine trabeculae in the subarachnoid space (10) connect the pia mater with the arachnoid (11); this space is normally filled with cerebrospinal fluid. Externally, there is a thick, fibrous dura mater (13), separated from the arachnoid by the subdural space (12). In this preparation, the subdural space is unusually large because of artificial retraction of the arachnoid.

PLATE 32 (Fig. 2)

NERVE CELLS OF SOME TYPICAL REGIONS OF THE CORD

Nerve cells, situated in the gray matter, present different characteristics according to the region they occupy and the function they carry out.

In this plate are shown several anterior horn cells (a), whose characteristics have been described in Plate 25, Fig. 1. Only the staining reaction is different here. The typical vesicular nucleus, with its prominent nucleolus, is centrally located. When the section passes through the superficial portion of a cell, the nucleus is not seen (2). Nissl substance appears as large clumps (1), uniformly distributed throughout the cytoplasm, and extends partway into the dendrites (4). The clear axon hillock and the beginning of the axon may be seen in some cells (3). These axons contribute to the formation of the ventral roots and terminate by innervating skeletal muscle (motor nerves).

The two cells in (b) are posterior horn cells from the substantia gelatinosa. They are much smaller than anterior horn cells, are ovoid or polygonal in shape, Nissl granules are fine, and the nucleus is usually deeply-stained. They are considered as association cells, especially for incoming pain and temperature impulses.

At (c) are represented two cells of the lateral sympathetic nucleus, located in the lateral gray column. These are also small cells, somewhat larger than those of the substantia gelatinosa, but show similar features. Their axons enter the ventral roots, and pass by way of white rami to vertebral or prevertebral ganglia.

The final group (d) represents cells from the nucleus dorsalis (column of Clarke); its location is seen at (22) in Fig. 1. They are large multipolar cells, similar in size to anterior horn cells. Nissl substance is in the form of clumps, which are characteristically situated at the periphery of the cell (5). The typical vesicular nucleus with its nucleolus is eccentrically placed (7). As usual, the nucleus is not seen when the section passes through the periphery of the cell (6). These cells receive incoming proprioceptive fibers.

—76—

PLATE 32

SPINAL CORD: MID-THORACIC REGION (TRANSVERSE SECTION)

1 Posterior spinal vessel (vein)

2 Dorsolateral sulcus

3 Dorsolateral fasciculus (of Lissauer)

4 Dorsal root fibers

5 Posterior gray horn

6 Lateral white column

7 Central canal

8 Anterior white commissure

9 Pia mater

10 Subarachnoid space

11 Arachnoid

12 Subdural space

13 Dura mater

14 Ventral root

15 Anterior spinal artery and vein

16 Posterior median sulcus and septum

17 Posterior intermediate septum

18 Fasciculus gracilis ⎫ Posterior white column

19 Fasciculus cuneatus ⎭

20 Substantia gelatinosa

21 Reticular process and reticular nucleus

22 Nucleus dorsalis (column of Clark)

23 Lateral (intermediate) column and lateral sympathetic nucleus

24 Medial and lateral motor nuclei in anterior gray horn

25 Filaments of ventral roots in anterior white column

26 Pia mater with blood vessels in anterior fissure

27 Anterior median sulcus

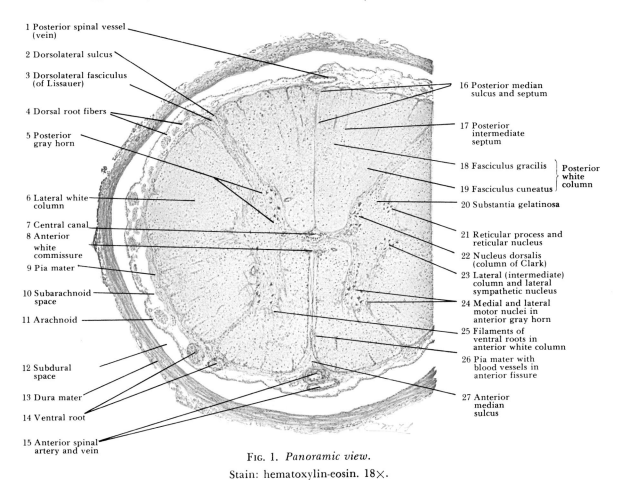

FIG. 1. *Panoramic view.*
Stain: hematoxylin-eosin. 18×.

b Cells of substantia gelatinosa

d Cells of nucleus dorsalis

1 Cytoplasm with Nissl substance

2 Cell sectioned through peripheral part

3 Axon hillock

4 Dendrites

5 Nissl substance at periphery

6 Cell sectioned through peripheral part

7 Eccentrically placed nucleus

a Anterior horn cells

d Cells of nucleus dorsalis

c Lateral sympathetic cells

FIG. 2. *Nerve cells of some typical regions of the spinal cord.*
Stain: hematoxylin-eosin. 380×.

PLATE 33 (Fig. 1)

CEREBELLUM (SECTIONAL VIEW, TRANSVERSE SECTION)

The cerebellum is composed of inner white matter (4) and outer gray matter (3).

The white matter (4) is made up of myelinated fibers; its ramifications (10) form the core of the numerous cerebellar folds. These fibers are incoming fibers to the cortex and efferent fibers of the cortex.

The gray matter constitutes the cortex. Three layers can be distinguished in the cortex: an outer molecular layer (6), with relatively few cells and with fibers directed horizontally; an inner granular layer (7) with numerous small cells with intensely stained nuclei; and an intermediate layer of Purkinje cells (8). The cells of Purkinje are pyriform and have ramified dendrites which extend into the molecular layer.

PLATE 33 (Fig. 2)

CEREBELLUM: CORTEX

Purkinje cells (pyriform cells) (9) are arranged typically in a single row at the junction of the molecular and granular layers. Their large flask-shaped cell bodies give off one or more thick dendrites (3) which extend through the molecular layer to the surface, giving off complex branchings along their course. The thin axon (5) leaves the base of the cell, passes through the granular layer and becomes a myelinated fiber as it enters the white matter (12).

In the molecular layer are scattered stellate cells (8). Their axons (unmyelinated fibers) course in a general horizontal direction. Descending collaterals of the more deeply placed stellate cells (basket cells) arborize around Purkinje cells (4) as "baskets" of terminal fibers. Axons of granule cells in the granular layer extend into the molecular layer and also course horizontally (2) as unmyelinated fibers.

In the granular layer are numerous small granule cells (6) with darkly staining nuclei (an exception to the usual vesicular nucleus of nerve cells) and very little cytoplasm. Also present are scattered larger stellate cells or Golgi II cells (7) with typical nuclei and more cytoplasm. Throughout the granular layer are small "clear" areas, the glomeruli (11) in which nerve cells are absent and synaptic connections occur.

PLATE 33

CEREBELLUM

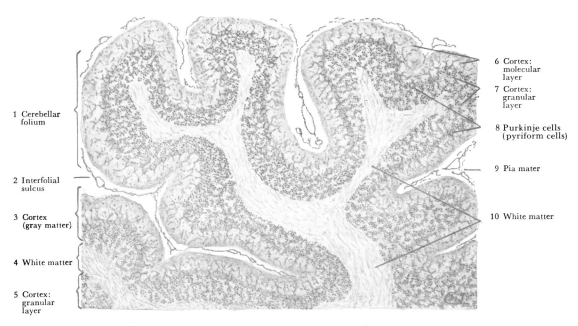

1 Cerebellar folium

2 Interfolial sulcus

3 Cortex (gray matter)

4 White matter

5 Cortex: granular layer

6 Cortex: molecular layer

7 Cortex: granular layer

8 Purkinje cells (pyriform cells)

9 Pia mater

10 White matter

FIG. 1. *Sectional view (transverse section).*
Silver impregnation: Cajal's method. 45×.

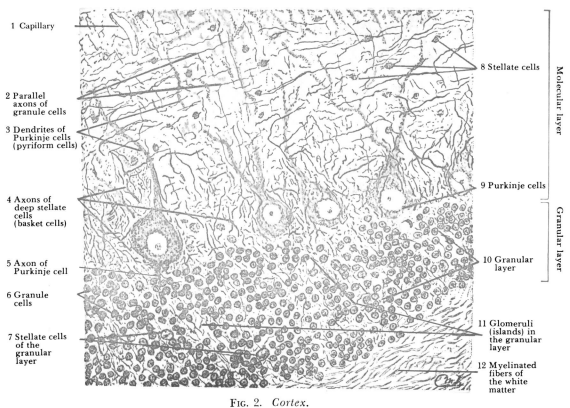

1 Capillary

2 Parallel axons of granule cells

3 Dendrites of Purkinje cells (pyriform cells)

4 Axons of deep stellate cells (basket cells)

5 Axon of Purkinje cell

6 Granule cells

7 Stellate cells of the granular layer

8 Stellate cells

9 Purkinje cells

10 Granular layer

11 Glomeruli (islands) in the granular layer

12 Myelinated fibers of the white matter

Molecular layer

Granular layer

FIG. 2. *Cortex.*
Silver impregnation: Cajal's method. 300×.

PLATE 34 (Fig. 1)

CEREBRAL CORTEX: SECTION PERPENDICULAR TO THE SURFACE OF THE CORTEX

The staining method demonstrates neurofibrils.

A variety of cell types is found in the cerebral cortex. These are not arranged at random but in layers, with one or more cell types predominant in each layer. Horizontal fibers associated with each layer also give a laminated appearance to the cortex. Fibers in radial arrangement (14) are also present.

Although there are variations in arrangement of cells in different parts of the cerebral cortex, six fundamental layers are recognized. These are indicated on the left side of the figure.

The outermost layer is the molecular layer (1). Its peripheral portion is composed exclusively of horizontally directed nerve fibers. In its deeper part lie the horizontal cells of Cajal (10) which are stellate or spindle-shaped cells; their axons give rise to the horizontal fibers. Overlying the molecular layer is the pia mater (8).

In the next four layers, the predominant cells are the characteristic pyramidal cells of the cerebral cortex. These vary in size. The figure indicates that they are progressively larger (11, 13) in layers 2, 3, 4, and 5. Their dendrites (13) are directed peripherally, the axon leaves from the base of the cell. In the internal granular layer (4), numerous small stellate or granule cells and some larger stellate cells (12) are intermingled with the pyramidal cells.

In the multiform layer (or layer of fusiform cells, layer of polymorphic cells) (6), pyramidal cells are lacking. Fusiform cells predominate, but granule cells, stellate cells and inverted cells of Martinotti are intermingled. All of these vary in size. Axons of the inverted cells are directed peripherally; axons of others enter the white matter (16).

PLATE 34 (Fig. 2)

CEREBRAL CORTEX: CENTRAL AREA OF THE CORTEX

Under higher magnification are seen large pyramidal cells (1, 8). Neurofibrils have the characteristic network arrangement in the cell bodies (1, 8) but are more in parallel in the dendrites (6) and definitely parallel in the axon (7). The typical large vesicular nucleus (3) with its prominent nucleolus (3, lower leader) is outlined. The outstanding cell process is the apical or main dendrite (6) which extends upward through the cortex toward the surface of the brain. Collaterals (5) are given off along its course. Smaller dendrites (6, middle leader) arise from other parts of the cell body. The axon (7) arises from the base of the cell and passes into the white matter.

The intercellular areas are occupied by nerve fibers (2) of various cells in the cortex, small cell bodies of astrocytes (4), and blood vessels.

PLATE 34

CEREBRAL CORTEX

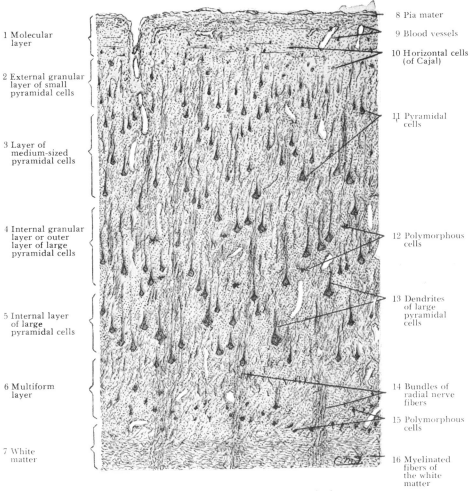

1 Molecular layer

2 External granular layer of small pyramidal cells

3 Layer of medium-sized pyramidal cells

4 Internal granular layer or outer layer of large pyramidal cells

5 Internal layer of large pyramidal cells

6 Multiform layer

7 White matter

8 Pia mater

9 Blood vessels

10 Horizontal cells (of Cajal)

11 Pyramidal cells

12 Polymorphous cells

13 Dendrites of large pyramidal cells

14 Bundles of radial nerve fibers

15 Polymorphous cells

16 Myelinated fibers of the white matter

FIG. 1.   *Section perpendicular to the cortical surface.*
Reduced silver nitrate method of Cajal. 80×.

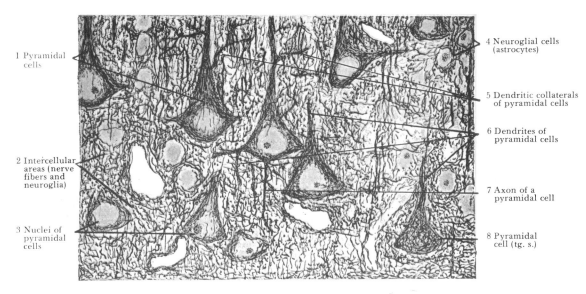

1 Pyramidal cells

2 Intercellular areas (nerve fibers and neuroglia)

3 Nuclei of pyramidal cells

4 Neuroglial cells (astrocytes)

5 Dendritic collaterals of pyramidal cells

6 Dendrites of pyramidal cells

7 Axon of a pyramidal cell

8 Pyramidal cell (tg. s.)

FIG. 2. *Central area of the cortex.*
Reduced silver nitrate method of Cajal. 300×.

PLATE 35 (Fig. 1)

BLOOD AND LYMPHATIC VESSELS

This plate illustrates various types of blood vessels and a lymphatic vessel, surrounded by loose connective tissue and numerous adipose cells (13, 28). Most vessels are in transverse or oblique sections.

An artery of small size, a terminal artery, is shown at the top center of the plate. It illustrates the basic structure of an artery. In contrast to a vein, an artery has a relatively thick wall and small lumen. The artery shows the following constituent layers:

a. Tunica intima, composed of the inner endothelium (16), a subendothelial layer of connective tissue (17), and an internal elastic membrane (19).

b. Tunica media (4), composed predominantly of circular smooth muscle fibers. Fine elastic fibers are interspersed.

c. Tunica adventitia (6), composed of connective tissue in which lie nerve fibers (14) and blood vessels (15). The latter are collectively called the vasa vasorum (15), or "blood vessels of blood vessels."

When arteries acquire about 25 or more layers of smooth muscle in the tunica media, they are referred to as medium-sized (muscular or distributing) arteries. Elastic fibers become more numerous, but are still present as thin fibers and networks.

A medium-sized vein (22) is shown at the lower center of the plate. It has a relatively thin wall and large lumen, the latter containing coagulated blood. The vein shows the following constituent layers:

a. Tunica intima, composed of endothelium (24) and a very thin layer of fine collagenous and elastic fibers which blend with the connective tissue of the media.

b. Tunica media (25) consisting of a thin layer of circularly arranged smooth muscle fibers loosely embedded in connective tissue.

c. Tunica adventitia (26) consisting of a wide layer of connective tissue.

Arterioles are illustrated (1, 5, 8). The smallest arteriole (1) has a thin internal elastic membrane and one layer of muscle in the media. One arteriole is sectioned longitudinally (8); a capillary is leaving it (9). Also illustrated are smaller veins (18, 27), venules (3, 10), capillaries (9, 11, 20) and small nerves (2, 23).

A lymphatic vessel (12) can be recognized by the thinness of its wall and the flaps of a valve in its lumen. Many veins have similar valves.

PLATE 35 (Fig. 2)

LARGE VEIN: PORTAL VEIN (TRANSVERSE SECTION)

In large veins, the outstanding feature is the thick, muscular adventitia, with its smooth muscle fibers oriented longitudinally. In this transverse section of the portal vein, the typical arrangement is noted: the muscle is in bundles, here seen mainly in cross sections (1), with varying amounts of connective tissue dispersed between them (2). Vasa vasorum (3, 7) are present in this intervening connective tissue.

In contrast, the media is a thinner layer of circularly arranged muscle (6), somewhat loosely arranged in connective tissue in this portal vein; in other large veins it may be a very thin, more compact layer. As in other vessels, the intima is of endothelium (4) supported by a small amount of connective tissue. In addition, large veins usually demonstrate an internal elastic membrane (5), not as well developed as in arteries.

—82—

PLATE 35

FIG. 1. BLOOD AND LYMPHATIC VESSELS

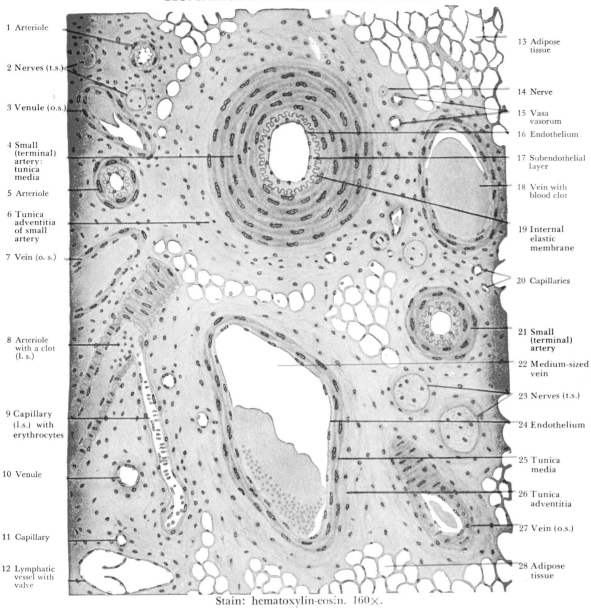

1 Arteriole

2 Nerves (t.s.)

3 Venule (o.s.)

4 Small (terminal) artery: tunica media

5 Arteriole

6 Tunica adventitia of small artery

7 Vein (o. s.)

8 Arteriole with a clot (l. s.)

9 Capillary (l.s.) with erythrocytes

10 Venule

11 Capillary

12 Lymphatic vessel with valve

13 Adipose tissue

14 Nerve

15 Vasa vasorum

16 Endothelium

17 Subendothelial layer

18 Vein with blood clot

19 Internal elastic membrane

20 Capillaries

21 Small (terminal) artery

22 Medium-sized vein

23 Nerves (t.s.)

24 Endothelium

25 Tunica media

26 Tunica adventitia

27 Vein (o.s.)

28 Adipose tissue

Stain: hematoxylin-eosin. 160×.

FIG. 2. LARGE VEIN: PORTAL VEIN (TRANSVERSE SECTION)

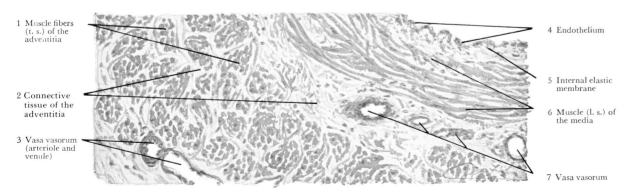

1 Muscle fibers (t. s.) of the adventitia

2 Connective tissue of the adventitia

3 Vasa vasorum (arteriole and venule)

4 Endothelium

5 Internal elastic membrane

6 Muscle (l. s.) of the media

7 Vasa vasorum

Stain: hematoxylin-eosin. 200×.

PLATE 36 (Fig. 1)

NEUROVASCULAR BUNDLE (TRANSVERSE SECTION)

In the center of the figure is a large, elastic artery (18) with a thick tunica media (16) made up mainly of concentric layers of elastic membranes (lamellae), between which are thin layers of smooth muscle. The intima consists of endothelium (19) whose rounded nuclei appear to project into the lumen of the artery, and a thin layer of subendothelial connective tissue (19) with fine collagenous and elastic fibers. The first elastic lamella is considered an internal elastic membrane (17). The tunica adventitia (15) is a thin layer of collagenous fibers; vasa vasorum and vasomotor nerves are present.

Several arterioles (3, 9, 26) are present, distinguished by their thin muscular wall and relatively narrow lumen. Numerous capillaries (21) are seen.

Veins show varied forms (4, 7, 22 and others) but each has a thin wall and a large lumen. Some contain a blood clot or hemolyzed blood (7, 22).

Nerves of various sizes (2, 8, 10, 25) accompany these blood vessels. Each is surrounded by a perineurium and is composed primarily of unmyelinated fibers. Also present is a sympathetic ganglion (1) surrounded by a capsule and containing nerve cells, nerve fibers and small blood vessels.

Part of a small lymph node (5) shows its hilus (5) and several efferent lymphatic vessels (6). In the larger node are seen its capsule (14) and its various component parts (11–13).

PLATE 36 (Fig. 2)

LARGE ARTERY: AORTA (TRANSVERSE SECTION)

The structure of this large artery is similar to that above, but it has been stained with orcein, which is specific for elastic fibers and stains them a dark brown color (2). Other tissues remain colorless or are only lightly stained. The size and arrangement of elastic lamellae in the media are well demonstrated. Smooth muscle (3) and fine elastic fibers between the lamellae remain unstained.

The intima (4) is indicated but unstained. The first elastic lamella is considered the internal elastic membrane (5). Sometimes smaller lamellae appear in the subendothelial connective tissue and a gradual transition is made to the larger lamellae of the media.

The adventitia (1), also unstained, is a narrow zone of collagenous fibers. In the aorta and pulmonary arteries, the media occupies most of the wall of the vessel; the adventitia is reduced to the proportion seen here.

PLATE 36

FIG. 1. NEUROVASCULAR BUNDLE (TRANSVERSE SECTION)

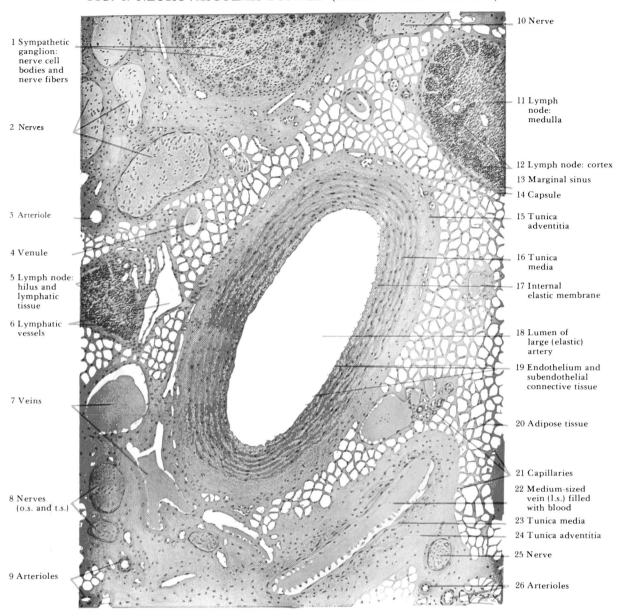

1 Sympathetic ganglion: nerve cell bodies and nerve fibers

2 Nerves

3 Arteriole

4 Venule

5 Lymph node: hilus and lymphatic tissue

6 Lymphatic vessels

7 Veins

8 Nerves (o.s. and t.s.)

9 Arterioles

10 Nerve

11 Lymph node: medulla

12 Lymph node: cortex

13 Marginal sinus

14 Capsule

15 Tunica adventitia

16 Tunica media

17 Internal elastic membrane

18 Lumen of large (elastic) artery

19 Endothelium and subendothelial connective tissue

20 Adipose tissue

21 Capillaries

22 Medium-sized vein (l.s.) filled with blood

23 Tunica media

24 Tunica adventitia

25 Nerve

26 Arterioles

Stain: hematoxylin-eosin. 50×.

FIG. 2. LARGE ARTERY: AORTA (TRANSVERSE SECTION)

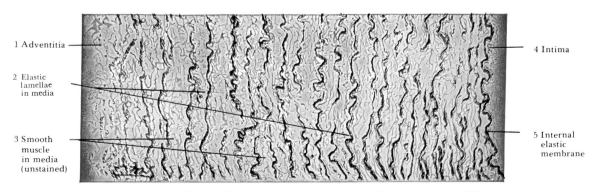

1 Adventitia

2 Elastic lamellae in media

3 Smooth muscle in media (unstained)

4 Intima

5 Internal elastic membrane

Orcein stain: aorta. Elastic fibers selectively stained dark brown. Approx. 300×.

PLATE 37

HEART: LEFT ATRIUM AND VENTRICLE
(PANORAMIC VIEW, LONGITUDINAL SECTION)

The plate represents a longitudinal section of the left heart showing the atrium, the atrioventricular (mitral) valve, and the ventricle.

In the atrium are seen the endocardium (1) consisting of endothelium and a thick subendothelial connective tissue, the myocardium (2) with the musculature arranged rather loosely, the epicardium (13), of mesothelium and a very thin layer of connective tissue, and the subepicardial connective tissue and fat (14) which varies in amount in different regions. This layer extends also into the atrioventricular groove and into the ventricle.

In the ventricle, the endocardium (6) is thin in comparison with that in the atrium, and the myocardium (7) is thick and more compact. The cardiac musculature is seen in various planes of section. The epicardium and subepicardial connective tissue (16) are continuous with those in the atrium.

Between the atrium and ventricle is seen the annulus fibrosus (3) of dense fibrous connective tissue, and a leaflet of the atrioventricular (mitral) valve (4), formed by a double membrane of endocardium (4a) and a core of dense connective tissue (4b) continuous with the annulus fibrosus. At (5) is shown the insertion of a chorda tendina into the valve.

On the inner surface of the ventricular wall, one can distinguish the characteristic prominences of the myocardium and endocardium: the apex of a papillary muscle (18) and two columnae carneae above this (17).

Purkinje fibers or conduction fibers (8), located in the loose subendocardial tissue, may be distinguished by their larger size and lighter staining. The small area within the rectangle (9) is shown at a higher magnification in Plate 38, Fig. 2.

The larger coronary vessels course in the subepicardial connective tissue. An artery is seen at (10). Below it is a section of the coronary sinus (11), and entering it, a coronary vein and its valve (12). Smaller coronary vessels may be seen in the subepicardial connective tissue and in the many perimysial septa extending into the myocardium (15).

PLATE 37

HEART: LEFT ATRIUM AND VENTRICLE
(PANORAMIC VIEW, LONGITUDINAL SECTION)

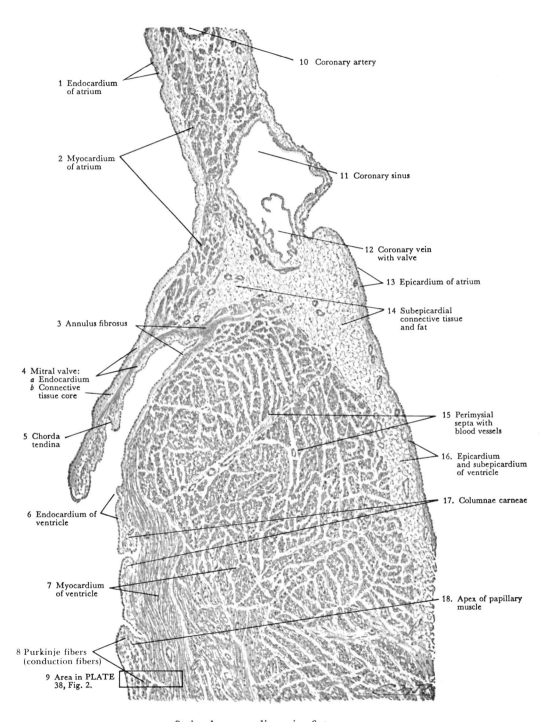

1 Endocardium of atrium

2 Myocardium of atrium

3 Annulus fibrosus

4 Mitral valve:
  a Endocardium
  b Connective tissue core

5 Chorda tendina

6 Endocardium of ventricle

7 Myocardium of ventricle

8 Purkinje fibers (conduction fibers)

9 Area in PLATE 38, Fig. 2.

10 Coronary artery

11 Coronary sinus

12 Coronary vein with valve

13 Epicardium of atrium

14 Subepicardial connective tissue and fat

15 Perimysial septa with blood vessels

16. Epicardium and subepicardium of ventricle

17. Columnae carneae

18. Apex of papillary muscle

Stain: hematoxylin-eosin. 6×.

Plate 38 (Fig. 1)

HEART: PULMONARY ARTERY, PULMONARY VALVE, RIGHT VENTRICLE (PANORAMIC VIEW, LONGITUDINAL SECTION)

A portion of the right ventricle, from which the pulmonary artery leaves, is represented in this plate.

A section of the wall of the pulmonary artery is seen at (6). The endothelium of its intima is distinguishable on its right surface. The media makes up the largest part of its wall; its thick elastic lamellae are not apparent at this magnification. A thin adventitia merges into the surrounding subepicardial connective tissue (2), which contains large amounts of fat in this specimen.

The pulmonary artery arises at (8) from the annulus fibrosus (9). One leaflet of the pulmonary (semilunar) valve is seen at (7). Like the mitral valve, it is covered with endocardium, and connective tissue from the annulus fibrosus extends into its base (10) and forms a central core.

The thick myocardium (4) of the right ventricle is covered on its internal surface by endocardium (11). The endocardium continues without interruption over the pulmonary valve and the annulus fibrosus, and becomes continuous with the intima of the pulmonary artery (in the region of 8).

The external surface of the pulmonary artery is covered with subepicardial connective tissue and fat (2), and this in turn is covered with epicardium (1). Both of these layers pass uninterruptedly over the external wall of the ventricle. Coronary vessels are seen in the subepicardium (3, 5).

Plate 38 (Fig. 2)

PURKINJE FIBERS (CONDUCTION FIBERS) (HEMATOXYLIN-EOSIN)

The area outlined by the rectangle (9) in Plate 37, is represented here at a high magnification (400×). Below the endocardium (1) are seen groups of Purkinje fibers, which are differentiated from typical cardiac muscle fibers (5) because of their larger size and their less intense staining. Some of the Purkinje fibers are sectioned transversally (2), others in longitudinal section (4). In the transverse sections, it is seen clearly that Purkinje fibers have fewer myofibrils, and that these are arranged peripherally, leaving a perinuclear zone of comparatively clear sarcoplasm. A nucleus is seen in some of the transverse sections; in others, a central area of sarcoplasm is seen, the section having passed above or below the nucleus.

Purkinje fibers merge with cardiac fibers. At (3) is seen a transitional fiber; the upper part corresponds to a Purkinje fiber, the lower part to an ordinary cardiac fiber.

Plate 38 (Fig. 3)

PURKINJE FIBERS (CONDUCTION FIBERS) (MALLORY-AZAN)

This figure is reproduced from a cardiac area where Purkinje fibers were abundant, in a preparation stained with Mallory-Azan, at the same high magnification as in Fig. 2.

The characteristic features of Purkinje fibers are well demonstrated in longitudinal and transverse sections (2).

With hematoxylin-eosin, connective tissue is not too apparent. In this preparation, blue staining of collagenous fibers shows conspicuously the subendocardial connective tissue (3) surrounding the Purkinje fibers. A capillary with red blood corpuscles is seen (1).

PLATE 38

FIG. 1. HEART:
PULMONARY ARTERY, PULMONARY VALVE, RIGHT
VENTRICLE (PANORAMIC VIEW, LONGITUDINAL SECTION)

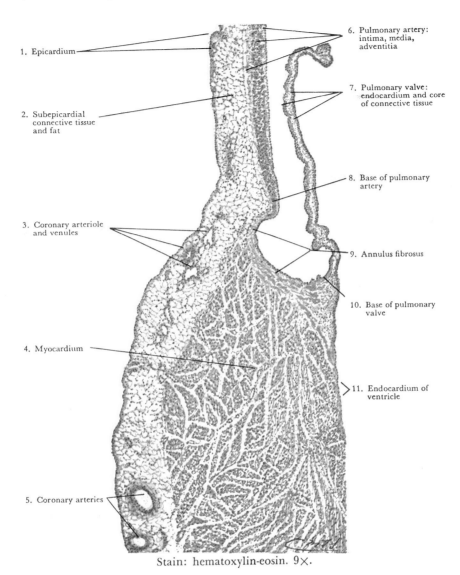

1. Epicardium

2. Subepicardial connective tissue and fat

3. Coronary arteriole and venules

4. Myocardium

5. Coronary arteries

6. Pulmonary artery: intima, media, adventitia

7. Pulmonary valve: endocardium and core of connective tissue

8. Base of pulmonary artery

9. Annulus fibrosus

10. Base of pulmonary valve

11. Endocardium of ventricle

Stain: hematoxylin-eosin. 9×.

FIGS. 2 AND 3: PURKINJE FIBERS (CONDUCTION FIBERS)

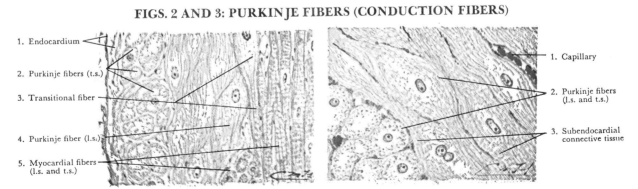

1. Endocardium

2. Purkinje fibers (t.s.)

3. Transitional fiber

4. Purkinje fiber (l.s.)

5. Myocardial fibers (l.s. and t.s.)

1. Capillary

2. Purkinje fibers (l.s. and t.s.)

3. Subendocardial connective tissue

Fig. 2. Stain: hematoxylin-eosin. 400×.   Fig. 3. Stain: Mallory-Azan. 400×.

PLATE 39

LYMPH NODE (PANORAMIC VIEW)

A lymph node is composed of varied aggregations of lymphocytes, intermeshed with lymphatic sinuses, supported in a framework of reticular connective tissue, and encased in a connective tissue capsule (2).

In the cortex of the node (5), the lymphocytes are aggregated into nodules (5, 15). In many of these cortical nodules, the centers are lightly stained; these are the germinal centers or light centers (17) in which proliferation of lymphocytes takes place.

In the medulla (6) of the node, the lymphocytes form cords of lymphatic tissue, the medullary cords (14). Medullary sinuses (13) surround these cords. Immediately under the capsule (2) is the marginal (subcapsular) sinus (9, 16). From it, trabecular sinuses extend along the trabeculae (7) into the medulla to pass into medullary sinuses. In the medulla, the trabeculae ramify and anastomose around the medullary cords and sinuses.

The capsule (2) is surrounded by connective tissue and fat (1). Afferent lymphatics (4) course in the connective tissue, and pierce the capsule at intervals to enter the subcapsular sinus.

At the upper right of the node is its hilus (12). In the hilus are efferent lymphatic vessels (11) which drain lymph from the node, arteries and veins (10) which supply and drain it, and nerves.

PLATE 39

LYMPH NODE (PANORAMIC VIEW)

1 Pericapsular
  fat and
  connective
  tissue

2 Capsule

3 Lymphatic
  tissue

4 Capsule and
  afferent
  lymphatics

5 Cortex

6 Medulla

7 Trabeculae

8 Blood
  vessels in
  trabeculae

9 Marginal
  (subcapsular)
  sinus

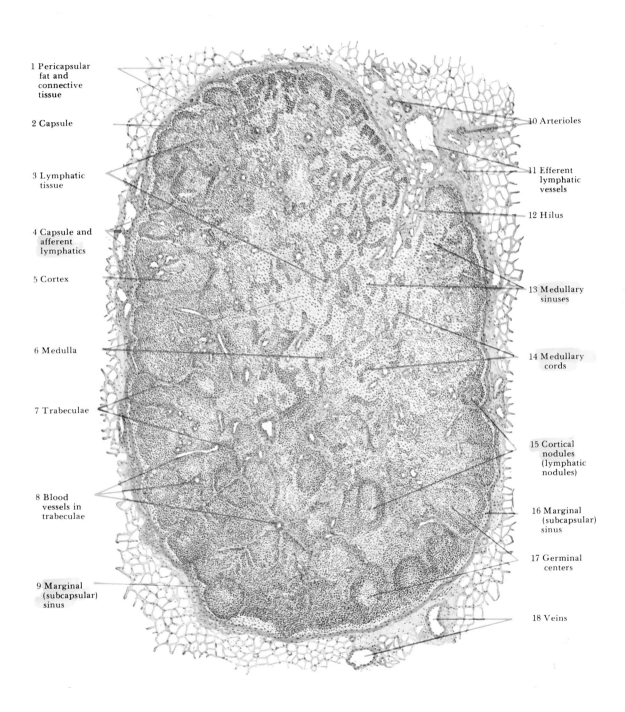

10 Arterioles

11 Efferent
  lymphatic
  vessels

12 Hilus

13 Medullary
  sinuses

14 Medullary
  cords

15 Cortical
  nodules
  (lymphatic
  nodules)

16 Marginal
  (subcapsular)
  sinus

17 Germinal
  centers

18 Veins

Stain: hematoxylin-eosin. 32×.

PLATE 40 (Fig. 1)

LYMPH NODE (SECTIONAL VIEW)

A small portion of a lymph node is shown here at a higher magnification.

The capsule (5) is surrounded by loose connective tissue (1) containing blood vessels (2, 3, 4) and afferent lymphatic vessels (13); the latter are lined with endothelium and contain valves (14). From the capsule (5), trabeculae (15) of fibrous connective tissue extend through the cortex and into the medulla. Blood vessels course in these partitions (18).

The cortex (7) is separated from the capsule (5) by the marginal (sub-capsular) sinus (6). The cortex consists of lymphatic nodules (cortical nodules) closely adjacent to each other but incompletely separated by trabeculae (15) and trabecular sinuses (16). In this figure, one complete cortical nodule is seen (7, lower leader; 8; 17, lower leader) and parts of two other nodules (7, upper leader; 17, upper leader). The medulla consists of anastomosing cords of lymphatic tissue, the medullary cords (12, 19), interspersed with medullary sinuses (11, 20). Trabeculae carrying blood vessels (18) course irregularly through the cortex and medulla.

Reticular connective tissue forms the stroma of the cortical nodules and medullary cords and of all the sinuses. Relatively few lymphocytes are seen in the sinuses (6, 11, 16, 20), thus it is possible to distinguish the reticular framework (20). In the nodules of the cortex (7, 17) and in the medullary cords (12, 19), lymphocytes are in such abundance that they obscure the reticulum unless special staining methods are used, as in Fig. 2. Most of the lymphocytes are small lymphocytes, with large nuclei containing dense accumulations of chromatin and showing little or no cytoplasm. The nuclei are deeply stained.

Cortical nodules often contain germinal centers (8) which stain less deeply than the surrounding peripheral portion of the nodule (7). In the germinal center (8), cells are not as densely aggregated, and the developing lymphocytes have larger, lighter nuclei and more cytoplasm than do small lymphocytes (see Plate 41, Fig. 1).

PLATE 40 (Fig. 2)

LYMPH NODE: RETICULAR FIBER STAIN

A portion of a lymph node has been stained with the Bielschowsky-Foot silver method which selectively stains reticular fibers.

The various zones seen in Fig. 1 are recognizable here: the cortex (1), the marginal or subcapsular sinus (2), capsule and a trabecula (3), medullary cords (5) and medullary sinuses (6). In all of these areas is demonstrated the stroma of delicate reticular fibers (4, 7) forming a fine meshwork.

PLATE 40

LYMPH NODE

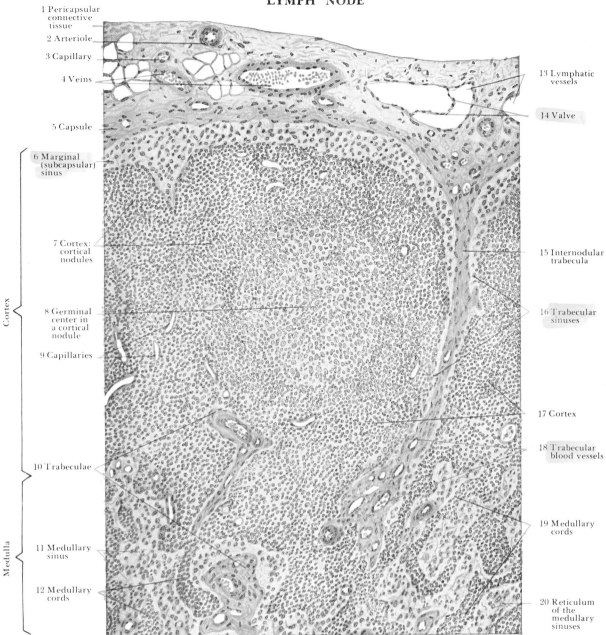

1 Pericapsular
  connective
  tissue

2 Arteriole

3 Capillary

4 Veins

5 Capsule

6 Marginal
  (subcapsular)
  sinus

7 Cortex:
  cortical
  nodules

8 Germinal
  center in
  a cortical
  nodule

9 Capillaries

10 Trabeculae

11 Medullary
  sinus

12 Medullary
  cords

Cortex

Medulla

13 Lymphatic
  vessels

14 Valve

15 Internodular
  trabecula

16 Trabecular
  sinuses

17 Cortex

18 Trabecular
  blood vessels

19 Medullary
  cords

20 Reticulum
  of the
  medullary
  sinuses

FIG. 1. *Sectional view.* Stain: hematoxylin-eosin. 150×.

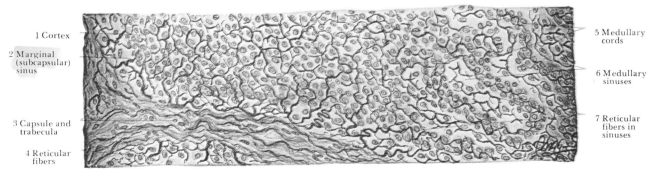

1 Cortex

2 Marginal
  (subcapsular)
  sinus

3 Capsule and
  trabecula

4 Reticular
  fibers

5 Medullary
  cords

6 Medullary
  sinuses

7 Reticular
  fibers in
  sinuses

FIG. 2. *Reticular fibers of the stroma.* Stain: Bielschowsky-Foot Silver method. 240×.

PLATE 41 (Fig. 1)

LYMPH NODE: PROLIFERATION OF LYMPHOCYTES

At a higher magnification than in Plate 40, this figure shows the capsule (1) of part of a lymph node, the marginal (subcapsular) sinus (2) and a cortical lymphatic nodule with its peripheral zone (5) and a germinal center (6) in which development of lymphocytes is taking place.

The reticular connective tissue of the stroma of the node is seen well in the marginal (subcapsular) sinus where reticular cells (9), their processes and associated delicate fibers are easily distinguishable. Small lymphocytes (11, upper leader) and free macrophages (3, 10) are also present. Reticular cells line up to form an incomplete covering over the surface of the node (4, limiting cells). In the dense portions of the node, reticular cells are obscured but may be seen at times (15). Free macrophages may be found anywhere in the node (3, 7, 10).

In the peripheral or marginal zone of the cortical nodule are seen dense accumulations of small lymphocytes (5; 11, lower leader) showing their darkly stained nuclei with prominent blocks of chromatin, and very little or no visible cytoplasm.

In the germinal center (6) the majority of cells are medium-sized lymphocytes (12) with larger, lighter nuclei than those of small lymphocytes, and more cytoplasm. The nuclei vary in size and in density of chromatin. The largest ones, with less concentrated chromatin, are derived from the large lymphocytes or lymphoblasts. With successive mitotic divisions (8), chromatin condenses and cell size decreases until small lymphocytes are formed.

Lymphoblasts or large lymphocytes (14) are seen in small numbers in the germinal center. Derived from reticular cells, they are large rounded cells with a broad band of cytoplasm and a large vesicular nucleus containing one or more nucleoli. Mitotic division of these (13) gives rise to other large lymphocytes and to medium-sized lymphocytes.

On Plate 43 are shown individual developing lymphocytes and other cells formed or found in lymphatic tissues.

PLATE 41 (Fig. 2)

PALATINE TONSIL

The surface of the palatine tonsil is covered with stratified squamous epithelium (1) which also lines the deep ramified invaginations or tonsillar crypts (3, 10). In the underlying connective tissue are numerous lymphatic nodules (2) distributed along the crypts. The nodules are embedded in a reticular connective tissue stroma and diffuse lymphatic tissue and frequently merge with each other (8). Germinal centers (7) are usually present.

Fibroelastic connective tissue underlies the tonsil, and forms a capsule for it (11). Septa (trabeculae) arise from this (5, 9) and pass upward as a core of connective tissue between the masses of lymphatic nodules that form the walls of the crypts. Skeletal muscle fibers (6, 12) from underlying muscles and glands (not illustrated) may be seen in the deeper connective tissue.

PLATE 41

FIG. 1. LYMPH NODE: PROLIFERATION OF LYMPHOCYTES

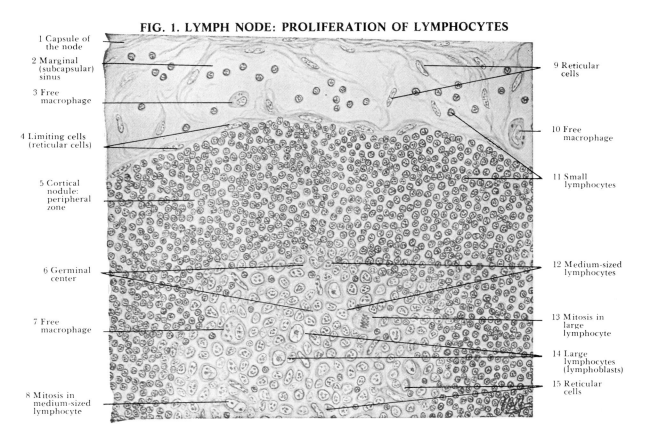

1 Capsule of the node

2 Marginal (subcapsular) sinus

3 Free macrophage

4 Limiting cells (reticular cells)

5 Cortical nodule: peripheral zone

6 Germinal center

7 Free macrophage

8 Mitosis in medium-sized lymphocyte

9 Reticular cells

10 Free macrophage

11 Small lymphocytes

12 Medium-sized lymphocytes

13 Mitosis in large lymphocyte

14 Large lymphocytes (lymphoblasts)

15 Reticular cells

Stain: hematoxylin-eosin. 450X.

FIG. 2. PALATINE TONSIL

1 Stratified squamous epithelium

2 Lymphatic nodules

3 Tonsillar crypts

4 Epithelium of crypt (tg. s.)

5 Internodular septum (trabecula)

6 Skeletal muscle fibers

7 Germinal center

8 Merging nodules

9 Internodular septum (trabecula)

10 Fundi of crypts

11 Blood vessel in the capsule

12 Skeletal muscle fibers

Stain: hematoxylin-eosin. 32X.

PLATE 42 (Fig. 1)

THYMUS (PANORAMIC VIEW)

The thymus has a lobular structure. From the capsule (1), trabeculae (2, 11) penetrate into the organ dividing it into lobules (5) in each of which there is a cortex (3) and a medulla (4). The lobular divisions are often incomplete (6) so that the medulla is continuous from one lobule to another (7).

The cells of the thymus are small lymphocytes (thymic lymphocytes). In the cortex they are densely aggregated (3) but do not form nodules. In the medulla (4, 7) they are less densely packed, thus giving a lighter appearance to this area. In the medulla are thymic corpuscles (Hassell's corpuscles) (9), which are spherical aggregations of flattened cells, often showing degenerative changes in the center.

The stroma resembles reticular connective tissue but is of endodermal-epithelial origin (see 6, 10 in Fig. 2). The stromal cells are referred to as epithelial reticular cells.

PLATE 42 (Fig. 2)

THYMUS (SECTIONAL VIEW)

Part of a lobule is illustrated, showing a small area of cortex and the central medulla. The dense aggregations of thymic lymphocytes in the cortex (4) contrast with the diffuse distribution of thymic lymphocytes in the medulla (5). The epithelial reticular cells of the stroma are more numerous, and more visible, in the medulla (6, 10) than in the cortex. Thin processes extend from the cell bodies, giving them a stellate appearance.

In the thymic corpuscles (7), epithelial reticular cells assume a concentric arrangement to form layers of cells. Continuity with the stroma of the medulla is often visible (9, also seen at the upper part of the corpuscle). Degenerative changes in the center of the corpuscle are indicated by a mass of acidophilic material (8).

An interlobular trabecula (3) with blood vessels (1, 2) is seen.

PLATE 42

THYMUS

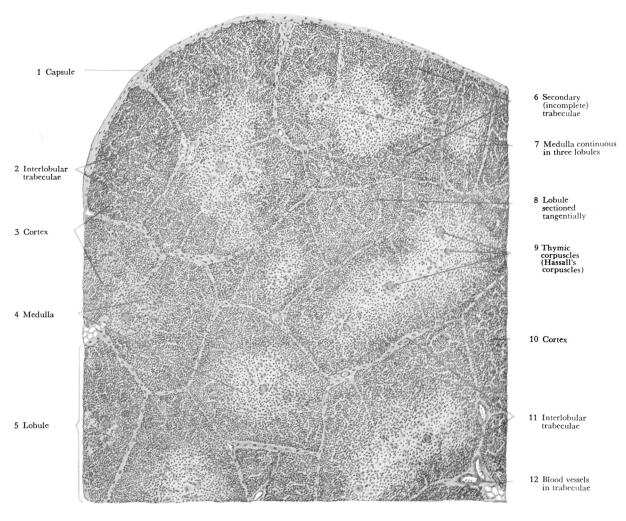

1 Capsule

2 Interlobular
trabeculae

3 Cortex

4 Medulla

5 Lobule

6 Secondary
(incomplete)
trabeculae

7 Medulla continuous
in three lobules

8 Lobule
sectioned
tangentially

9 Thymic
corpuscles
(Hassall's
corpuscles)

10 Cortex

11 Interlobular
trabeculae

12 Blood vessels
in trabeculae

FIG. 1. *Panoramic view.*
Stain: hematoxylin-eosin. 40×.

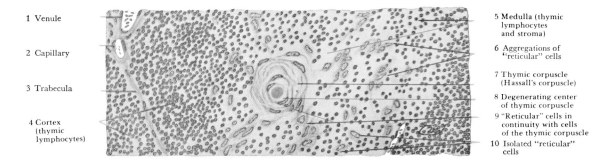

1 Venule

2 Capillary

3 Trabecula

4 Cortex
(thymic
lymphocytes)

5 Medulla (thymic
lymphocytes
and stroma)

6 Aggregations of
"reticular" cells

7 Thymic corpuscle
(Hassall's corpuscle)

8 Degenerating center
of thymic corpuscle

9 "Reticular" cells in
continuity with cells
of the thymic corpuscle

10 Isolated "reticular"
cells

FIG. 2. *Sectional view.*
Stain: hematoxylin-eosin. 250×.

PLATE 43 (Fig. 1)

SPLEEN (PANORAMIC VIEW)

From the capsule (1), trabeculae (3) extend into the body of the spleen. However, the principal trabeculae enter at the hilus, are distributed throughout the spleen, and carry with them trabecular arteries (4) and trabecular veins (11). Trabeculae seen in transverse sections may look like nodules of connective tissue (12).

Throughout the spleen are lymphatic nodules, the splenic nodules (2, 8). In young individuals, they contain germinal centers (7). Through each splenic nodule passes an arteriole, the central artery (6, 9), which is usually placed eccentrically within the nodule. Central arteries are branches of trabecular arteries. They become ensheathed with lymphatic tissue as they leave the trabeculae. This sheath expands to form the splenic nodule. This lymphatic tissue constitutes the white pulp of the spleen.

Surrounding the splenic nodules and intermeshed with trabeculae is a diffuse mass of cells which collectively forms the red pulp or splenic pulp; it appears as a reddish paste in fresh tissue. This mass contains the venous sinuses or splenic sinuses (10) and the splenic cords (of Billroth) (5). The cords are diffuse strands of lymphatic tissue between the venous sinuses. They form a spongy network spread on a mesh of reticular connective tissue, which is usually obscured by the density of other tissues. (The sinuses are actually sinusoids.)

It is to be noted that the spleen does not have a cortex and medulla as do lymph nodes; splenic nodules are found throughout the spleen. The spleen has venous sinuses in contrast to lymphatic sinuses in the node. The spleen does not have marginal sinuses or trabecular sinuses. Capsule and trabeculae in spleen are thicker than in nodes and contain smooth muscle.

PLATE 43 (Fig. 2)

SPLEEN: RED AND WHITE PULP

Illustrated here is a small area of red pulp and white pulp and their relationship to each other.

The splenic nodule represents the white pulp. Each nodule has a peripheral or marginal zone of densely packed small lymphocytes (8), a germinal center (9) which may not always be present, and an eccentrically placed central artery (10). In the more lightly stained germinal center are developing lymphocytes (9), mainly medium-sized lymphocytes, some small lymphocytes and large lymphocytes (lymphoblasts), as in any other lymphatic nodule where development of lymphocytes is in progress.

In the red pulp are the splenic cords (6) (of Billroth) and venous sinuses (2, 7) everywhere between the splenic cords. Splenic cords (6) are thin aggregations of lymphatic tissue containing small lymphocytes and other associated cells, as well as free red blood corpuscles (in sections of spleen). Venous sinuses (2, 7) are dilated vessels lined with reticuloendothelium (modified reticular cells which have lined up to simulate endothelium).

Also in the red pulp are pulp arteries (11) which are small arterioles; they are the divisions of the central artery just after it leaves the splenic nodule. Divisions of these, sheathed arteries, are not illustrated but one is seen in Fig. 1: 13. Capillaries and pulp veins (venules) are also present.

Trabeculae (1, 4) carrying trabecular arteries (1) and trabecular veins (4, 5) are seen. These vessels have an intima and media but no apparent adventitia; connective tissue of the trabecula surrounds the media.

PLATE 43 (Fig. 3).

DEVELOPMENT OF LYMPHOCYTES AND RELATED CELLS

The cells shown here may be found in lymph nodes, spleen and other lymphatic tissues, originating from reticular cells or a progenitor derived from reticular cells.

The large, highly phagocytic macrophage (1), usually ranging from $25-35\mu$, shows an eccentric nucleus, vacuoles in the cytoplasm (due to dissolved lipid inclusions), fragments of ingested nuclei, and a larger unidentified inclusion.

The lymphoblast (2), about $15-20\mu$ in diameter, has basophilic cytoplasm, a rounded nucleus with delicate chromatin filaments and two or more nucleoli. In the medium sized lymphocyte (prolymphocyte, $12-15\mu$ in diameter) (3), cytoplasm is less basophilic, nuclear chromatin is condensing, nucleoli are indistinct or absent. In the small lymphocyte ($6-12\mu$ in diameter) (4), cytoplasm is reduced; it may contain azurophilic granules. Nuclear chromatin is in small clusters which stain deeply.

In a plasmablast ($16-20\mu$ in diameter) (5), nuclear chromatin forms a heavier reticulum than in a lymphoblast. In a proplasmacyte ($12-18\mu$ in diameter) (6), cytoplasm is more deeply basophilic than in a prolymphocyte, the nucleus is eccentric, its chromatin clumps are heavier. The plasma cell (mature plasmacyte) (7) is oval, has abundant deeply basophilic cytoplasm except for a light halo near the small, ececntrically placed nucleus. The "cart wheel" arrangement of chromatin is distinctive.

A monoblast ($18-20\mu$) (8) is much like a lymphoblast. The monocyte ($15-18\mu$) (9) has a bean-shaped or deeply indented nucleus with chromatin in filaments and strands. The ample cytoplasm may contain fine azurophilic granules (10).

PLATE 43

SPLEEN

1 Peritoneum
  and
  capsule

2 Splenic
  nodules
  (white
  pulp)

3 Trabeculae

4 Trabecular
  artery

5 Splenic
  cords in
  the red
  pulp

6 Central
  artery (l.s.)

7 Germinal
  center

8 Tangential
  section of a
  splenic
  nodule

9 Central
  arteries (t.s.)
  in splenic
  nodules

10 Venous
   sinuses in the
   red pulp

11 Trabecular
   veins

12 Trabeculae (t.s.)

13 Sheathed artery

14 Pulp arteries
   (arterioles)

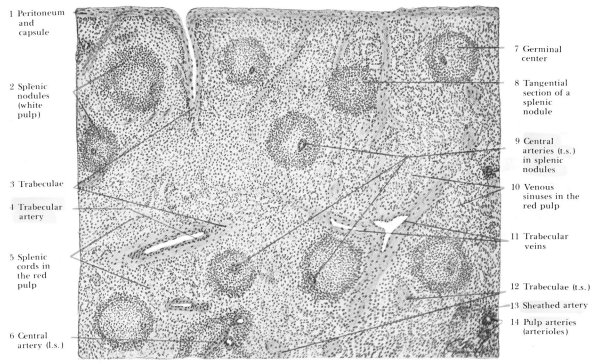

Fig. 1 Panoramic view. Stain: hematoxylin-eosin. 50×.

1 Trabecula
  with a
  trabecular
  artery

2 Venous
  sinuses

3 Pulp arteries
  (arterioles) in
  the red pulp

4 Trabecula
  with
  trabecular
  veins

5 Endothelium
  of trabecular
  veins

6 Splenic cord

7 Venous
  sinuses

8 Small
  lymphocytes
  in the marginal
  area of a
  splenic nodule

9 Germinal center
  with developing
  lymphocytes

10 Central artery in
   a splenic nodule

11 Pulp arteries

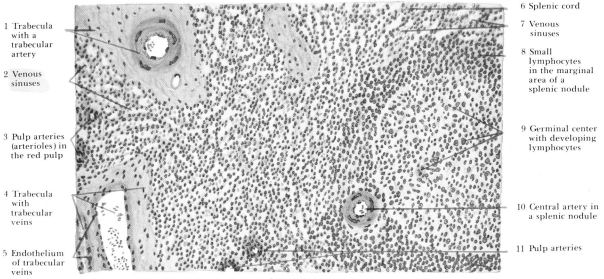

Fig. 2 Red and white pulp. Stain: hematoxylin-eosin. 250×.

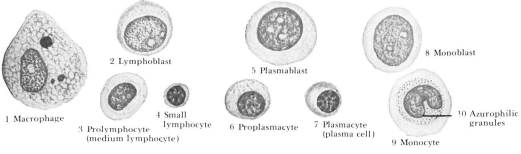

1 Macrophage

2 Lymphoblast

3 Prolymphocyte
  (medium lymphocyte)

4 Small
  lymphocyte

5 Plasmablast

6 Proplasmacyte

7 Plasmacyte
  (plasma cell)

8 Monoblast

9 Monocyte

10 Azurophilic
   granules

Fig. 3 Development of lymphocytes and related cells. Stain: May-Grünwald-Giemsa. 800×.

PLATE 44 (Fig. 1)

INTEGUMENT: THIN SKIN, GENERAL BODY SURFACE
(CAJAL'S TRICHROME STAIN)

The skin is composed of two principal layers: epidermis and dermis or corium. In this illustration is seen a section of skin such as occurs on the general body surface where there is not much wear and tear. The epidermis (1), of stratified squamous epithelium, is thin, and shows only a stratum corneum (5) and a stratum germinativum (6). The narrow zone of fine-fibered dense irregular connective tissue is the papillary layer or subepithelial layer (2) of the dermis. Its projections into the basal epidermis are the dermal papillae (7). The reticular layer (3), of heavy, dense, irregular connective tissue, comprises the bulk of the dermis. A small portion of hypodermis, the superficial region of the underlying subcutaneous tissue (4), is seen.

The accessory structures of the skin lie, for the most part, in the dermis. Shown here are scattered hair follicles and a sweat gland (sudoriferous gland), whose structure is seen in more detail in Plate 45. The lower part of a hair follicle in longitudinal section (12) shows its papilla and hair bulb at its base in the deepest part of the dermis. The upper part of another follicle (8) shows its erector muscle (arrector pili muscle) (9) which is smooth muscle, and a sebaceous gland (10). At (13) is an oblique section of a hair follicle in the subcutaneous tissue.

A group of tubules in the deep dermis are cross-sections through the coiled portion of a sweat gland (sudoriferous gland); those sections with lightly-stained epithelium (11a) are through the secreting portion; those with more deeply-stained epithelium (11b) are through the duct.

Cajal's trichrome stain emphasizes the variations in density of collagenous fibers, and distinguishes clearly between muscle and connective tissue. Aniline dyes are used to stain the nuclei and cytoplasm. The nuclei are stained bright red by basic fuchsin. Indigo carmine in picric acid solution is used to stain the cytoplasm, which takes on an orange hue. Collagenous fibers stain deep blue.

PLATE 44 (Fig. 2)

THICK SKIN, PALM: SUPERFICIAL LAYERS

A section of the skin of the palm is shown. Here both epidermis and dermis are much thicker than in Fig. 1 above. The epidermis, in addition to being thicker, has a more complex structure, in that five layers or zones are recognizable. The outer stratum corneum (1) is a wide zone of layers of dead, flattened cells which are constantly desquamating off the surface (10). Beneath it, stained red, is the thin stratum lucidum (2). At a higher magnification, one can sometimes distinguish faint outlines of flattened clear cells and eleidin droplets. Under the stratum lucidum is the stratum granulosum (3); its cells have keratohyalin granules, stained darkly, which can be observed more clearly at higher magnification (7).

Below this is the thick stratum germinativum which is subdivided into the stratum spinosum (4) composed of layers of polyhedral cells, and a basal layer, the stratum basale or stratum cylindricum (5) of columnar cells which rests on a basement membrane.

Cells of the stratum spinosum (4) appear to be connected by spinous processes or intercellular bridges (8, 9) which are actually desmosomes (maculae adherens). Mitosis (12) occurs in the deeper layers of the stratum spinosum and in the stratum basale.

Ducts of sweat glands (sudoriferous glands) penetrate the epidermis in the area between two dermal papillae, lose their epithelial wall, and spiral through the epidermis (11) as channels which have only a thin cuticular lining.

Dermal papillae (subepithelial papillae) are prominent in thick skin. In some of these papillae are located tactile corpuscles (Meissner's corpuscles) (13). In others are loops of large capillaries.

—100—

PLATE 44

INTEGUMENT

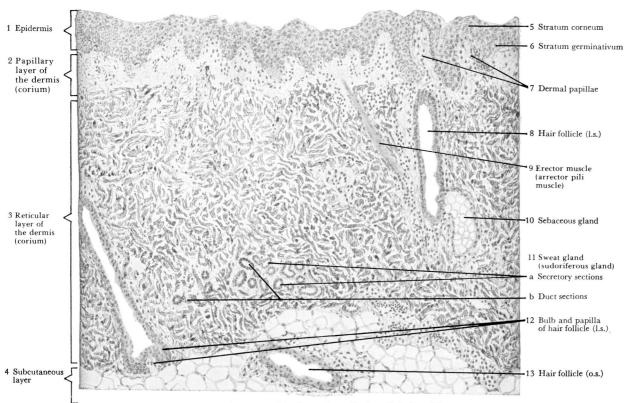

1 Epidermis

2 Papillary
layer of
the dermis
(corium)

3 Reticular
layer of
the dermis
(corium)

4 Subcutaneous
layer

5 Stratum corneum

6 Stratum germinativum

7 Dermal papillae

8 Hair follicle (l.s.)

9 Erector muscle
(arrector pili
muscle)

10 Sebaceous gland

11 Sweat gland
(sudoriferous gland)
a Secretory sections

b Duct sections

12 Bulb and papilla
of hair follicle (l.s.)

13 Hair follicle (o.s.)

FIG. 1. *Thin skin, general body surface*. Stain: Cajal's trichrome.

Cytoplasm: orange; nuclei: bright red; collagenous fibers: deep blue. About 50×.

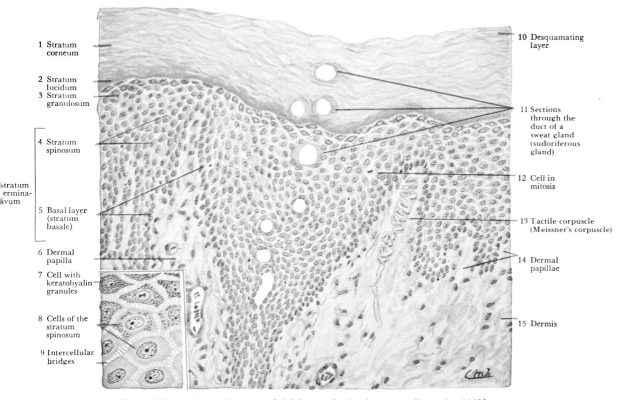

1 Stratum
corneum

2 Stratum
lucidum
3 Stratum
granulosum

4 Stratum
spinosum

stratum
ermina-
ivum

5 Basal layer
(stratum
basale)

6 Dermal
papilla

7 Cell with
keratohyalin
granules

8 Cells of the
stratum
spinosum

9 Intercellular
bridges

10 Desquamating
layer

11 Sections
through the
duct of a
sweat gland
(sudoriferous
gland)

12 Cell in
mitosis

13 Tactile corpuscle
(Meissner's corpuscle)

14 Dermal
papillae

15 Dermis

FIG. 2. *Thick skin, palm: superficial layers*. Stain: hematoxylin-eosin. 200X.

PLATE 45

INTEGUMENT
Fig. 1. SKIN: SCALP

This section of skin shows a stratum corneum (1) with extensive cornification of the superficial cells, and a stratum germinativum (2).

Characteristic dermal papillae are seen (3). The thin papillary layer of the dermis or corium is not readily apparent at this magnification. The thick reticular layer (4) extends from just above (4) to the region of abundant adipose tissue (23) which is in the subcutaneous layer. Beneath this is skeletal muscle (13).

Hair follicles are numerous, close together, and are placed at an angle with respect to the free surface of the skin. A complete hair follicle, in longitudinal section (17), traverses the center of the plate. Parts of other follicles, sectioned in various planes, are seen (5, 8, 18, 20). A hair follicle includes the following structures: cuticle, internal root sheath (18), external root sheath (20), connective tissue sheath (19), hair bulb (10), and a connective tissue papilla (11). The hair passes up through the follicle (17, 21).

Sebaceous glands (6, 15) are sac-like aggregations of clear cells provided with a duct which opens into the hair follicle. (See Fig. 2 below.)

Erector muscles (arrector pili muscles) (7) are smooth muscle, originating in the papillary layer of the dermis and inserting into the connective tissue sheath of the hair follicle. Their contraction is responsible for the erection of the hair.

The basal portions of sweat glands lie in the deep dermis or in the subcutaneous layer (see also Plate 46). Sections with lightly stained columnar epithelium (12) through the secretory portion of a gland are distinct from sections through the duct (9) with its two layers of smaller, more darkly stained epithelial cells (stratified cuboidal epithelium). Each duct is coiled (9) in its deep portion, becomes more or less straight in the upper dermis (16), and follows a spiral course through the epidermis (14).

Lamellar corpuscles (Pacinian corpuscles) (22), found in the subcutaneous tissue, are deep pressure receptors.

Fig. 2. A SEBACEOUS GLAND AND ADJACENT HAIR FOLLICLE

The sebaceous gland, an alveolar gland, is sectioned through its central or interior part. The potential lumen is filled with secretory cells in the process of cytolysis (3). The gland is lined with a stratified epithelium which is continuous with the external root sheath (1) of a hair follicle. Its epithelium is greatly modified. Along the base of the gland is a single row of columnar or cuboidal cells (5), the basal cells, whose nuclei may be flattened as here. This rests on a basement membrane, and is surrounded by connective tissue of the dermis. Mitosis occurs in these cells. The polyhedral cells acquire progressively more secretory material, enlarging and becoming rounded (4) during this process. The cells in the interior of the alveolus undergo cytolysis (3) (holocrine secretion), and, together with the secretion, pass into the short duct (2) of the gland into the lumen of the hair follicle.

The sebaceous gland lies in dermal connective tissue in the angle between the hair follicle and the erector muscle (11).

The various layers of a hair follicle at the level of a sebaceous gland may be identified. The follicle is surrounded by a connective sheath (7), a condensation of dermal connective tissue. The external root sheath (8), composed of several layers of cells, is continuous with the stratum germinativum of the epidermis. The internal root sheath (9) is composed of a very thin, pale epithelial stratum, Henle's layer (9) and a thin granular epithelial stratum, Huxley's layer. This layer is in direct contact with the cortex of the hair (10), shown here in pale yellow, which also has layers of cells.

Fig. 3. THE BULB OF THE HAIR FOLLICLE AND ADJACENT SWEAT GLANDS

The bulb of a hair follicle is shown. The various layers may be identified. A sheath of fibrous connective tissue (7) surrounds the bulb. The external root sheath (1) at this level is a single layer of cells which are columnar above the bulb but become flattened toward the base of the bulb where they cannot be distinguished from the cells of the matrix of the follicle (13). Above the bulb can be distinguished the internal root sheath, composed, as at a higher level, of a thin, pale epithelial stratum, Henle's layer (2) and a thin granular stratum, Huxley's layer (3). These layers also lose their identity as their cells merge with those of the bulb. Internal to these layers are the cuticles (4), cortex (5) and medulla (6) of the hair. These layers merge, in the bulb, into undifferentiated cells of the matrix of the hair (12) which caps the papilla (11) of connective tissue of the hair follicle. Mitosis (10) is seen in the cells of the matrix.

In the dermal connective tissue adjacent to the hair follicle are seen sections through the basal coiled portion of a sweat gland. The secretory cells (9) are tall columnar, staining lightly. Along their bases may be seen the flattened nuclei of myoepithelial cells (14). Sections of the duct (8) are smaller in diameter than the secretory tubule, and are lined with a two-layered stratified cuboidal epithelium.

PLATE 45

INTEGUMENT

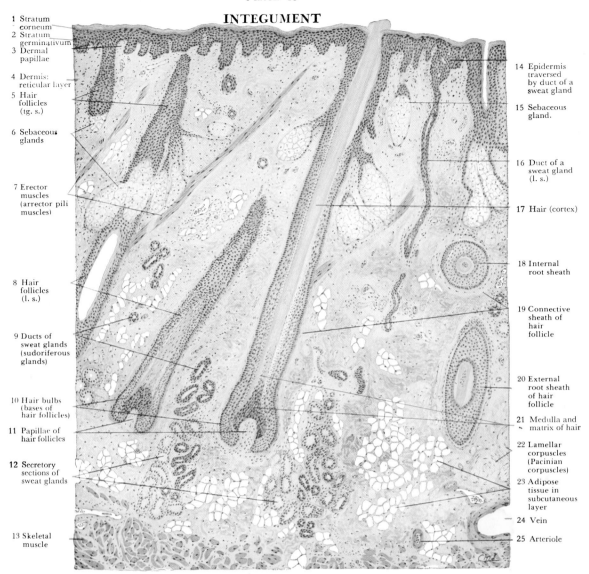

1 Stratum corneum
2 Stratum germinativum
3 Dermal papillae
4 Dermis: reticular layer
5 Hair follicles (tg. s.)
6 Sebaceous glands
7 Erector muscles (arrector pili muscles)
8 Hair follicles (l. s.)
9 Ducts of sweat glands (sudoriferous glands)
10 Hair bulbs (bases of hair follicles)
11 Papillae of hair follicles
12 Secretory sections of sweat glands
13 Skeletal muscle

14 Epidermis traversed by duct of a sweat gland
15 Sebaceous gland.
16 Duct of a sweat gland (l. s.)
17 Hair (cortex)
18 Internal root sheath
19 Connective sheath of hair follicle
20 External root sheath of hair follicle
21 Medulla and matrix of hair
22 Lamellar corpuscles (Pacinian corpuscles)
23 Adipose tissue in subcutaneous layer
24 Vein
25 Arteriole

FIG. 1. *Skin: scalp.* Stain: hematoxylin-eosin. 50×.

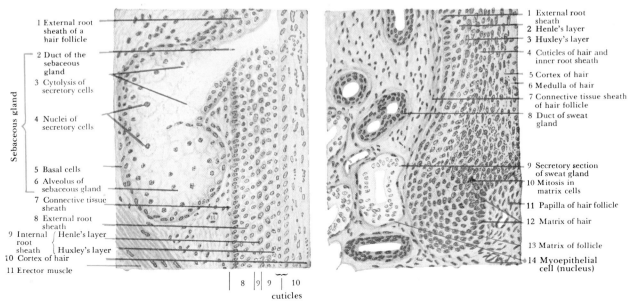

Sebaceous gland

1 External root sheath of a hair follicle
2 Duct of the sebaceous gland
3 Cytolysis of secretory cells
4 Nuclei of secretory cells
5 Basal cells
6 Alveolus of sebaceous gland
7 Connective tissue sheath
8 External root sheath
9 Internal root sheath { Henle's layer / Huxley's layer
10 Cortex of hair
11 Erector muscle

1 External root sheath
2 Henle's layer
3 Huxley's layer
4 Cuticles of hair and inner root sheath
5 Cortex of hair
6 Medulla of hair
7 Connective tissue sheath of hair follicle
8 Duct of sweat gland
9 Secretory section of sweat gland
10 Mitosis in matrix cells
11 Papilla of hair follicle
12 Matrix of hair
13 Matrix of follicle
14 Myoepithelial cell (nucleus)

8 |9| 9 ⌢ 10
cuticles

FIG. 2. *A sebaceous gland and adjacent hair follicle.*   FIG. 3. *The bulb of a hair follicle and adjacent sweat gland.*

Stain: hematoxylin-eosin. 200×.

PLATE 46

SWEAT GLAND (DIAGRAM)

In the midline of the plate is a reconstruction of a coiled tubular sweat gland. The coiled portion (B) is embedded in the deep dermis or in the subcutaneous tissue. This comprises the secretory portion, indicated in light pink in this diagram, and the thinner proximal portion of the duct, indicated in the deeper pink.

The duct straightens out as it passes through the dermis (7). It then penetrates the epidermis, loses its epithelial wall, and pursues a spiral course (6) through the epidermis.

Areas A, B and C show the appearance of different parts of the gland, as seen in histological sections, when cuts are made through the gland along lines a-a', b-b' and c-c'. Secretory portions of the gland are lined with large columnar cells (3, 5, 8) which stain rather lightly. Myoepithelial cells are present but not indicated here. The proximal excretory ducts are smaller in diameter, and lined with two rows of small, deeply staining cuboidal cells (4, 9). The duct cells increase somewhat in size as the duct approaches the epidermis (2), and its wall is gradually lost in the epidermis (1).

PLATE 46

SWEAT GLAND (DIAGRAM)

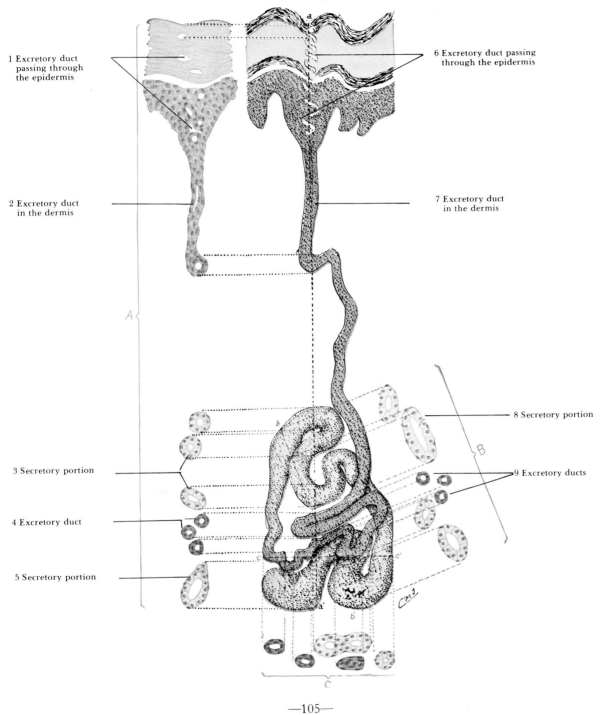

1 Excretory duct
passing through
the epidermis

6 Excretory duct passing
through the epidermis

2 Excretory duct
in the dermis

7 Excretory duct
in the dermis

8 Secretory portion

3 Secretory portion

9 Excretory ducts

4 Excretory duct

5 Secretory portion

PLATE 47

LIP (LONGITUDINAL SECTION)

The central area of the lip is occupied by the striated fibers of the orbicularis oris muscle (8). Special stains would also reveal the presence of intertwining dense fibroelastic connective tissue. To the right of the muscle tissue is the skin of the lower lip. To the left is the mucosal lining of the mouth.

Of the skin, the outer layer is epidermis (9), composed of keratinized, stratified squamous epithelium. Beneath the epidermis lies the dermis (10). In the dermis lie sebaceous glands (11), hair follicles (12), and sweat glands (14), all of which are derivatives of the epidermis. Also seen are erector muscles (arrector pili muscles) (13, 15) and the neurovascular bundle of the edge of the lip (7).

Of the mucosa, the outer layer is nonkeratinized, stratified squamous epithelium (1). The surface cells of this epithelium, without becoming cornified, slough off in the fluids of the mouth (see Plate 1, Fig. 1). Beneath the mucosal epithelium is the lamina propria (2), the counterpart of the dermis to the epidermis. Labial mucous glands (4) embedded in the lamina propria keep the oral mucosa moist. Their small ducts (4, lower leader) open into the oral cavity.

Transition of the epidermis of the skin to the epithelium of the oral mucosa illustrates one of the main muco-cutaneous junctions of the body. The "red line," or border of the lip, is at (6). The surface of the epithelium of the lip and oral mucosa is relatively more smooth than that of the epidermis. The underlying papillae of the lip and oral mucosa are high, numerous, and abundantly supplied with capillaries. The color of the blood shows through the overlying cells, resulting in the characteristic red appearance. It should be noted that the epithelium of the labial mucosa (1) is thicker than the epidermis of the skin (9).

PLATE 47

LIP (LONGITUDINAL SECTION)

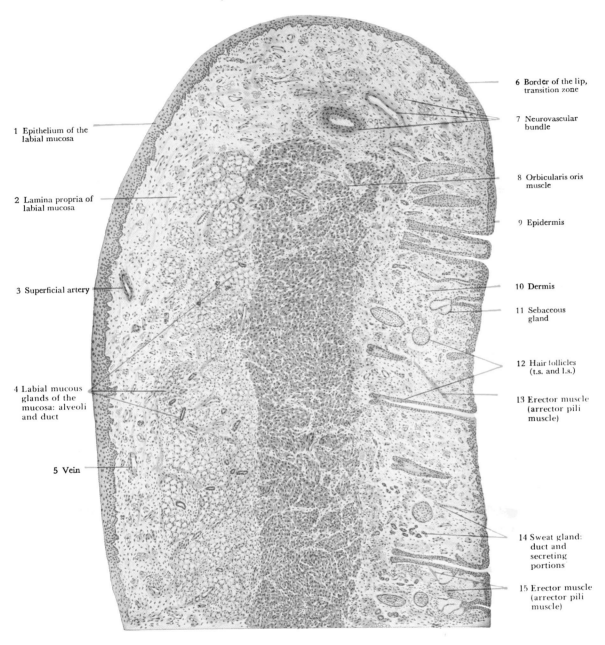

1 Epithelium of the labial mucosa

2 Lamina propria of labial mucosa

3 Superficial artery

4 Labial mucous glands of the mucosa: alveoli and duct

5 Vein

6 Border of the lip, transition zone

7 Neurovascular bundle

8 Orbicularis oris muscle

9 Epidermis

10 Dermis

11 Sebaceous gland

12 Hair follicles (t.s. and l.s.)

13 Erector muscle (arrector pili muscle)

14 Sweat gland: duct and secreting portions

15 Erector muscle (arrector pili muscle)

Stain: Hematoxylin-eosin. 20×.

PLATE 48

TONGUE: APEX (LONGITUDINAL SECTION, PANORAMIC VIEW)

The mucosa of the tongue consists of stratified squamous epithelium and a thin papillated lamina propria (1, 18) in which may be seen diffuse lymphatic tissue. The dorsal upper surface of the tongue is characterized by mucosal projections forming papillae: numerous, slender, filiform papillae with cornified tips (6) and fewer fungiform papillae (4, 7), each of which has a broad, rounded surface of non-cornified epithelium and a prominent core of lamina propria (4). Papillae are still present on the dorsal apex of the tongue (fungiform papillae in this section) (7) but are absent on the entire ventral (lower) surface (18).

Compact masses of skeletal muscle occupy the interior of the tongue. The muscle is seen typically as groups of fibers sectioned in various planes, longitudinally (2), in transverse section (3) and obliquely (5). In the inter-fascicular connective tissue, which is continuous with the lamina propria, may be seen numerous blood vessels (9, 10, 15, 16) and nerves (8, 17).

In the lower half of the tongue, near the apex, embedded in the muscle, is seen part of the anterior lingual gland, a mixed gland of serous alveoli (11), mucous alveoli (13) and mucous alveoli with demilunes (not illustrated). Inter-lobular ducts (12) pass into excretory ducts (14) which open on the ventral surface of the tongue.

PLATE 48

TONGUE: APEX (LONGITUDINAL SECTION, PANORAMIC VIEW)

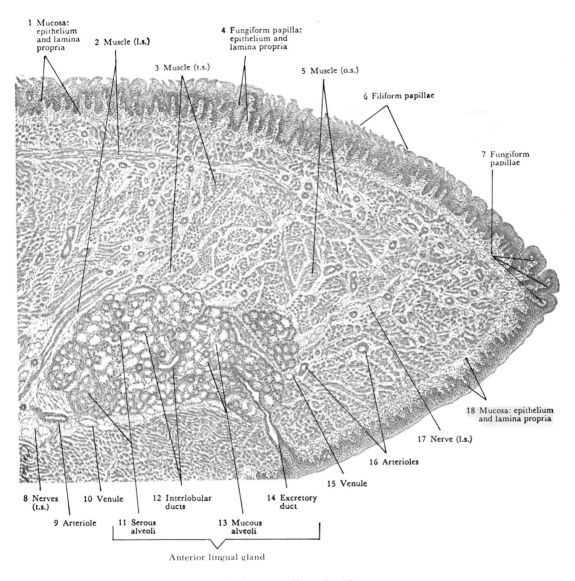

1 Mucosa: epithelium and lamina propria

2 Muscle (l.s.)

3 Muscle (t.s.)

4 Fungiform papilla: epithelium and lamina propria

5 Muscle (o.s.)

6 Filiform papillae

7 Fungiform papillae

8 Nerves (t.s.)

9 Arteriole

10 Venule

11 Serous alveoli

12 Interlobular ducts

13 Mucous alveoli

14 Excretory duct

15 Venule

16 Arterioles

17 Nerve (l.s.)

18 Mucosa: epithelium and lamina propria

Anterior lingual gland

Stain: hematoxylin-eosin. 25✕.

PLATE 49 (Fig. 1)

TONGUE: VALLATE (CIRCUMVALLATE) PAPILLA
(VERTICAL SECTION)

A vertical section through a vallate or circumvallate papilla of the tongue is illustrated. The lamina propria or core of connective tissue of the papilla has numerous secondary papillae (3), which project into the overlying stratified squamous epithelium (8). Blood vessels (4) in the stroma are abundant. The upper part of the vallate papilla does not usually project above the level of the adjacent lingual epithelium (1). A narrow trench, the circular furrow or sulcus (9) surrounds the papilla.

Barrel-shaped taste buds (5, 11) are located in the epithelium of the lateral surfaces of the papilla; some may also be present in the epithelium of the outer wall of the furrow.

Many serous alveoli composing the tubuloalveolar glands of the vallate papillae (von Ebner's glands) (12) are located among the bundles of skeletal muscle fibers (6, 14). Their ducts (7, 13) open into the base of the circular furrow.

PLATE 49 (Fig. 2)

POSTERIOR TONGUE (LONGITUDINAL SECTION)

This section illustrates posterior tongue about 2 cm behind the circumvallate papillae, approaching the area occupied by lingual tonsils. The dorsal surface of the posterior tongue typically shows large mucosal ridges (1), and rounded elevations (6) or folds which may somewhat resemble large fungiform papillae. Lymphatic nodules of the lingual tonsils will be seen in such elevations. Typical filiform and fungiform papillae are absent.

The lamina propria of the mucosa is wider but similar to that in the anterior two-thirds of the tongue, with diffuse lymphatic tissue in the subepithelial zone (2), groups of adipose cells (3), many blood vessels and nerves. A large nerve is seen coursing along the vertical axis of the mucosal fold (9).

Numerous alveoli of the posterior lingual mucous glands (4) lie in the deep lamina propria and in connective tissue trabeculae between groups of skeletal muscle fibers (5, 10), extending deep down into the muscular mass. The excretory ducts (7) open onto the dorsal surface of the tongue, usually between bases of the mucosal ridges and folds, but in this figure, at the apex of a ridge. Anteriorly these glands come in contact with the serous glands of the vallate papilla (von Ebner's glands); posteriorly they extend through the root of the tongue.

PLATE 49

TONGUE

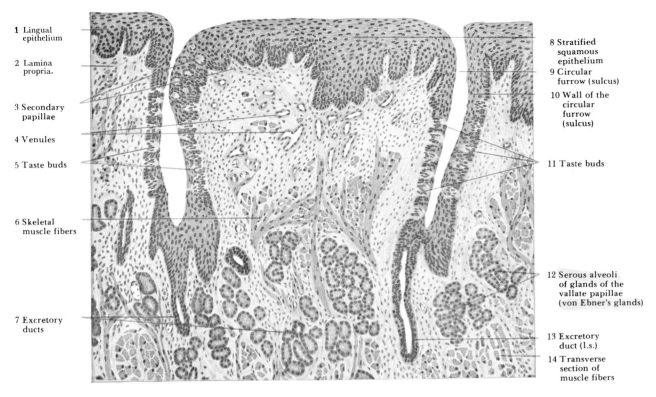

1 Lingual epithelium

2 Lamina propria.

3 Secondary papillae

4 Venules

5 Taste buds

6 Skeletal muscle fibers

7 Excretory ducts

8 Stratified squamous epithelium

9 Circular furrow (sulcus)

10 Wall of the circular furrow (sulcus)

11 Taste buds

12 Serous alveoli of glands of the vallate papillae (von Ebner's glands)

13 Excretory duct (l.s.)

14 Transverse section of muscle fibers

FIG. 1. *Vallate (circumvallate) papilla (vertical section)*.

Stain: hematoxylin-eosin. 115×.

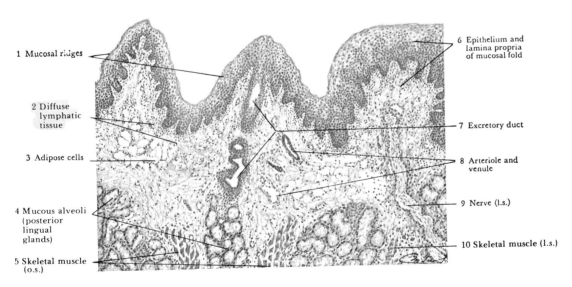

1 Mucosal ridges

2 Diffuse lymphatic tissue

3 Adipose cells

4 Mucous alveoli (posterior lingual glands)

5 Skeletal muscle (o.s.)

6 Epithelium and lamina propria of mucosal fold

7 Excretory duct

8 Arteriole and venule

9 Nerve (l.s.)

10 Skeletal muscle (l.s.)

FIG. 2. *Posterior tongue (longitudinal section)*.

Stain: hematoxylin-eosin. 85×.

PLATE 50 (Fig. 1)

DRIED TOOTH (PANORAMIC VIEW, LONGITUDINAL SECTION)

Dentin (3, 5) surrounds the pulp cavity (4) and its extension, the root canal (6). In the living tooth, the pulp cavity and root canal are filled with fine connective tissue which contains fibroblasts, histiocytes, odontoblasts, blood vessels and nerves. Dentin (3) has wavy, parallel, dentinal tubules. The oldest or primary dentin lies at the periphery of the tooth (3); the later or secondary dentin lies along the pulp cavity (5), where it is formed throughout life by odontoblasts. In the crown of a dried tooth, at the periphery of the dentin close to its junction with the enamel, there are many irregular spaces filled with air which appear black. These are the interglobular spaces (12) which, in the living tooth, are filled with incompletely calcified dentin (interglobular dentin). Similar areas, but smaller and closer together, are present in the root, close to the dentinal-cementum junction, where they form the granular layer (of Tomes) (13).

Dentin of the crown is covered by a thick layer of enamel (1) composed of enamel rods or prisms held together by a small amount of interprismatic cementing substance. With adequate lighting it is possible to see the incremental growth lines or dark striae (lines of Retzius) (8), which represent variations in the rate of enamel deposition, and the light striae (bands of Schreger) (9). Light rays passing through dried sections of tooth are refracted by twists which occur in the enamel rods as they course toward the surface of the tooth. These refracted rays appear to the eye as the light striae or bands of Schreger. At the dentinal-enamel junction may be seen enamel spindles (10) and enamel tufts (11), which are shown at a higher magnification in Fig. 2.

Cementum (7) covers the dentin of the root. In it are lacunae with canaliculi (14), which contain cementocytes (osteocytes) in the living tooth.

PLATE 50 (Fig. 2)

DRIED TOOTH (LAYERS OF THE CROWN)

Enamel and dentin are shown. In the enamel are elongated enamel rods (1). In the enamel near the dentinal junction are seen enamel spindles (2), extensions of dentinal matrix penetrating for short distances into the enamel. Enamel tufts (3), which extend from the dentinal-enamel junction (4) into the enamel, are groups of poorly calcified, twisted enamel rods. Dentin with dentinal canals is shown (6). In the dentin are the interglobular spaces (5) filled with air and appearing black.

PLATE 50 (Fig. 3)

DRIED TOOTH (LAYERS OF THE ROOT)

Dentin (1) and cementum (4) are shown. In the dentin, near the dentinal-cementum junction, is the granular layer (of Tomes) (2). Internal to this are the large, irregular interglobular spaces (3) which are commonly seen in the crown of the tooth but may also be present in the root. In the cementum (4) are lacunae (5) with their canaliculi.

PLATE 50

DRIED TOOTH

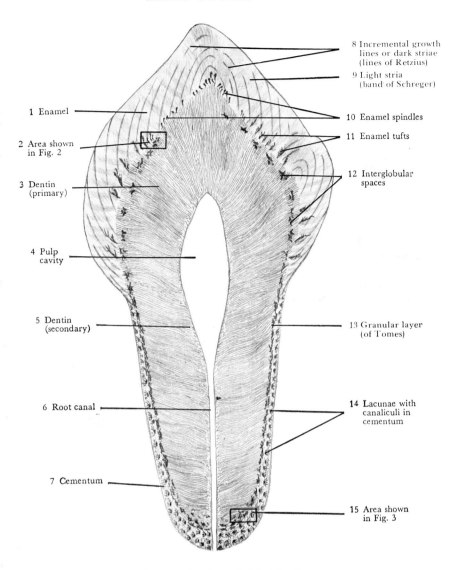

8 Incremental growth lines or dark striae (lines of Retzius)

9 Light stria (band of Schreger)

1 Enamel

10 Enamel spindles

2 Area shown in Fig. 2

11 Enamel tufts

3 Dentin (primary)

12 Interglobular spaces

4 Pulp cavity

5 Dentin (secondary)

13 Granular layer (of Tomes)

6 Root canal

14 Lacunae with canaliculi in cementum

7 Cementum

15 Area shown in Fig. 3

FIG. 1. *Panoramic view of dried tooth.*

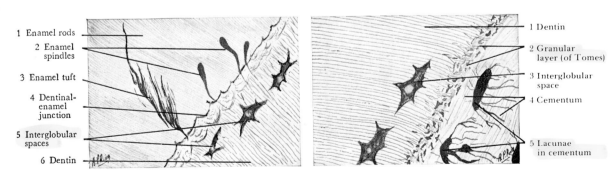

1 Enamel rods
2 Enamel spindles
3 Enamel tuft
4 Dentinal-enamel junction
5 Interglobular spaces
6 Dentin

1 Dentin
2 Granular layer (of Tomes)
3 Interglobular space
4 Cementum
5 Lacunae in cementum

FIG. 2. *Layers of the crown. Area corresponding to (2) in Fig. 1. 160×.*

FIG. 3. *Layers of the root. Area corresponding to (15) in Fig. 1. 160×.*

Plate 51 (Fig. 1)

DEVELOPING TOOTH (PANORAMIC VIEW)

A developing deciduous tooth is shown embedded in a socket, the dental alveolus, in the bone of the jaw (4, 22). Connective tissue (3) surrounds the developing tooth; it forms a compact layer immediately around the tooth, the dental sac (5). Enclosed within the sac is the enamel organ, composed of the external enamel epithelium (18), the stellate reticulum or enamel pulp (6, 19), the intermediate stratum (20) and the ameloblasts or inner enamel epithelium (7). All of these were differentiated from an epithelial downgrowth from the epithelium of the gum. The ameloblasts secrete enamel around the dentin. The enamel (8, 15) is the narrow deep pink band in the figure.

The dental pulp (21) of primitive connective tissue forms the core of the developing tooth. Blood vessels and nerves grow into it from below. A layer of modified fibroblasts, odontoblasts (11), form the outer margin of the pulp. Odontoblasts secrete predentin (10, 17) or uncalcified dentin. As it calcifies, it forms a layer of dentin (9, 16) next to the enamel.

The oral mucosa (1, 13) covers the developing tooth. An epithelial downgrowth from the oral epithelium is seen, probably the germ of a permanent tooth (2).

At the base of the tooth, the outer enamel epithelium and the ameloblasts come together and form the epithelial root sheath (of Hertwig) (12).

Plate 51 (Fig. 2)

DEVELOPING TOOTH (SECTIONAL VIEW)

At the left of the figure is a small area of dental pulp; fibroblasts (1) and fine fibers are seen. Odontoblasts (2) at the margin of the pulp are epithelioid cells (modified fibroblasts) which secrete the uncalcified predentin (3). This calcifies to become dentin (4). Processes of odontoblasts remain in the predentin and dentin as the dentinal fibers (of Tomes) (3).

At the right of the figure is a small area of stellate reticulum (7) showing nuclei and processes of its modified epithelial cells; the intermediate stratum (8), a transition region; and the tall columnar ameloblasts (6) which secrete the enamel (5, 10) in the form of enamel rods (prisms). In the process of enamel formation, the apical end of each ameloblast becomes transformed into a terminal granular portion (process of Tomes). These processes then appear collectively, in advanced enamel formation, as a separate layer of enamel processes (of Tomes) (9).

—114—

PLATE 51

DEVELOPING TOOTH

1 Epithelium of gum

2 Germ of permanent tooth

3 Connective tissue

4 Bone

5 Dental sac

6 Stellate reticulum (enamel pulp)

7 Ameloblasts (inner enamel epithelium)

8 Enamel

9 Dentin

10 Predentin

11 Odonto-blasts

12 Epithelial root sheath (of Hertwig)

13 Lamina propria of the buccal mucosa (gum)

14 Muscle

15 Enamel

16 Dentin

17 Predentin

18 External enamel epithelium

19 Stellate reticulum (enamel pulp)

20 Intermediate stratum

21 Dental pulp

22 Bone of dental alveolus

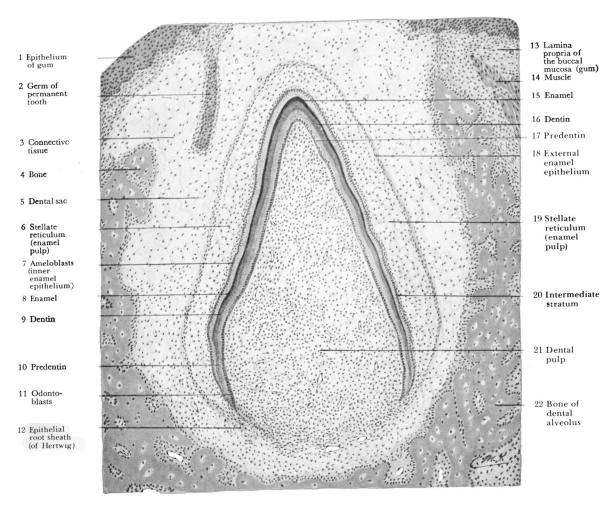

Fig. 1. *Panoramic view.*
Stain: hematoxylin-eosin. 50×.

1 Fibroblasts of dental pulp

2 Odontoblast; nucleus and cytoplasm

3 Predentin and dentinal fibers (of Tomes)

4 Dentin

5 Enamel (enamel rods or prisms)

6 Ameloblasts (inner enamel epithelium)

7 Stellate reticulum

8 Intermediate stratum

9 Layer of enamel processes (of Tomes)

10 Enamel rods (prisms)

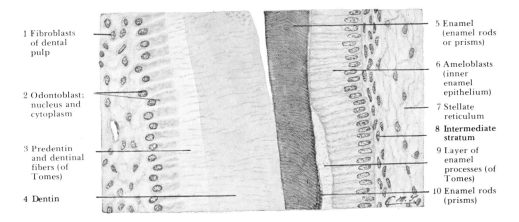

Fig. 2. *Sectional view.*
Stain: hematoxylin-eosin. 300×.

Plate 52

SALIVARY GLAND: PAROTID

The parotid gland is a purely serous gland with a well developed capsule and septa (trabeculae) which divide the gland into lobes and lobules. Parts of several lobules are illustrated in this figure.

Within each lobule are masses of serous alveoli (1, 15) supported by thin partitions of connective tissue. Each alveolus is formed by pyramidal cells arranged around a small, scarcely visible lumen (I). In sections, the lumen is not seen in all alveoli. The serous cells show a small, rounded nucleus in the deeper part of the cell, a basal zone of basophilic cytoplasm, and a lighter apical portion (15). With higher magnification (I) basal filaments (chromophilic material) are often visible in the deep zone (22) and small acidophilic secretory granules (zymogen granules) (21) are seen in the apical area, their number varying with the state of activity of the cell. Myoepithelial basal or basket cells (23) lie between the basement membrane and the epithelial cells; usually only the nucleus is visible.

Also within the lobules, among the alveoli, are small blood vesesls (18), groups of adipose cells (2, 19), striated ducts (5, 7), and intercalated ducts (8, 17, 25). Intercalated ducts drain the alveoli (17), are of small diameter and are lined with low cuboidal cells (II). Striated ducts (5, 7) have a larger lumen and are lined with columnar epithelium. The nucleus is centrally placed. Basal filaments (striations) are prominent (III, 24).

Striated ducts drain into a series of interlobular excretory ducts (6, 9, 12, 14) coursing in the connective septa (11, 13, 16). The lumen becomes progressively wider as the ducts increase in size. The epithelium varies from low simple columnar (6, IV) to pseudostratified in the larger ducts (9, 12).

Also in the interlobular connective tissue are seen blood vessels (3, 4, 10) of various sizes, nerves, and occasional parasympathetic ganglia (20).

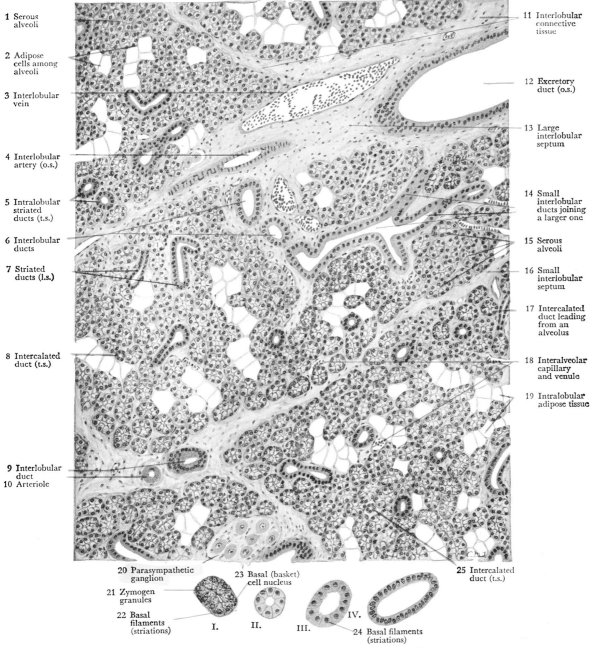

PLATE 52

SALIVARY GLAND: PAROTID

1 Serous alveoli

2 Adipose cells among alveoli

3 Interlobular vein

4 Interlobular artery (o.s.)

5 Intralobular striated ducts (t.s.)

6 Interlobular ducts

7 Striated ducts (l.s.)

8 Intercalated duct (t.s.)

9 Interlobular duct
10 Arteriole

11 Interlobular connective tissue

12 Excretory duct (o.s.)

13 Large interlobular septum

14 Small interlobular ducts joining a larger one

15 Serous alveoli

16 Small interlobular septum

17 Intercalated duct leading from an alveolus

18 Interalveolar capillary and venule

19 Intralobular adipose tissue

20 Parasympathetic ganglion

21 Zymogen granules

22 Basal filaments (striations)

23 Basal (basket) cell nucleus

24 Basal filaments (striations)

25 Intercalated duct (t.s.)

I.   II.   III.   IV.

I. serous alveolus; II. intercalated duct; III. striated duct; IV. excretory duct.

Stain: hematoxylin-eosin. 120×.

—117—

PLATE 53

SALIVARY GLAND: SUBMANDIBULAR

The figure demonstrates parts of several lobules of the submandibular gland.

The submandibular is a mixed gland, but is composed primarily of serous alveoli. Intermingled with these are small numbers of mucous or mixed alveoli. The presence of these distinguishes the submandibular from the parotid gland, since in other respects they are generally similar.

The serous alveoli (3, 10, II), like those in the parotid gland, can be recognized by their comparatively smaller size, the intense staining of their pyramidal cells which show the deeply basophilic zone of cytoplasm surrounding the rounded nucleus and a more lightly staining apical area, and the narrow almost obliterated lumen (3, II). The mucous alveoli (4, 9, IV) are larger and more variable in size and shape. They differ also from serous alveoli in the larger size and often more columnar form of the mucous cells, the pale, almost colorless staining reaction, the oval or flattened nuclei at the bases of the cells, and a somewhat larger more apparent lumen.

Mixed alveoli (8, V) are, typically, mucous alveoli surrounded by one or more groups of serous cells, the serous demilunes (14, 15). Myoepithelial cells (basal cells, basket cells) (16) may be present.

The duct system is similar to that in the parotid gland. Intralobular intercalated ducts (I, 12) of small caliber and striated ducts (7, III, 13) are present. A longitudinal section (IV) shows an alveolus opening into an intercalated duct (12) which is passing into a striated duct (13). Interlobular ducts (1, 5) course in the interlobular septa. Adipose cells (11) are scattered among the alveoli but are not as numerous as in the parotid gland.

PLATE 53

SALIVARY GLAND: SUBMANDIBULAR

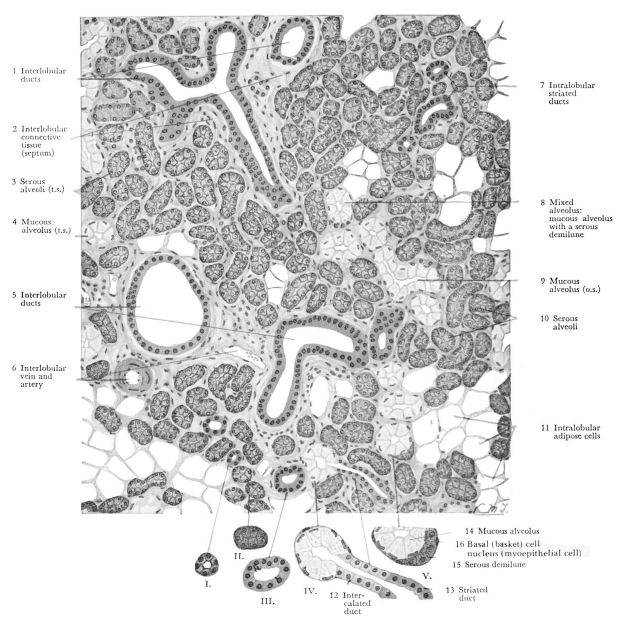

1 Interlobular ducts

2 Interlobular connective tissue (septum)

3 Serous alveoli (t.s.)

4 Mucous alveolus (t.s.)

5 Interlobular ducts

6 Interlobular vein and artery

7 Intralobular striated ducts

8 Mixed alveolus: mucous alveolus with a serous demilune

9 Mucous alveolus (o.s.)

10 Serous alveoli

11 Intralobular adipose cells

14 Mucous alveolus

16 Basal (basket) cell nucleus (myoepithelial cell)

15 Serous demilune

13 Striated duct

12 Intercalated duct

I.   II.   III.   IV.   V.

I. intercalated duct; II. serous alveolus; III. striated duct; IV. mucous alveolus with intercalated and striated ducts (l.s.); V. mixed alveolus.

Stain: hematoxylin-eosin. 170×.

PLATE 54

SALIVARY GLAND: SUBLINGUAL

The sublingual gland, also a mixed gland, is predominantly mucous in character, consisting largely of mucous alveoli (4, 6, I) and mucous alveoli with serous demilunes (2, 7, II). Purely serous alveoli are scarce, but the composition of the gland varies in its different parts. In this figure, serous alveoli are comparatively numerous (3); in other sections, they might be absent. Basal cells (basket cells) may be present (16, 19, 21) around any of the alveoli, situated as usual between the basement membrane and the base of the cell.

Typical intralobular intercalated ducts (8, IV) are infrequent or absent. Typical striated ducts (1, 9, V) are seen only occasionally; poorly developed striated ducts or non-striated intralobular ducts are more prevalent.

Interlobular connective tissue (13) is characteristically more abundant than in the parotid and submandibular glands, since the body of the sublingual is not as compact. Epithelial lining of interlobular excretory ducts varies from low columnar in the smaller ducts to pseudostratified columnar in the larger ones (15, VI), as in the parotid and submandibular glands. Blood vessels (5, 11, 12), nerves (10), and parasympathetic ganglia (14) are seen in the interlobular connective tissue.

PLATE 54

SALIVARY GLAND: SUBLINGUAL

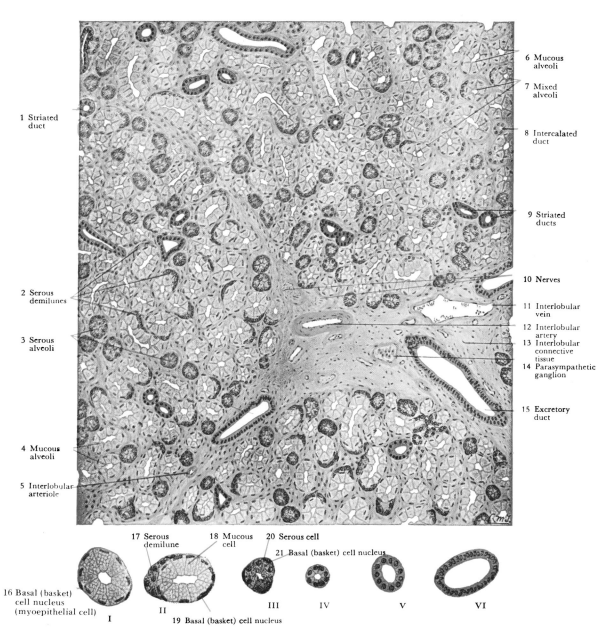

1 Striated
duct

2 Serous
demilunes

3 Serous
alveoli

4 Mucous
alveoli

5 Interlobular
arteriole

6 Mucous
alveoli

7 Mixed
alveoli

8 Intercalated
duct

9 Striated
ducts

10 Nerves

11 Interlobular
vein

12 Interlobular
artery

13 Interlobular
connective
tissue

14 Parasympathetic
ganglion

15 Excretory
duct

16 Basal (basket)
cell nucleus
(myoepithelial cell)

17 Serous
demilune

18 Mucous
cell

19 Basal (basket) cell nucleus

20 Serous cell

21 Basal (basket) cell nucleus

I   II   III   IV   V   VI

I. mucous alveolus; II. mixed alveolus; III. serous alveolus; IV. intercalated duct; V. striated duct;
VI. excretory duct.

Stain: hematoxylin-eosin. 85×.

PLATE 55

UPPER ESOPHAGUS: WALL (TRANSVERSE SECTION)

The esophagus is a tubular organ whose wall is composed of four distinct parts: a mucosa, submucosa, muscularis externa and adventitia (fibrosa).

The mucosa consists of an inner lining of non-cornified stratified squamous epithelium (1), an adjacent thin layer of fine connective tissue, the lamina propria (2) and a muscularis mucosae (3). Connective tissue papillae of the lamina propria indent the epithelium. Present in the lamina propria are small blood vessels, scanty diffuse lymphatic tissue, and occasional small lymphatic nodules (9). The muscularis mucosae (3) is formed by longitudinal smooth muscle fibers, which are seen here as cross or oblique sections.

The submucosa (4) is a wide layer of loose or moderately dense irregular connective tissue which often contains groups of adipose cells (14). Tubulo-alveolar mucous glands, the esophageal glands (11) are present here, and occur at intervals throughout the esophagus. Ducts (12) arising from the alveoli pass through the muscularis mucosae (10) and lamina propria and open into the lumen of the esophagus. Their epithelium merges with the stratified squamous epithelium (see Plate 56). Larger blood vessels (13) course in the submucosa.

Adjacent to the submucosa is the muscularis externa composed of two broad, well-defined layers, an inner circular layer (5) which is sectioned longitudinally in this transverse section of esophagus, and an outer longitudinal layer (7) in which the fibers are seen mainly in transverse sections. A thin layer of connective tissue lies between the two muscle layers (6). In the upper esophagus, the musculature is wholly or predominantly skeletal muscle. The peripheral location of nuclei in the muscle fibers is seen best in those fibers cut transversally (7).

The adventitia (8) or most peripheral layer of the esophagus is a connective tissue layer which blends with the adventitia of the trachea and other surrounding structures. Adipose cells or adipose tissue (16) are frequently present. In the adventitia are larger blood vessels (17, 18) and nerves (19) forming neuro-vascular bundles, as well as smaller divisions of these.

PLATE 55

UPPER ESOPHAGUS: WALL (TRANSVERSE SECTION)

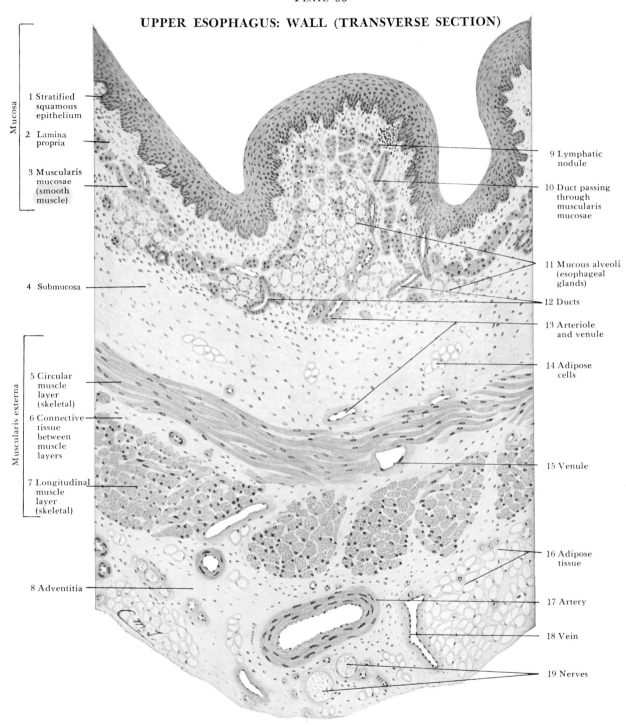

Mucosa

1 Stratified squamous epithelium

2 Lamina propria

3 Muscularis mucosae (smooth muscle)

4 Submucosa

Muscularis externa

5 Circular muscle layer (skeletal)

6 Connective tissue between muscle layers

7 Longitudinal muscle layer (skeletal)

8 Adventitia

9 Lymphatic nodule

10 Duct passing through muscularis mucosae

11 Mucous alveoli (esophageal glands)

12 Ducts

13 Arteriole and venule

14 Adipose cells

15 Venule

16 Adipose tissue

17 Artery

18 Vein

19 Nerves

Stain: hematoxylin-eosin. 50×.

PLATE 56

UPPER ESOPHAGUS: MUCOSA AND SUBMUCOSA
(TRANSVERSE SECTION)

At a higher magnification are seen the mucosa (1, 2, 3) and submucosa (4). In the stratified squamous epithelium (1) are seen the typical cell layers of this type of epithelium: squamous cells (6) forming the outer layers, rows of polyhedral cells (7) of the intermediate layers, and low columnar cells (9) of the basal layer. Mitosis occurs in the deeper layers (8).

In the lamina propria (2, 10) are seen blood vessels (11), scattered lymphocytes and a small lymphatic nodule (12). The muscularis mucosae (which is always smooth muscle) is seen as small bundles sectioned transversally (13).

In the submucosa, the alveoli of the esophageal glands (15) show the typical characteristics of mucous alveoli whose cells are filled with mucigen. Small ducts from the glands (16, lower leaders) lined with simple epithelium pass into larger excretory ducts (16, upper leader) lined with stratified epithelium. At (14), the duct is sectioned tangentially. Its epithelium becomes continuous with the stratified squamous epithelium.

Also seen in the submucosa (4) are blood vessels (17, 18), nerves (19) and adipose cells (20). A small area of skeletal muscle fibers from the circular layer of the muscularis externa (5) is present.

PLATE 56

UPPER ESOPHAGUS: MUCOSA AND SUBMUCOSA
(TRANSVERSE SECTION)

Mucosa

1 Stratified
squamous
epithelium

2 Lamina
propria

3 Muscularis
mucosae

4 Submucosa

5 Circular
layer of
the
muscularis
externa

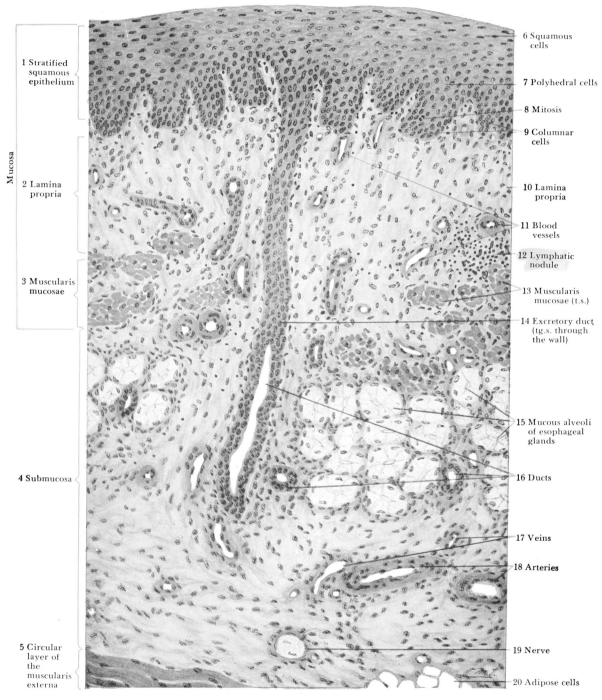

6 Squamous
cells

7 Polyhedral cells

8 Mitosis

9 Columnar
cells

10 Lamina
propria

11 Blood
vessels

12 Lymphatic
nodule

13 Muscularis
mucosae (t.s.)

14 Excretory duct
(tg.s. through
the wall)

15 Mucous alveoli
of esophageal
glands

16 Ducts

17 Veins

18 Arteries

19 Nerve

20 Adipose cells

Stain: hematoxylin-eosin. 250×.

PLATE 57 (Fig. 1)

UPPER ESOPHAGUS

This section of upper esophagus is generally similar to that on Plate 55, but is stained with one of Heidenhain's modifications of Mallory's trichrome (Mallory-Azan). Azocarmine is employed to stain nuclei an intense red. A mixture of aniline blue and orange G then selectively stains other tissues or tissue components. Collagenous fibers stain bright blue (1, 4, 5, 7, 9), cytoplasm of epithelial cells and muscle stains orange to red (2, 3, 6, 8).

The layers of the wall are easily distinguishable. Since this is upper esophagus (as in Plate 55), the outermost layer is an adventitia (1) and the external muscle layers are skeletal muscle (2, 3). Aniline blue stains not only the large amounts of connective tissue in the submucosa (9) and adventitia (1) but also demonstrates the smaller amounts between layers of muscle (4) and still lesser amounts within the muscle layers (5). The connective tissue of the lamina propria (7) is distinct from the smooth muscle of the muscularis mucosae (8).

PLATE 57 (Fig. 2)

LOWER ESOPHAGUS

This section of lower esophagus is stained with Van Gieson's trichrome which employs iron hematoxylin (Weigert's or Heidenhain's) as a nuclear stain and picrofuchsin for other components. Cellular detail is not well revealed, but it is useful for differentiating between connective tissue and muscle. Nuclei are dark brown. Collagenous fibers are stained red with acid fuchsin (3, 5, 7), whereas muscle (and other tissues) are stained yellow with picric acid (2, 4, 6, 8, 9).

The layers of the wall of the lower esophagus are generally similar to those in the upper esophagus, with regional modifications, however. The outer layer of the wall is a serosa (visceral peritoneum) (1) rather than a fibrosa. The external muscle layers are entirely smooth muscle (2, 4), although this is not apparent with this stain at this magnification. Distribution of the mucous glands in the submucosa is variable; some are present in this section (9), but they may be absent altogether.

In addition to the abundant collagenous fibers in the submucosa (5), distribution of finer fibers in lesser amounts may be seen between and around bundles of smooth muscle fibers (3, 8), in the serosa (1) and in the lamina propria (7).

PLATE 57

ESOPHAGUS (TRANSVERSE SECTIONS)

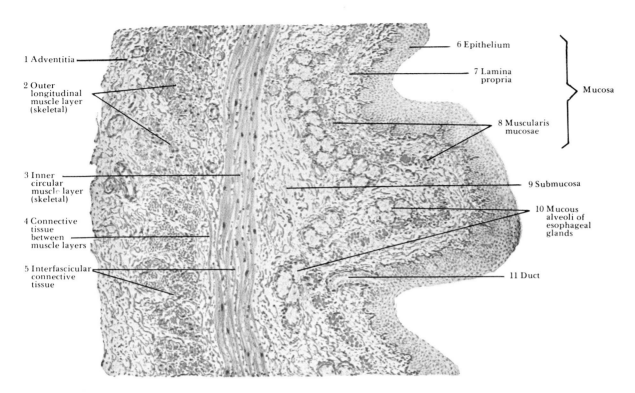

1 Adventitia

2 Outer longitudinal muscle layer (skeletal)

3 Inner circular muscle layer (skeletal)

4 Connective tissue between muscle layers

5 Interfascicular connective tissue

6 Epithelium

7 Lamina propria

8 Muscularis mucosae

Mucosa

9 Submucosa

10 Mucous alveoli of esophageal glands

11 Duct

FIG. 1. *Upper esophagus.* Stain: Mallory's trichrome. 40×. (Nuclei, red; connective tissue, blue; epithelium and muscle, orange to red.)

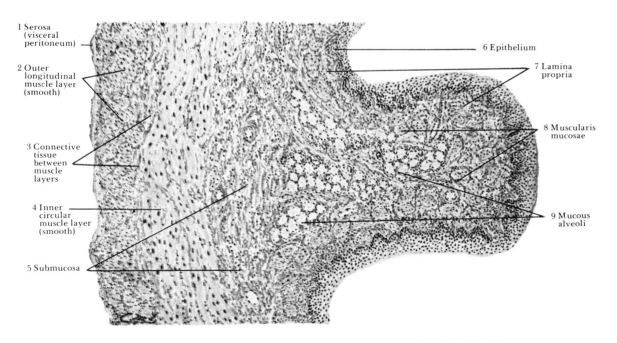

1 Serosa (visceral peritoneum)

2 Outer longitudinal muscle layer (smooth)

3 Connective tissue between muscle layers

4 Inner circular muscle layer (smooth)

5 Submucosa

6 Epithelium

7 Lamina propria

8 Muscularis mucosae

9 Mucous alveoli

FIG. 2. *Lower esophagus.* Stain: Van Gieson's trichrome. 40×. (Nuclei, dark brown; connective tissue, red; epithelium and muscle, yellow.)

PLATE 58

CARDIA (LONGITUDINAL SECTION)

At the lower end of the esophagus, esophageal (submucosal) glands may still be present (11). As in the upper region, ducts (13) leading from these glands penetrate the muscularis mucosae, course through the lamina propria (15) and empty into the lumen of the esophagus. The lamina propria (14) may contain a few cardiac glands (12).

At the cardia, or esophageal-stomach junction, the stratified squamous epithelium of the esophagus is replaced abruptly by simple columnar mucus-secreting epithelium of the stomach. The boundary between the two organs is thus sharply defined.

The lamina propria of the stomach (16) is continuous with that of the esophagus but it becomes a wide layer containing diffuse lymphatic tissue and glands. The lamina propria is indented by shallow foveolae or gastric pits (19) into which the mucosal glands empty.

The glands are of two types. Simple tubular cardiac glands (17), limited to the transition region (cardia), are lined with a single type of cell, a mucus-secreting columnar cell. Cardiac glands are replaced quickly by simple tubular gastric glands (20). They may branch somewhat at their bases. They are lined principally by two types of cells, chief cells (21) and parietal cells (23). A third type, mucous neck cells (22), are found at the distal ends of the glands just before they open into the foveolae or gastric pits.

The muscularis mucosae (8) is continuous from esophagus to stomach. In the esophagus, it is usually a single layer of longitudinal fibers. In the stomach, a second inner circular layer is added (8).

Submucosa (7) and muscularis externa (6) are continuous. Many blood vessels are seen throughout the length of the submucosa (1, 2, 3, 4, 5, 9). The larger of these distribute smaller vessels to other regions.

PLATE 58

CARDIA (LONGITUDINAL SECTION)

Muscularis externa | Submucosa | Mucosa

m.m. lamina propria | epithelium

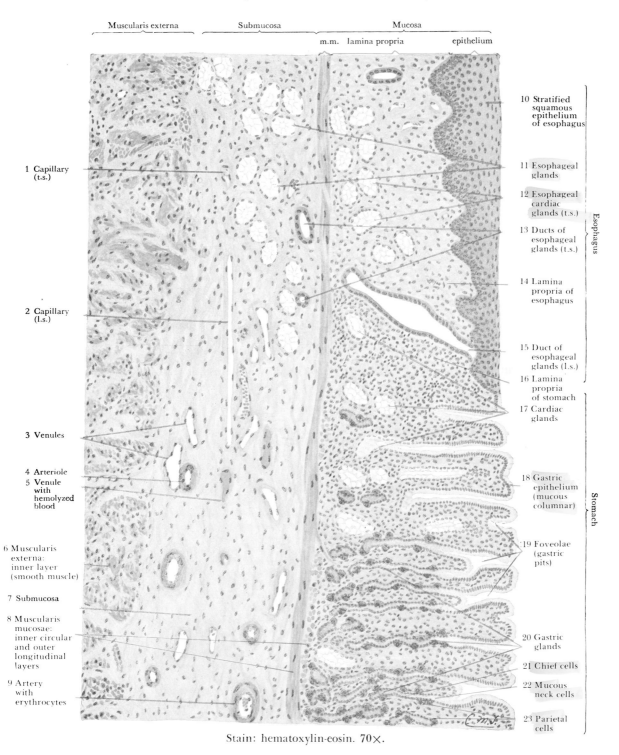

1 Capillary (t.s.)

2 Capillary (l.s.)

3 Venules

4 Arteriole
5 Venule with hemolyzed blood

6 Muscularis externa: inner layer (smooth muscle)

7 Submucosa

8 Muscularis mucosae: inner circular and outer longitudinal layers

9 Artery with erythrocytes

10 Stratified squamous epithelium of esophagus

11 Esophageal glands

12 Esophageal cardiac glands (t.s.)

13 Ducts of esophageal glands (t.s.)

14 Lamina propria of esophagus

15 Duct of esophageal glands (l.s.)
16 Lamina propria of stomach

17 Cardiac glands

18 Gastric epithelium (mucous columnar)

19 Foveolae (gastric pits)

20 Gastric glands

21 Chief cells

22 Mucous neck cells

23 Parietal cells

Esophagus

Stomach

Stain: hematoxylin-eosin. 70×.

— 129 —

PLATE 59

STOMACH: FUNDUS OR BODY (TRANSVERSE SECTION)

Under low magnification, a section through the wall of the fundus or body of the stomach illustrates the following general areas: mucosa (1, 2, 3), submucosa (4), muscularis externa (5, 6) and serosa (7).

The outermost layer of the mucosa is the lining epithelium of the stomach (1), a simple columnar mucous epithelium. This epithelium is continued as the lining of the foveolae or gastric pits (8), which extend into the body of the mucosa to a distance about one-fourth its thickness. Extensions of the lamina propria proper, the mucosal ridges (9), surround the foveolae.

Into the bases of the foveolae open the gastric glands (10) which occupy the lamina propria proper (2) and extend downward almost to the muscularis mucosae (3). The glands contain mainly chief (principal) cells and parietal cells. The lamina propria (2) comprises the supporting connective tissue of the mucosa. The muscularis mucosae (3) is a thin band of smooth muscle (two layers), forming the deepest layer of the mucosa. From it, small bundles of muscle pass upward into the lamina propria. In the subglandular lamina propria, small lymphatic nodules are noted at the right (11) and left of the section.

The submucosa (4) is a broad layer of connective tissue. In it are seen small blood vessels (12, 13, 14, 15). At the left is a vein filled with a clot and hemolyzed blood.

In the muscularis externa, the inner layer of circular fibers (5) has been sectioned longitudinally and the outer longitudinal muscle layer (6) has been sectioned transversely. A third inner layer of obliquely arranged muscle fibers is not always apparent, since the bundles of circular muscle fibers tend to course in various directions (as indicated in this figure) (16) rather than in a regular circular manner. Parasympathetic ganglia of the myenteric plexus (Auerbach's plexus) (17) are seen in the connective tissue between the muscle layers. Similar but smaller parasympathetic ganglia are found in the submucosa (submucosal plexus or Meissner's plexus).

Serosa (7) covers the outer surface of the stomach. It is visceral peritoneum, consisting of mesothelium and a thin lamina propria of loose connective tissue.

PLATE 59

STOMACH: FUNDUS OR BODY (TRANSVERSE SECTION)

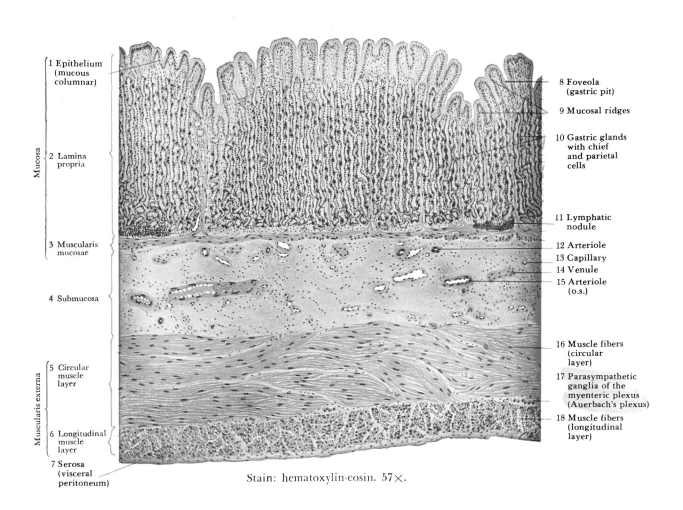

1 Epithelium (mucous columnar)

Mucosa

2 Lamina propria

3 Muscularis mucosae

4 Submucosa

Muscularis externa

5 Circular muscle layer

6 Longitudinal muscle layer

7 Serosa (visceral peritoneum)

8 Foveola (gastric pit)

9 Mucosal ridges

10 Gastric glands with chief and parietal cells

11 Lymphatic nodule

12 Arteriole

13 Capillary

14 Venule

15 Arteriole (o.s.)

16 Muscle fibers (circular layer)

17 Parasympathetic ganglia of the myenteric plexus (Auerbach's plexus)

18 Muscle fibers (longitudinal layer)

Stain: hematoxylin-eosin. 57×.

PLATE 60

STOMACH: MUCOSA OF THE FUNDUS OR BODY
(TRANSVERSE SECTION)

The gastric mucosa and the adjacent submucosa are shown under medium magnification. The foveolae or gastric pits (13) are now seen to better advantage as depressions in the lamina propria, with extensions of lamina propria, the mucosal ridges (2), surrounding them. The simple columnar mucous epithelium (1) which lines the stomach becomes lower as it approaches the bases of the foveolae.

The gastric glands (15, 16, 17) are close together but are separated from each other by interglandular lamina propria (7). The structure of the lamina propria is seen better in the mucosal ridges (2); it consists of fine connective tissue with diffuse lymphatic tissue and scattered smooth muscle fibers (14).

The tubular structure of the gastric glands (15, 16, 17) is apparent; the basal branching is indicated by transverse and oblique sections in this area (17, fundus). The greater part of the gland is the body (16); the basal portion is the fundus (17). Body and fundus are made up of chief or zymogenic cells (5) which take a basophilic stain, and parietal cells (6) which take an acidophilic stain (and argentaffine cells, not illustrated). The distal part of the gland is the short, constricted neck (15), lined with mucous neck cells (3), which become continuous with the mucous cells lining the foveola as the gland empties into its base.

A subglandular region of lamina propria (9) may be present between the bases of the glands and the muscularis mucosae (10, 11). Diffuse lymphatic tissue and a small lymphatic nodule (18) are seen here.

Single or small bundles of smooth muscle fibers, arising from the inner layer of the muscularis mucosae (10), may be seen passing upward through the lamina propria (8) between glands and into mucosal ridges (14).

In this transverse section of gastric mucosa, the circular layer of the muscularis mucosae is sectioned longitudinally (10) and the outer longitudinal layer (11) is sectioned transversally.

PLATE 60

STOMACH: MUCOSA OF THE FUNDUS OR BODY
(TRANSVERSE SECTION)

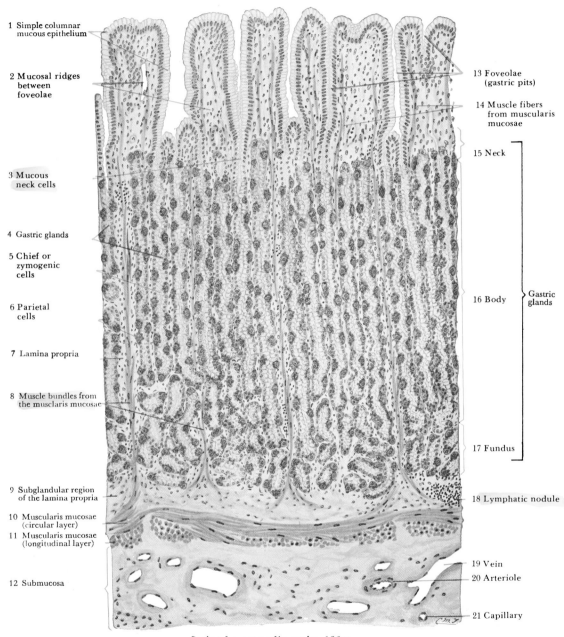

1 Simple columnar mucous epithelium

2 Mucosal ridges between foveolae

3 Mucous neck cells

4 Gastric glands

5 Chief or zymogenic cells

6 Parietal cells

7 Lamina propria

8 Muscle bundles from the muscularis mucosae

9 Subglandular region of the lamina propria

10 Muscularis mucosae (circular layer)

11 Muscularis mucosae (longitudinal layer)

12 Submucosa

13 Foveolae (gastric pits)

14 Muscle fibers from muscularis mucosae

15 Neck

16 Body

17 Fundus

Gastric glands

18 Lymphatic nodule

19 Vein

20 Arteriole

21 Capillary

Stain: hematoxylin-eosin. 180×.

PLATE 61 (Fig. 1)

STOMACH: SUPERFICIAL REGION OF THE MUCOSA OF THE FUNDUS AND BODY OF THE STOMACH

At a higher magnification are seen the characteristic features of the various cells which compose the superficial region of the gastric mucosa of the fundus and body.

The tall columnar surface epithelium (1) is lightly stained (due to solution of mucigen droplets), has basally-placed oval nuclei, and a thin but distinct basement membrane (2). This epithelium extends into the foveolae (4). The bordering lamina propria (3) is fibroreticular connective tissue.

Gastric glands lie in the lamina propria (11) below the foveolae. Necks of the gastric glands (5) are lined with low columnar mucous neck cells (6) with rounded, basal nuclei. The constricted neck of the gland (10) opens by a short transition region or mouth (9) into the base of a foveola (8).

Parietal cells (7) are interspersed among mucous neck cells; their free surfaces border on the lumen. They are large, rounded acidophilic cells with a rounded nucleus. They may be binucleated.

Deeper in the gland, below the neck region, mucous neck cells are replaced by basophilic chief or zymogenic cells (13) which border on the lumen. Parietal cells are now displaced peripherally and lie against the basement membrane but do not reach the lumen.

PLATE 61 (Fig. 2)

DEEP REGION OF THE MUCOSA

Gastric glands are branched tubular glands; the branching occurs at the base (or fundus) of the gland. A section through the deep region of the mucosa therefore shows basal portions of glands sectioned in various planes (1, 10).

As in the body of the gland, chief (zymogenic) cells are seen bordering the lumen of the gland (4, 9, 12). Parietal cells are wedged against the basement membrane (3, 8, 11) and are not in contact with the lumen. This is especially well demonstrated in a transverse section (3, lower leader).

Also illustrated are the small amount of lamina propria between glands (2) and a narrow zone of subglandular lamina propria (5) which is not always distinguishable.

The two layers of the muscularis mucosae are seen (13, 14).

PLATE 61

STOMACH: FUNDUS OR BODY

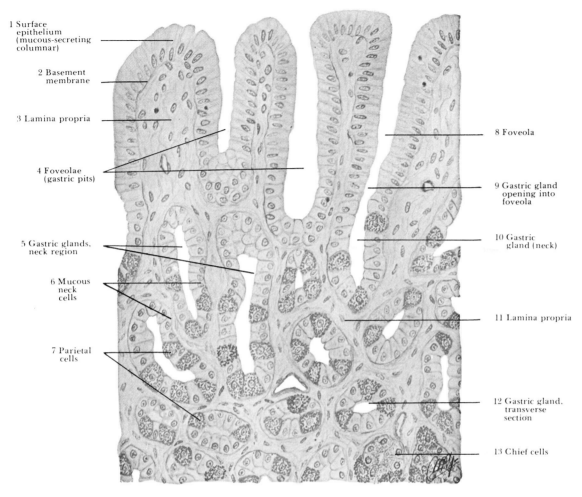

1 Surface
epithelium
(mucous-secreting
columnar)

2 Basement
membrane

3 Lamina propria

4 Foveolae
(gastric pits)

5 Gastric glands,
neck region

6 Mucous
neck
cells

7 Parietal
cells

8 Foveola

9 Gastric gland
opening into
foveola

10 Gastric
gland (neck)

11 Lamina propria

12 Gastric gland,
transverse
section

13 Chief cells

FIG. 1. *Superficial region of the gastric mucosa.* Stain: hematoxylin-eosin. 350×.

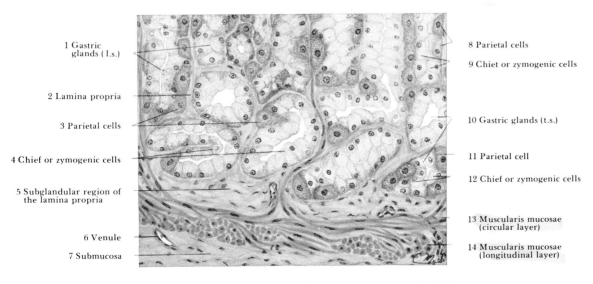

1 Gastric
glands (l.s.)

2 Lamina propria

3 Parietal cells

4 Chief or zymogenic cells

5 Subglandular region of
the lamina propria

6 Venule

7 Submucosa

8 Parietal cells

9 Chief or zymogenic cells

10 Gastric glands (t.s.)

11 Parietal cell

12 Chief or zymogenic cells

13 Muscularis mucosae
(circular layer)

14 Muscularis mucosae
(longitudinal layer)

FIG. 2. *Deep region of the mucosa.* Stain: hematoxylin-eosin. 350×.

PLATE 62

STOMACH: MUCOSA OF THE PYLORIC REGION

In the mucosa of the pyloric region, the foveolae (4, 12) are deeper than those in the body, extending into the mucosa to one-half or more of its thickness. The simple columnar mucous epithelium (10) which lines the stomach continues into the foveolae.

The gastric glands of the body of the stomach are replaced by pyloric glands (5, 6, 14). These are branched or coiled tubular mucous glands. Typically, these have only one type of cell, a tall columnar cell with slightly granular cytoplasm, lightly stained because of solution of mucigen droplets, and a flattened or oval nucleus at the base. The glands open into the bases of the foveolae (4, lower leader).

Other structures are like those in the upper stomach. The lamina propria contains diffuse lymphatic tissue (13) and occasional lymphatic nodules (16) in its deeper part. These may increase in size and penetrate through the muscularis mucosae into the submucosa. Smooth muscle fibers from the circular layer of the muscularis mucosae pass into the lamina propria (7) extending between glands and into mucosal ridges (2, 3).

PLATE 62

STOMACH: MUCOSA OF THE PYLORIC REGION

1 Lymphocyte migrating through the epithelium

2 Muscle fibers from the muscularis mucosae

3 Mucosal ridges

4 Foveolae (gastric pits)

5 Pyloric glands (l. s.)

6 Pyloric glands (t.s.)

7 Muscle fibers passing into lamina propria

8 Arteriole

9 Venule

10 Epithelium (mucous columnar)

11 Epithelium (h.s.)

12 Foveolae (gastric pits)

13 Lamina propria

14 Pyloric glands

15 Muscle fibers from muscularis mucosae

16 Lymphatic nodule

17 Capillary

18 Muscularis mucosae

19 Venule

20 Submucosa

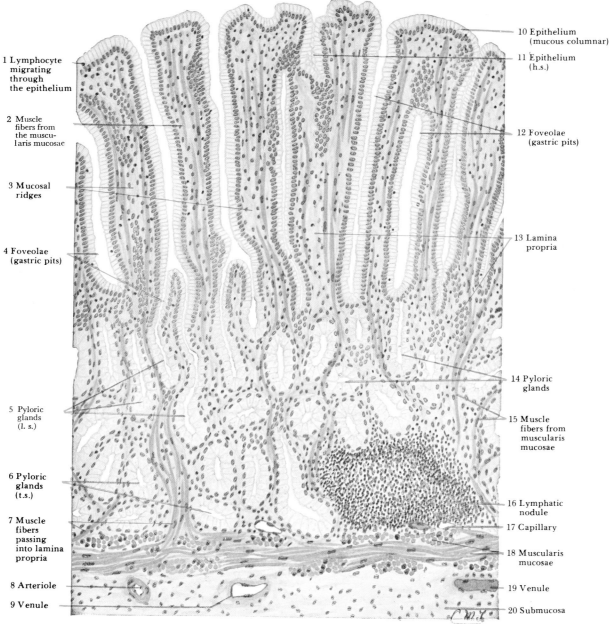

Stain: hematoxylin-eosin. 100×.

—137—

PLATE 63

PYLORIC-DUODENAL JUNCTION (LONGITUDINAL SECTION)

In the pyloric stomach (1), just before its junction with the duodenum (2), is the pyloric sphincter (7), formed primarily by great thickening of the circular layer of the muscularis externa. Several other features serve to differentiate pyloric stomach from duodenum.

As the pylorus approaches the duodenum, the mucosal ridges (5) which surround the foveolae (6) become broader and more irregular in outline, often assuming varied shapes in sectioned material. Coiled tubular pyloric mucous glands (4) are still present in the lamina propria proper, and open into foveolae. Lymphatic nodules (10) occur frequently at the transition region.

In the duodenum (2), mucosal evaginations, villi (13), make their appearance. Each villus is a leaf-shaped projection (13) with a somewhat pointed tip. Between the villi are intervillous spaces (16), continuations of the intestinal lumen. The mucus-secreting epithelium of the stomach (3) makes a sudden transition (11) to intestinal epithelium, consisting of goblet cells and columnar cells with striated borders (microvilli) which continue to be present throughout the length of the small intestine.

Short simple tubular intestinal glands (crypts of Lieberkühn) (12) in the lamina propria proper replace pyloric glands. They are lined mainly with goblet cells and striated-bordered cells continued in from the surface epithelium. One or more intestinal glands open into an intervillous space (17).

Duodenal glands (Brunner's glands) (14) occupy most of the submucosa in the upper duodenum, and frequently extend through the muscularis mucosae into the deep mucosa. The muscularis mucosae is disrupted (15) and strands of muscle may be dispersed among the mucous tubules of the glands. Aside from the esophageal (submucosal) glands, the duodenal glands are the only submucosal glands in the digestive tract proper.

PLATE 63

PYLORIC-DUODENAL JUNCTION (LONGITUDINAL SECTION)

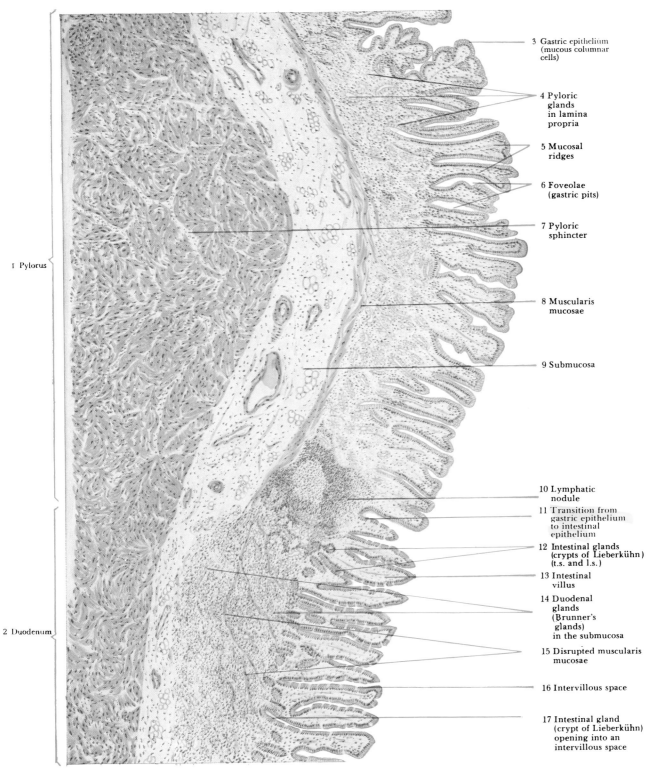

3 Gastric epithelium
(mucous columnar
cells)

4 Pyloric
glands
in lamina
propria

5 Mucosal
ridges

6 Foveolae
(gastric pits)

7 Pyloric
sphincter

8 Muscularis
mucosae

9 Submucosa

10 Lymphatic
nodule

11 Transition from
gastric epithelium
to intestinal
epithelium

12 Intestinal glands
(crypts of Lieberkühn)
(t.s. and l.s.)

13 Intestinal
villus

14 Duodenal
glands
(Brunner's
glands)
in the submucosa

15 Disrupted muscularis
mucosae

16 Intervillous space

17 Intestinal gland
(crypt of Lieberkühn)
opening into an
intervillous space

1 Pylorus

2 Duodenum

Stain: Hematoxylin-eosin. 25×.

PLATE 64

SMALL INTESTINE: DUODENUM
(LONGITUDINAL SECTION)

The wall of the duodenum is made up of four layers: mucosa (13, 14, 15), submucosa (17), muscularis externa (18) and serosa (visceral peritoneum) (19). These are continuous with the same layers of the stomach and continue uninterruptedly into the rest of the small intestine and the large intestine.

Distinctive features of the small intestine are villi (3, 13), a lining epithelium of columnar cells with striated borders and goblet cells (1), and short tubular intestinal glands (crypts of Lieberkühn) (6, 7) in the lamina propria proper. The presence of mucous glands in the submucosa (17) indicates that this figure is upper duodenum. Submucosal glands are absent elsewhere in the intestine.

Villi (3, 13) are mucosal evaginations with intervillous spaces (2) between them. The lining epithelium (1) covers the villi and lines the spaces, and continues into the intestinal glands (5). Each villus has a core of lamina propria (3, 13), some smooth muscle fibers (4) extending in from the muscularis mucosae (15), and a central lacteal which is not indicated in this figure. (See Plate 66, Fig. 2, for detailed structure of a villus.)

In the lamina propria proper (14) are the intestinal glands (crypts of Lieberkühn) (6, 7) which open into intervillous spaces (5), and sometimes extensions of the submucosal duodenal glands (Brunner's glands) (8, upper leader, and 16). The lamina propria is fine connective tissue with reticular cells and diffuse lymphatic tissue. Lymphatic nodules may be present in the deep lamina propria.

The submucosa (17) is almost completely filled with highly branched tubular duodenal glands (Brunner's glands) (8, 17). The muscularis mucosae may be disrupted if these glands penetrate into the deep lamina propria of the mucosa, and strands of muscle may be seen throughout the glandular layer (9). The duodenal glands open into the bases of intestinal glands.

The muscularis externa (18) consists of an inner circular and an outer longitudinal layer. Parasympathetic ganglion cells of the myenteric plexus (Auerbach's plexus) (12) are seen in the thin layer of connective tissue between the two muscle layers; they continue to be found in this location throughout the small and large intestines. Similar but smaller ganglion cells are likewise found in the submucosa throughout the small and large intestine (submucosal plexus or Meissner's plexus).

Serosa or visceral peritoneum (19) forms the outermost layer.

PLATE 64

SMALL INTESTINE: DUODENUM
(LONGITUDINAL SECTION)

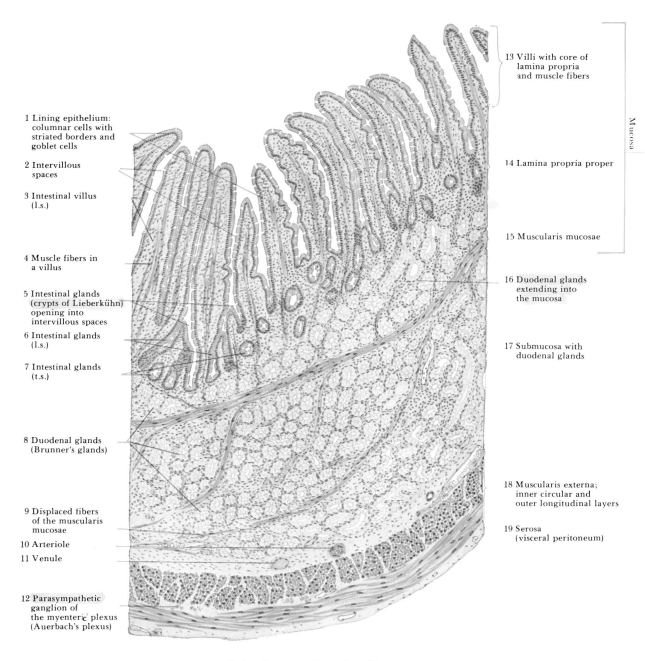

1 Lining epithelium:
columnar cells with
striated borders and
goblet cells

2 Intervillous
spaces

3 Intestinal villus
(l.s.)

4 Muscle fibers in
a villus

5 Intestinal glands
(crypts of Lieberkühn)
opening into
intervillous spaces

6 Intestinal glands
(l.s.)

7 Intestinal glands
(t.s.)

8 Duodenal glands
(Brunner's glands)

9 Displaced fibers
of the muscularis
mucosae

10 Arteriole

11 Venule

12 Parasympathetic
ganglion of
the myenteric plexus
(Auerbach's plexus)

13 Villi with core of
lamina propria
and muscle fibers

14 Lamina propria proper

15 Muscularis mucosae

16 Duodenal glands
extending into
the mucosa

17 Submucosa with
duodenal glands

18 Muscularis externa;
inner circular and
outer longitudinal layers

19 Serosa
(visceral peritoneum)

Mucosa

Stain: hematoxylin-eosin. 50×.

PLATE 65 (Fig. 1)

SMALL INTESTINE: JEJUNUM-ILEUM
(TRANSVERSE SECTION)

Structure of the lower duodenum, jejunum and ileum between aggregated nodules is basically similar to that already seen in the upper duodenum on Plate 64 (except for duodenal glands, which are usually limited to the upper part of the duodenum). Villi differ somewhat in shape and in length in the different regions but this is not usually apparent in sections. Aggregated nodules (Peyer's patches) occur at intervals in the ileum (see Plate 66, Fig. 1).

In this figure, villi are seen sectioned longitudinally (1), obliquely (13), and transversally (12, 16). A contracted villus (14) appears shorter and broader. Each villus shows its typical structure, a surface epithelium of striated-bordered cells and goblet cells (11), a core of lamina propria with diffuse lymphatic tissue and groups of smooth muscle fibers (15). The central lacteal and small blood vessels are not indicated (see Plate 66, Fig. 2).

Intestinal glands (crypts of Lieberkühn) (3, 17) in the lamina propria proper are close together. They open into intervillous spaces (3, middle leader).

A lymphatic nodule (21), seen here in the submucosa, had its origin in the mucosa, then penetrated through the muscularis mucosae into the submucosa.

Muscularis mucosae (6), submucosa (7), muscularis externa (8, 9) and serosa (10) are typical although adipose tissue (19) is not always present in the serosa. Ganglion cells of the myenteric plexus (18) are seen in the connective tissue between the muscle layers. Submucosal plexuses are also present.

PLATE 65 (Fig. 2)

INTESTINAL GLANDS WITH PANETH CELLS

In the basal region of the jejunal mucosa, adjacent to the muscularis mucosae (4), are represented the deep portions of several intestinal glands. The characteristic goblet cells (1) and cells with striated borders (2) are seen in the glands. In addition, at the base of each gland, is found a group of pyramidal-shaped cells with large acidophilic granules, the Paneth cells (3). These coarse granules, which stain a reddish-orange in this preparation, fill most of the cytoplasm. The nucleus and ordinary cytoplasm are displaced toward the base of the cell.

Paneth cells are apparently secretory and have the appearance of zymogenic cells, but their specific function is not yet known. Several varied functions have been indicated.

Paneth cells are found throughout the small intestine and occasionally in the large intestine.

PLATE 65 (Fig. 3)

INTESTINAL GLANDS WITH ARGENTAFFIN CELLS

This section was prepared from an operative specimen of ileum. Transverse or oblique sections of intestinal glands are shown. Cytoplasm and nuclei of goblet and striated-bordered cells are stained with Darrow red. Special silver technique demonstrates fine granules in the basal portions of some cells; nuclei lie above these argyrophilic granules. These are the argentaffin cells or enterochromaffin cells (2). They secrete serotonin. They are found in the small intestine (duodenum mainly), in the appendix and in the stomach.

The silver staining also reveals argyrophilic reticular fibers (1) in the connective tissue of the lamina propria.

PLATE 65

FIG. 1. SMALL INTESTINE: JEJUNUM-ILEUM
(TRANSVERSE SECTION)

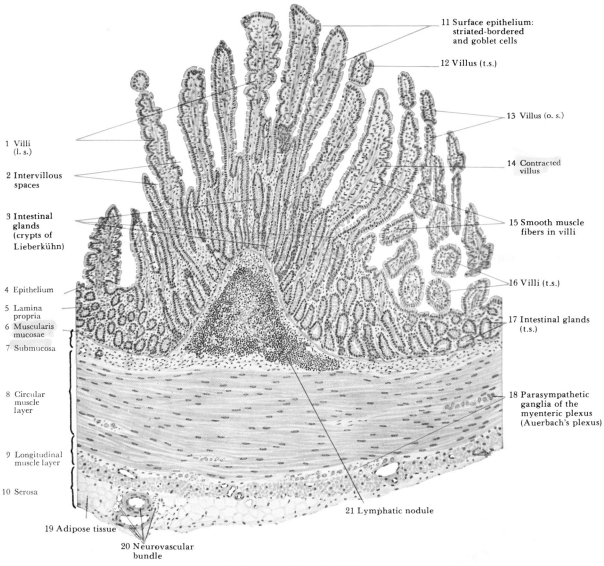

11 Surface epithelium: striated-bordered and goblet cells

12 Villus (t.s.)

13 Villus (o. s.)

14 Contracted villus

15 Smooth muscle fibers in villi

16 Villi (t.s.)

17 Intestinal glands (t.s.)

18 Parasympathetic ganglia of the myenteric plexus (Auerbach's plexus)

1 Villi (l. s.)

2 Intervillous spaces

3 Intestinal glands (crypts of Lieberkühn)

4 Epithelium

5 Lamina propria

6 Muscularis mucosae

7 Submucosa

8 Circular muscle layer

9 Longitudinal muscle layer

10 Serosa

19 Adipose tissue

20 Neurovascular bundle

21 Lymphatic nodule

Stain: hematoxylin-eosin. 50×.

FIG. 2. PANETH CELLS   FIG. 3. ARGENTAFFIN CELLS

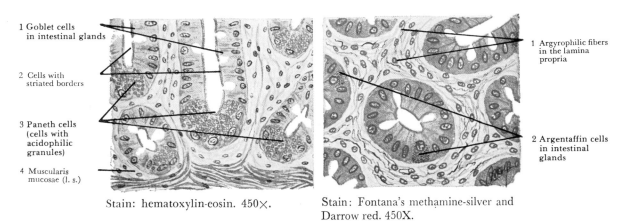

1 Goblet cells in intestinal glands

2 Cells with striated borders

3 Paneth cells (cells with acidophilic granules)

4 Muscularis mucosae (l. s.)

1 Argyrophilic fibers in the lamina propria

2 Argentaffin cells in intestinal glands

Stain: hematoxylin-eosin. 450×.

Stain: Fontana's methamine-silver and Darrow red. 450X.

PLATE 66 (Fig. 1)

SMALL INTESTINE: ILEUM WITH AGGREGATED NODULES
(PEYER'S PATCH)

Again, the typical four coats of wall are indicated (9–16 inclusive). Villi are seen in various planes of section (1, 2, 9) and intestinal glands (crypts of Lieberkühn) (3, 10) are seen in the lamina propria proper; two of these are opening into an intervillous space (upper 3, upper 10).

Characteristic of the ileum are aggregated nodules or Peyer's patches, each patch being an aggregation of ten or more lymphatic nodules. These are located in the wall of the ileum opposite the attachment of the mesentery. The portion of a Peyer's patch illustrated here shows nine nodules (4, 5, and others), most of which have germinal centers (5). The nodules tend to coalesce, so that boundaries between them are not usually visible.

The nodules originate in the diffuse lymphatic tissue of the lamina propria. Villi are absent in the area where they reach the surface of the mucosa (4). Typically, they extend into the submucosa (7), disrupting the muscularis mucosae (6) in doing so, and spread out in the loose connective tissue of the submucosa.

PLATE 66 (Fig. 2)

SMALL INTESTINE: VILLI

The distal parts of three villi are shown here at a higher magnification. Two are sectioned longitudinally (left and right). The central one had been folded, thus is seen in two parts: the apex has been sectioned transversally (1), the lower portion tangentially (7) and longitudinally (8).

The surface epithelium (2) shows goblet cells (9, 10, 13) and columnar cells with striated borders (14, 15). The thin basement membrane is visible in places (5). In the core of lamina propria (12) are seen reticular cells of the stroma, lymphocytes and smooth muscle fibers (4, 16). Present in each villus (but not always seen in sections) is a central lacteal, a dilated lymphatic vessel lined with endothelium (3, 17). Blood vessels in a villus consist of an arteriole, one or more venules, and capillaries (11).

—144—

PLATE 66

FIG. 1. SMALL INTESTINE: ILEUM WITH AGGREGATED NODULES (PEYER'S PATCH)
(TRANSVERSE SECTION)

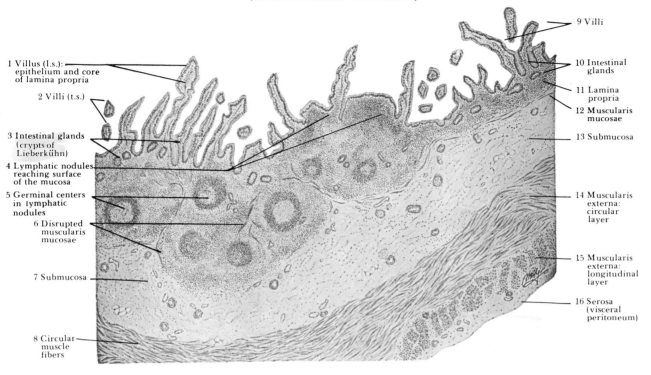

1 Villus (l.s.): epithelium and core of lamina propria

2 Villi (t.s.)

3 Intestinal glands (crypts of Lieberkühn)

4 Lymphatic nodules reaching surface of the mucosa

5 Germinal centers in lymphatic nodules

6 Disrupted muscularis mucosae

7 Submucosa

8 Circular muscle fibers

9 Villi

10 Intestinal glands

11 Lamina propria

12 Muscularis mucosae

13 Submucosa

14 Muscularis externa: circular layer

15 Muscularis externa: longitudinal layer

16 Serosa (visceral peritoneum)

Stain: hematoxylin-eosin. 25×.

FIG. 2. SMALL INTESTINE: VILLI

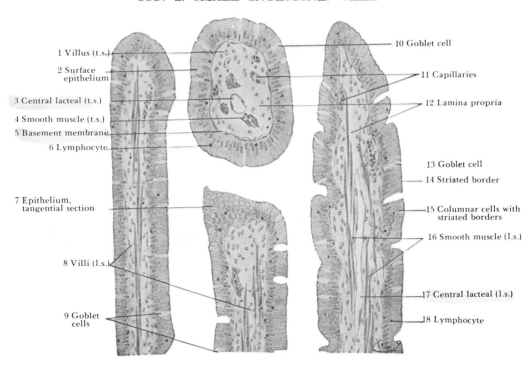

1 Villus (t.s.)

2 Surface epithelium

3 Central lacteal (t.s.)

4 Smooth muscle (t.s.)

5 Basement membrane

6 Lymphocyte

7 Epithelium, tangential section

8 Villi (l.s.)

9 Goblet cells

10 Goblet cell

11 Capillaries

12 Lamina propria

13 Goblet cell

14 Striated border

15 Columnar cells with striated borders

16 Smooth muscle (l.s.)

17 Central lacteal (l.s.)

18 Lymphocyte

Stain: hematoxylin-eosin. 200×.

PLATE 67

LARGE INTESTINE: COLON (WALL, TRANSVERSE SECTION)

Like the small intestine, the large intestine has a mucosa (27), submucosa (26), muscularis externa (25) and serosa (24), all of which are continuous with those of the small intestine.

Villi are absent in the large intestine. The free surface appears smooth, and is indented at close intervals by long tubular intestinal glands (crypts of Lieberkühn) (20) which extend to the muscularis mucosae.

In the colon, the surface epithelium is principally columnar cells with thin striated borders (14) and some goblet cells. This continues into the glands (15, 20) but goblet cells now become the principal cells. Parts of glands may be seen sectioned longitudinally (20), transversally (21), or tangentially (16).

The lamina propria (19), as in the small intestine, contains abundant diffuse lymphatic tissue. Lymphatic nodules (17, 23) occur in the deep lamina propria. They may extend through the muscularis mucosae into the submucosa.

Structure of the muscularis mucosae (10), submucosa (9), muscularis externa (5, 6) and serosa (1) is typical. However, the external longitudinal muscle layer is modified so that the muscle is arranged in three, thick flat bands, the taeniae coli, with little or no muscle between them (best illustrated in transverse sections).

Serosa (1) covers the entire transverse colon, but parts of the ascending and descending colon have adventitia.

PLATE 67

LARGE INTESTINE: COLON (WALL, TRANSVERSE SECTION)

24 Serosa · 25 Muscularis externa 26 Submucosa : 27 Mucosa

m.m. Lamina propria Epithelium

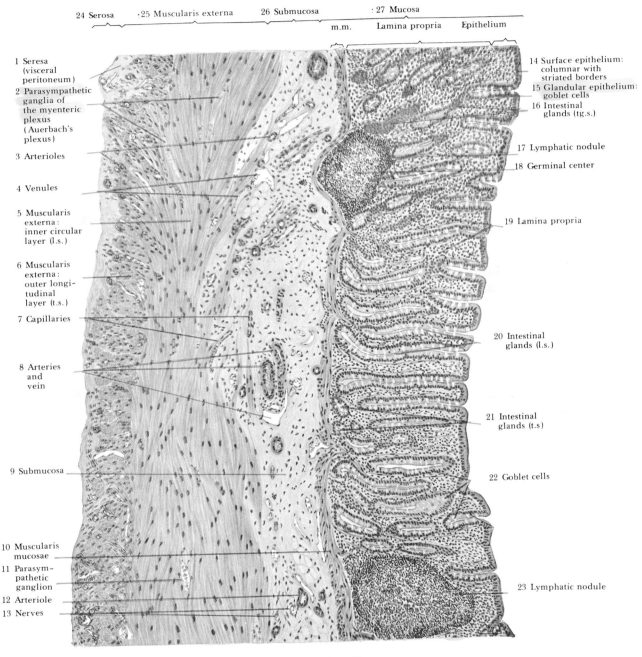

1 Seresa (visceral peritoneum)

2 Parasympathetic ganglia of the myenteric plexus (Auerbach's plexus)

3 Arterioles

4 Venules

5 Muscularis externa: inner circular layer (l.s.)

6 Muscularis externa: outer longitudinal layer (t.s.)

7 Capillaries

8 Arteries and vein

9 Submucosa

10 Muscularis mucosae

11 Parasympathetic ganglion

12 Arteriole

13 Nerves

14 Surface epithelium: columnar with striated borders

15 Glandular epithelium: goblet cells

16 Intestinal glands (tg.s.)

17 Lymphatic nodule

18 Germinal center

19 Lamina propria

20 Intestinal glands (l.s.)

21 Intestinal glands (t.s)

22 Goblet cells

23 Lymphatic nodule

Stain: hematoxylin-eosin. 53×.

Plate 68

APPENDIX (PANORAMIC VIEW, TRANSVERSE SECTION)

The illustration presents a panoramic view of a cross section of the cecal or vermiform appendix. Its structure is basically that of the colon, but several modifications are characteristic of the appendix.

Components of the mucosa are like those of the colon: a similar lining epithelium (9), lamina propria (5, 11) with intestinal glands (crypts of Lieberkühn) (6, 10), and a muscularis mucosae (12). The intestinal glands (6, 10) are less well developed, are shorter or irregular, and often farther apart than in the colon. Diffuse lymphatic tissue in the lamina propria is abundant, and often continues into the adjacent submucosa.

Lymphatic nodules (1, 7, 19) are numerous and often contain large germinal centers (7). As always, the lymphatic nodules originate in the lamina propria (19) where they may become large enough to reach the surface epithelium (19, lower leader). Characteristically, they extend into the submucosa, disrupting the muscularis mucosae (16), where they expand to increase greatly in size.

The submucosa is very vascular (8). The muscularis externa (14) has the usual inner circular and outer longitudinal layers (17, 18) but they may vary in thickness. Serosa (15) covers the muscle layers.

PLATE 68

APPENDIX (PANORAMIC VIEW, TRANSVERSE SECTION)

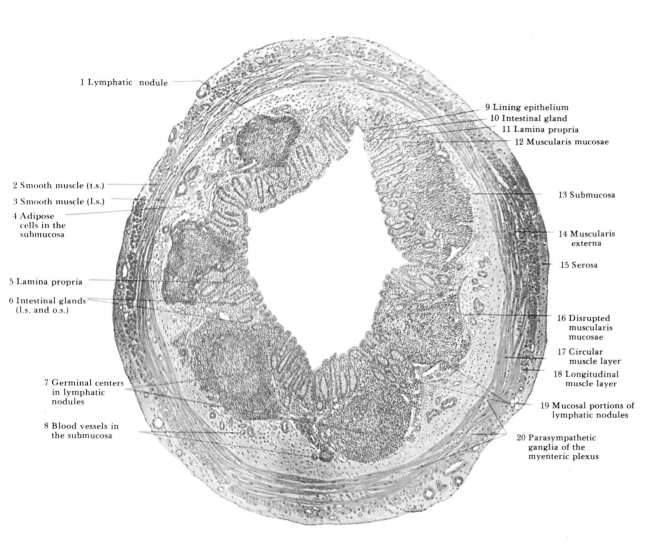

1 Lymphatic nodule

9 Lining epithelium
10 Intestinal gland
11 Lamina propria
12 Muscularis mucosae

2 Smooth muscle (t.s.)

3 Smooth muscle (l.s.)

4 Adipose cells in the submucosa

13 Submucosa

14 Muscularis externa

15 Serosa

5 Lamina propria

6 Intestinal glands (l.s. and o.s.)

16 Disrupted muscularis mucosae

17 Circular muscle layer

18 Longitudinal muscle layer

7 Germinal centers in lymphatic nodules

8 Blood vessels in the submucosa

19 Mucosal portions of lymphatic nodules

20 Parasympathetic ganglia of the myenteric plexus

Stain: hematoxylin-eosin. 25×.

PLATE 69

LARGE INTESTINE: RECTUM
(PANORAMIC VIEW, TRANSVERSE SECTION)

This figure represents a transverse section through the upper rectum or rectum proper, whose histological structure is generally similar to that of the colon, having the same layers in its wall (3, 8–15) and the same components in each layer. Except for a difference in the longitudinal muscle layer, this figure could be that of colon.

Surface epithelium (8) continues to have columnar cells with striated borders and goblet cells. Intestinal glands (10, 11) in the wide lamina propria are like those in the colon but are longer, closer together, and have more goblet cells; virtually all cells in the gland are goblet cells.

Temporary longitudinal folds (4) may be present in the upper rectum and also in the colon. These have a core of submucosa and are covered by mucosa (4). Permanent transverse folds of the rectum (plicae transversalis), if present in a section, would also contain smooth muscle fibers from the circular layer of the muscularis externa.

Permanent longitudinal folds (rectal columns) appear in the lowermost rectum, in the anal canal. At this level, the circular muscle layer will be greatly thickened, and the longitudinal layer will be thinned (see Plate 70).

Taeniae coli of the colon are not continued into the rectum, therefore the muscularis externa (13, 14) again has the typical inner circular and outer longitudinal layers.

Adventitia (15) covers part of the rectum, serosa the remainder.

PLATE 69

RECTUM (PANORAMIC VIEW, TRANSVERSE SECTION)

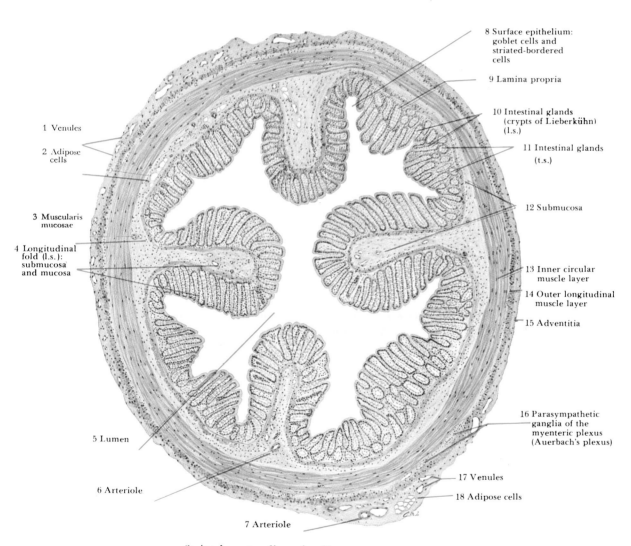

1 Venules

2 Adipose cells

3 Muscularis mucosae

4 Longitudinal fold (l.s.): submucosa and mucosa

5 Lumen

6 Arteriole

7 Arteriole

8 Surface epithelium: goblet cells and striated-bordered cells

9 Lamina propria

10 Intestinal glands (crypts of Lieberkühn) (l.s.)

11 Intestinal glands (t.s.)

12 Submucosa

13 Inner circular muscle layer

14 Outer longitudinal muscle layer

15 Adventitia

16 Parasympathetic ganglia of the myenteric plexus (Auerbach's plexus)

17 Venules

18 Adipose cells

Stain: hematoxylin-eosin. 40×.

PLATE 70

ANAL CANAL (LONGITUDINAL SECTION)

The upper part of the anal canal (A), above the anal valves (11), is the lowermost part of the rectum. The lower part of the anal canal (B), below the anal valves (11), is the transition area to skin. The change from rectal mucosa to anal mucosa takes place at the apex of the anal valves (10), and is called the anorectal line.

Rectal mucosa (4–8) is typical in structure but intestinal glands (7) become shorter and are farther apart, thus there is more lamina propria (8) between glands, diffuse lymphatic tissue is more abundant, and solitary lymphatic nodules (6) are numerous. The muscularis mucosae (5) terminates at the anal valve (12).

At the apex of the anal valve, the columnar epithelium of the rectum is replaced abruptly by non-cornified stratified squamous epithelium (10) of the anal canal. Intestinal glands terminate at this point. The lamina propria of the rectum is replaced by the dense irregular connective tissue of the lamina propria of the anal canal (13, lower leader). The submucosa of the rectum (9) merges with the lamina propria of the anal canal.

Both submucosa and lamina propria are very vascular in this region. The internal hemorrhoidal plexus of veins (15) lies in the mucosa of the anal canal and vessels extend from this into the submucosa of the rectum. Internal hemorrhoids result from pathological dilation of these vessels. External hemorrhoids develop from vessels of the external venous plexus (not illustrated) at the lip of the anus.

The circular muscle layer of the muscularis externa (1) increases greatly in thickness and forms the internal anal sphincter (1, 14). Lower, this is replaced by skeletal muscle fibers forming the external anal sphincter (16). Above and external to this sphincter is the levator ani muscle (skeletal), a small part of which is seen at (3). The longitudinal muscle layer of the muscularis externa (2) is thin laterally; it fades out in the connective tissue around the external anal sphincter.

Plate 70

ANAL CANAL (LONGITUDINAL SECTION)

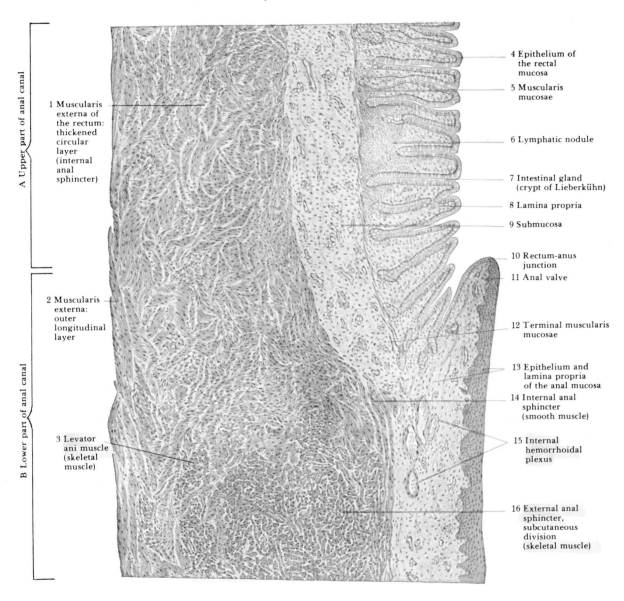

A Upper part of anal canal

B Lower part of anal canal

1 Muscularis externa of the rectum: thickened circular layer (internal anal sphincter)

2 Muscularis externa: outer longitudinal layer

3 Levator ani muscle (skeletal muscle)

4 Epithelium of the rectal mucosa

5 Muscularis mucosae

6 Lymphatic nodule

7 Intestinal gland (crypt of Lieberkühn)

8 Lamina propria

9 Submucosa

10 Rectum-anus junction

11 Anal valve

12 Terminal muscularis mucosae

13 Epithelium and lamina propria of the anal mucosa

14 Internal anal sphincter (smooth muscle)

15 Internal hemorrhoidal plexus

16 External anal sphincter, subcutaneous division (skeletal muscle)

Stain: hematoxylin-eosin. 25×.

PLATE 71

LIVER LOBULE (PANORAMIC VIEW, TRANSVERSE SECTION)

From the hilus of the liver, connective tissue passes between lobes and is distributed throughout the liver as interlobular septa (2). These partially outline the small hepatic lobules. In the interlobular septa course the interlobular branches of the portal vein, hepatic artery and bile ducts (hepatic triads), also small lymphatics and nerves.

In this figure are seen one complete hepatic lobule in the center and parts of several adjacent lobules (1, and others) all in transverse section. The boundaries between lobules are conspicuous only where three lobules come together at an interlobular septum (portal areas). In transverse sections, the septum at these corners appears somewhat triangular in shape (7, 18). Here are seen the hepatic triads: the interlobular branches of the portal vein, hepatic artery and bile duct (4, 5, 6; 16, 17, 19; and others). No well defined separation between lobules occurs elsewhere, the liver tissue and sinusoids being continuous from one lobule to the adjacent one (10).

In the center of each hepatic lobule is a central or intralobular vein (9, 13). Around the periphery of each lobule are several hepatic triads and their interlobular connective tissue (portal areas). For the lobule in the center of the figure, hepatic triads and connective tissue are seen at 4–7, 11–12, 16–19, forming a partial boundary. Any one portal area forms a partial boundary for more than one lobule.

Within the lobule, laminae or plates of hepatic cells (14, 20) radiate from the central vein toward the periphery. Between the laminae are hepatic sinusoids (15, 21). These are formed from small distributing branches of the interlobular vein. Bile formed in the liver cells drains through bile canaliculi into interlobular bile ducts (Plate 72, Fig. 3).

Interlobular vessels and bile ducts continually give off smaller branches during their course. Thus, in a section of liver, it is possible to see more than one section of each of these within a hepatic triad, as in the triad and connective tissue (4–7), where there are five sections of bile ducts, three portal vein branches, and one artery. Conversely, all three structures may not be seen in any one triad, as in (11–12), where no artery is present because of the plane of the section. Lymphatics and nerves are small and inconspicuous and are seen only occasionally.

PLATE 71

LIVER LOBULE (PANORAMIC VIEW, TRANSVERSE SECTION)

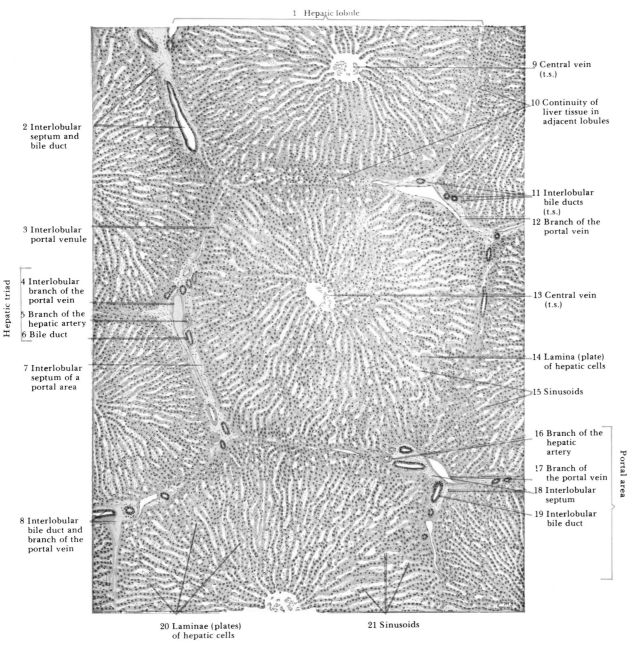

1 Hepatic lobule

9 Central vein (t.s.)

10 Continuity of liver tissue in adjacent lobules

2 Interlobular septum and bile duct

11 Interlobular bile ducts (t.s.)

12 Branch of the portal vein

3 Interlobular portal venule

Hepatic triad

4 Interlobular branch of the portal vein

5 Branch of the hepatic artery

6 Bile duct

13 Central vein (t.s.)

14 Lamina (plate) of hepatic cells

7 Interlobular septum of a portal area

15 Sinusoids

16 Branch of the hepatic artery

17 Branch of the portal vein

18 Interlobular septum

19 Interlobular bile duct

Portal area

8 Interlobular bile duct and branch of the portal vein

20 Laminae (plates) of hepatic cells

21 Sinusoids

Stain: hematoxylin-eosin. 45×.

PLATE 72 (Fig. 1)

LIVER LOBULE (SECTIONAL VIEW, TRANSVERSE SECTION)

Part of a hepatic lobule between the central vein (1) and the peripheral interlobular septum (8) is shown. The section shows in more detail structures already seen on Plate 71.

The central vein (1), a venule, is lined with endothelium. At the periphery of the lobule is seen an interlobular septum (8) with its hepatic triad, showing a branch of the portal vein (7), two hepatic artery branches (5, 11), four sections of bile duct (6, 13 and two others) and a lymphatic vessel (12).

Within the lobule are seen the laminae or plates of hepatic cells (10). The laminae branch and anastomose, except at the periphery of the lobule, where they form a solid lamina of hepatic cells, the limiting lamina or plate (9) which separates the laminae and sinusoids from the interlobular connective tissue. Distributing venules and arterioles penetrate through this to give rise to sinusoids.

The hepatic cells are of polygonal shape. They vary in size, have a large round vesicular nucleus or are sometimes binucleated, and have a granular acidophilic cytoplasm which varies, however, with the functional states of the cells (see Fig. 2 also).

The sinusoids (2, 3, 4) are between the laminae, and follow their branchings and anastomoses. They are lined incompletely with reticuloendothelium which has fixed macrophages (the stellate cells of Kupffer) and smaller cells resembling endothelial cells which are inactive fixed macrophages. The sinusoids open into the central vein (1). Erythrocytes (3) and leukocytes may be seen in some of them.

PLATE 72 (Fig. 2)

LIVER: RETICULOENDOTHELIUM (INDIA INK PREPARATION)

To demonstrate the reticuloendothelial system, a rabbit was injected intravenously with India ink. A section of the rabbit's liver is illustrated. Hepatic laminae (3) and sinusoids (2) are shown.

The reticuloendothelial stellate cells (Kupffer cells) (1, 4) which line the sinusoids incompletely are prominent because of the engorged carbon particles. They are seen as large cells with several processes, giving them an irregular or stellate outline. The nucleus is obscured by the carbon particles. Most of the otherwise inactive lining cells have become stellate cells.

PLATE 72 (Fig. 3)

LIVER: BILE CANALICULI (OSMIC ACID PREPARATION)

A small block of liver tissue was fixed with osmic acid, sections were prepared and stained with hematoxylin-eosin. Penetration of osmic acid into the liver tissue reveals the presence of bile canaliculi (2, 7, 8) which exist as minute channels between cells of the hepatic laminae (1, 6). The canaliculi are seen following the irregular course of the rows of hepatic cells within the laminae, and branching laterally between cells. Some canaliculi are seen in transverse section (8).

In the sinusoids (4, 5) are seen the small nuclei of inactive reticuloendothelial cells and an occasional stellate cell (lower center).

PLATE 72

LIVER

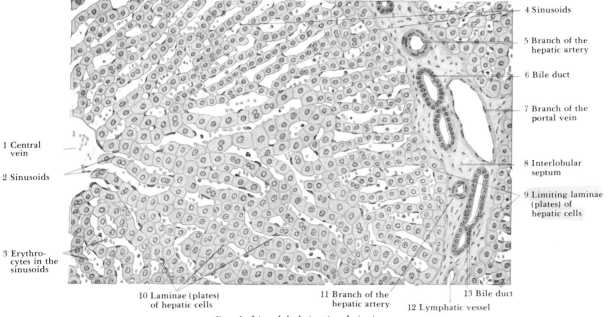

1 Central vein

2 Sinusoids

3 Erythro-cytes in the sinusoids

4 Sinusoids

5 Branch of the hepatic artery

6 Bile duct

7 Branch of the portal vein

8 Interlobular septum

9 Limiting laminae (plates) of hepatic cells

10 Laminae (plates) of hepatic cells

11 Branch of the hepatic artery

12 Lymphatic vessel

13 Bile duct

FIG. 1. *Liver lobule (sectional view)*
Stain: hematoxylin-eosin. 285×.

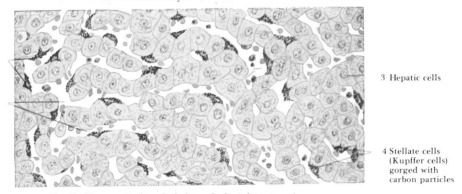

1 Stellate cells (Kupffer cells) gorged with carbon particles

2 Sinusoids

3 Hepatic cells

4 Stellate cells (Kupffer cells) gorged with carbon particles

FIG. 2. *Liver: reticuloendothelium. India ink preparation.*
Stain: hematoxylin-eosin. 350×.

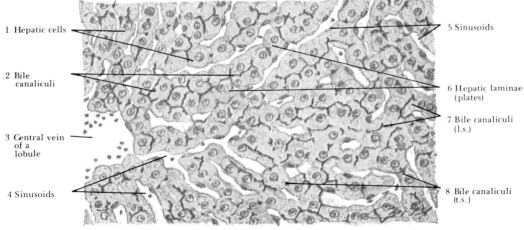

1 Hepatic cells

2 Bile canaliculi

3 Central vein of a lobule

4 Sinusoids

5 Sinusoids

6 Hepatic laminae (plates)

7 Bile canaliculi (l.s.)

8 Bile canaliculi (t.s.)

FIG 3. *Liver: bile canaliculi (osmic acid preparation).*
Stain: hematoxylin-eosin. 300×.

PLATE 73 (Fig. 1)

MITOCHONDRIA AND FAT DROPLETS IN LIVER CELLS (ALTMANN'S STAIN)

The specimen has been fixed in potassium bichromate and osmic acid, stained with acid fuchsin and differentiated with picric acid. The mitochondria stain red. The fat droplets usually stain black by the reduction of osmic acid by fat, but in this specimen they are blue.

PLATE 73 (Fig. 2)

GLYCOGEN IN LIVER CELLS (BEST'S CARMINE STAIN)

In sections stained with an alcohol and ammonia solution of carmine, glycogen is demonstrated in the form of red granules irregularly distributed in the cytoplasm. If the sections are stained previously with Meyer's hemalum, the nuclei take on a violet color.

PLATE 73 (Fig. 3)

RETICULAR FIBERS IN A HEPATIC LOBULE (DEL RIO HORTEGA'S STAIN)

Del Rio Hortega uses a modification of his ammonium silver carbonate method for silver impregnation to demonstrate the finest fibrillar structure of the stroma of tissues. Reticular fibers are stained black and the liver cells a pale violet.

Reticular fibers form most of the supporting connective tissue of the liver. They line the sinusoids in part (1), where they are between the liver cells and the incomplete lining of reticuloendothelial cells. They form a dense network around the central veins (3, 2).

The collagenous fibers in the dense irregular connective tissue of the interlobular septa stain a dark brown color (4). Reticular fibers merge with these.

—158—

PLATE 73

LIVER

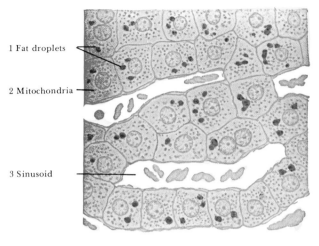

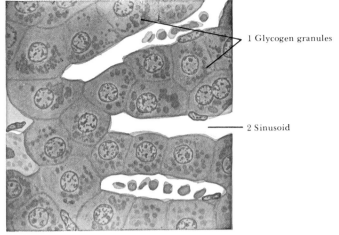

1 Fat droplets

2 Mitochondria

3 Sinusoid

1 Glycogen granules

2 Sinusoid

FIG. 1. *Altmann's stain: mitochondria (red) and fat droplets (blue) in liver cells.* Fixation in Champy's fluid. 800X.

FIG. 2. *Best's carmine stain: glycogen in liver cells.* 800X.

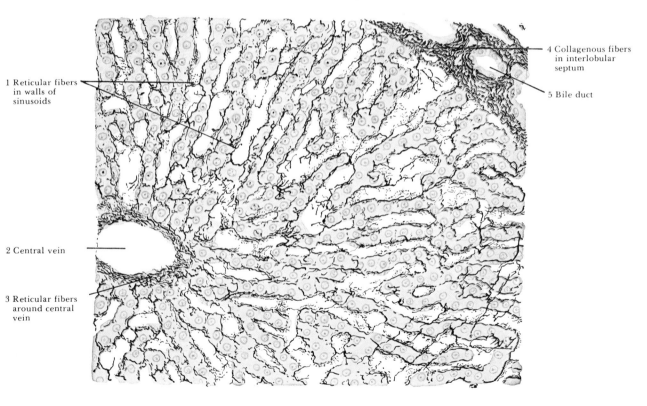

1 Reticular fibers in walls of sinusoids

2 Central vein

3 Reticular fibers around central vein

4 Collagenous fibers in interlobular septum

5 Bile duct

FIG. 3. *Reticular fibers in a hepatic lobule.* 300X.

PLATE 74

GALL BLADDER

The wall of the gall bladder consists of a mucosa (3, 4, 5), a fibromuscular layer (2), a perimuscular connective tissue layer (1, 10), and a serosa (6) on its free surface. Elsewhere, an adventitia attaches it to the liver.

The mucosa is thrown into temporary folds (15) which disappear when the gall bladder is distended. These folds may resemble villi somewhat but are actually different because of their varying sizes and shapes and irregular arrangement. The crypts or diverticula between the folds often form deep indentations (16). When seen in transverse sections in the lamina propria they resemble tubular glands (18) but no glands are present in the gall bladder proper (only in the neck).

The lining epithelium (5, 14, 20) is simple tall columnar whose cells have a lightly-stained cytoplasm and basally placed nuclei. The lamina propria (4, 17) of loose connective tissue has some diffuse lymphatic tissue.

In the fibromuscular layer (2), the smooth muscles (7) do not form a compact layer but are interspersed with layers of loose connective tissue which is rich in elastic fibers (8). In contrast to other organs where a serosa or adventitia covers the muscle layer, the gall bladder has a wide layer of perimuscular loose connective tissue (1, 10) in which are numerous blood vessels (11, 13), lymphatics, and nerves (12). Serosa (6) covers this.

PLATE 74

GALL BLADDER

1 Perimuscular connective tissue layer

2 Fibromuscular coat

3 Mucosa

4 Lamina propria 5 Epithelium

6 Serosa

7 Smooth muscle fibers

8 Elastic fibers in intermuscular connective tissue

9 Veins

10 Perimuscular connective tissue

11 Capillary (l.s.)

12 Nerves

13 Artery

14 Columnar epithelium

15 Fold in mucosa: epithelium and lamina propria

16 Diverticulum or crypt of mucosa (l.s.)

17 Lamina propria

18 Diverticula or crypts (t.s.)

19 Arterioles

20 Columnar epithelium

21 Lymphocyte migrating through the epithelium

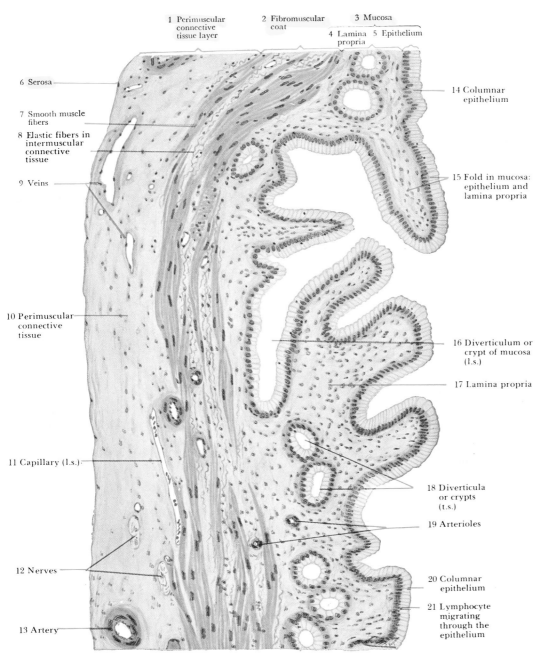

Stain: hematoxylin-eosin. 120X.

PLATE 75 (Fig. 1)

PANCREAS (SECTIONAL VIEW)

The pancreas is composed of masses of serous acini (2, 15) arranged into many small, indistinct lobules and lobule groups, intralobular and interlobular connective tissue and corresponding ducts (1, 5, 20; 10, 11), and the characteristic pancreatic islets (of Langerhans) (4, 8, 9).

A pancreatic acinus (2, 15, I) is composed of pyramidal secretory zymogenic cells (I, 21) and small centroacinar cells (22) along its lumen. Occasional basal or myoepithelial cells (basal cells, basket cells) (23) may be seen between the bases of the glandular cells and the basement membrane.

The acini are drained by long, narrow intercalated ducts (intralobular ducts) (1, 5, 20, II) which have a small lumen and are lined with low cuboidal cells (II). This epithelium narrows to extend into the acini as centroacinar cells (22).

Intercalated ducts drain into larger interlobular ducts (11, 19, III) lined with columnar epithelium. These ducts course in the connective tissue septa (10, 11).

The pancreatic islets (of Langerhans) (4, 8, 9) are rounded structures of varying sizes but always larger than acini. Under high magnification (IV), they are seen to be made up of anastomosing cell columns (24) between which are capillaries (25).

In the connective tissue septa are blood vessels (6, 7, 12, 13, 18), nerves (14, 17), occasional small ganglia and lamellar corpuscles (Pacinian corpuscles) (16).

PLATE 75 (Fig. 2)

PANCREATIC ACINI (SPECIAL PREPARATION)

A small field of pancreas is represented, showing cellular detail in acini after staining with Gomori's chrome hematoxylin-phloxine. Zymogen granules are stained red (1), and the basophilic substance (chromophilic substance, chromidial substance, etc.) is stained blue (2).

The upper triangle of the figure can be compared with Fig. 1 above (90×). In the lower triangle, at a higher magnification (450×), zymogen granules (1) are seen clearly, filling the apical portion of the cells (storage phase).

In the basal portion of the cells, concentration of basophilic substance and its striated appearance (2) are emphasized by the staining reaction. The nucleus lies within this zone.

PLATE 75 (Fig. 3)

PANCREATIC ISLETS (SPECIAL PREPARATION)

Here is illustrated a pancreatic islet (of Langerhans), its surrounding connective tissue (4) and a few adjacent pancreatic acini (5). Staining with Gomori's chrome hematoxylin-phloxine differentiates alpha and beta cells of the islets. Granules of A or alpha cells stain red (1), granules of B or beta cells are blue (2). Cell membranes are usually more distinguishable in alpha cells. Alpha cells tend to be situated more peripherally in the islet, beta cells, in general, lie deeper.

Capillaries (3) stand out clearly, demonstrating the rich blood supply to the islet.

—162—

PLATE 75

FIG. 1. PANCREAS (SECTIONAL VIEW)

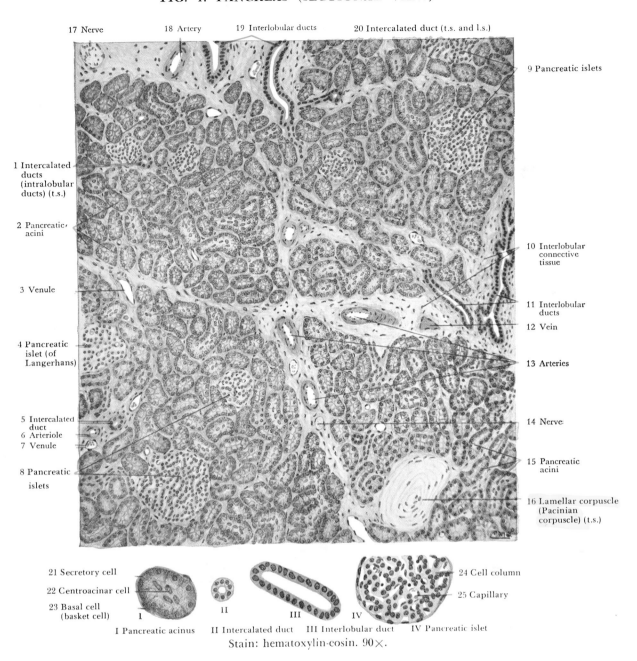

17 Nerve   18 Artery   19 Interlobular ducts   20 Intercalated duct (t.s. and l.s.)

9 Pancreatic islets

1 Intercalated ducts (intralobular ducts) (t.s.)

2 Pancreatic acini

3 Venule

4 Pancreatic islet (of Langerhans)

5 Intercalated duct
6 Arteriole
7 Venule

8 Pancreatic islets

10 Interlobular connective tissue

11 Interlobular ducts
12 Vein

13 Arteries

14 Nerve

15 Pancreatic acini

16 Lamellar corpuscle (Pacinian corpuscle) (t.s.)

21 Secretory cell
22 Centroacinar cell
23 Basal cell (basket cell)

24 Cell column
25 Capillary

I   II   III   IV

I Pancreatic acinus   II Intercalated duct   III Interlobular duct   IV Pancreatic islet

Stain: hematoxylin-eosin. 90×.

FIG. 2. PANCREATIC ACINI (SPECIAL PREPARATION)

FIG. 3. PANCREATIC ISLETS (SPECIAL PREPARATION)

1 Zymogen granules

2 Basophilic (chromophilic) substance

1 Alpha cells

2 Beta cell

3 Capillaries

4 Connective tissue

5 Pancreatic acinus

Stain: Gomori's chrome hematoxylin-phloxine.
90× and 450×   350×.

PLATE 76

LARYNX (FRONTAL SECTION)

The larynx has been sectioned vertically, showing its two prominent folds (13, 18–20), the supporting cartilages (8, 11) and muscles (10, 20).

The superior, or false vocal fold (13), is formed only by mucosa. It is continuous with the posterior surface of the epiglottis (12). The covering epithelium is pseudostratified ciliated columnar (14) with goblet cells. Mixed glands, predominantly mucous in character (15), lie in the lamina propria below the epithelium. Sections of excretory ducts (16) are seen among the alveoli; these ducts open onto the epithelial surface. Lymphatic nodules (7) occur in the lamina propria on the ventricular side of the fold.

The ventricle (17) is a deep indentation and recess separating the false vocal fold (13) from the true vocal fold (18–20). The mucosa of its lateral wall (3, 4, 5, 6) is similar in structure to that of the false vocal fold. Lymphatic nodules are more numerous, however, and are sometimes called the "laryngeal tonsils" (7). The lamina propria (3) blends with the perichondrium of the thyroid cartilage (8); there is no distinct submucosa. The lower wall of the ventricle makes a transition to the true vocal fold.

The mucosa of the true vocal fold consists of non-cornified stratified squamous epithelium (18) and a thin, dense lamina propria devoid of glands, lymphatic tissue and blood vessels. At the apex of the true vocal fold is the vocal ligament (19), a mass of dense elastic fibers. Its marginal fibers spread out into the adjacent lamina propria and into the vocalis muscle (20). The thyroarytenoid muscle (10) and the thyroid cartilage (8) comprise the remaining wall.

Passing into the lower larynx, the epithelium again becomes pseudostratified ciliated columnar (21). In the lamina propria are mixed glands (22). The cricoid cartilage (11) is the lowermost cartilage of the larynx.

PLATE 76

LARYNX (FRONTAL SECTION)

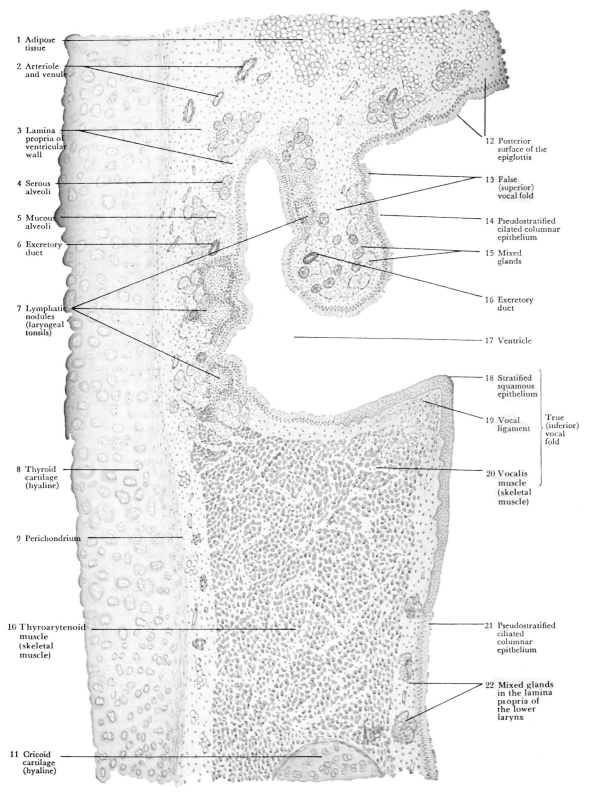

1 Adipose tissue

2 Arteriole and venule

3 Lamina propria of ventricular wall

4 Serous alveoli

5 Mucous alveoli

6 Excretory duct

7 Lymphatic nodules (laryngeal tonsils)

8 Thyroid cartilage (hyaline)

9 Perichondrium

10 Thyroarytenoid muscle (skeletal muscle)

11 Cricoid cartilage (hyaline)

12 Posterior surface of the epiglottis

13 False (superior) vocal fold

14 Pseudostratified ciliated columnar epithelium

15 Mixed glands

16 Excretory duct

17 Ventricle

18 Stratified squamous epithelium

19 Vocal ligament

20 Vocalis muscle (skeletal muscle)

True (inferior) vocal fold

21 Pseudostratified ciliated columnar epithelium

22 Mixed glands in the lamina propria of the lower larynx

Stain: hematoxylin-eosin. 35×.

PLATE 77 (Fig. 1)

TRACHEA (PANORAMIC VIEW, TRANSVERSE SECTION)

The wall of the trachea consists of a mucosa, submucosa, fibrocartilaginous layer, and adventitia. The cartilages are C-shaped. Between their ends lies the trachealis muscle (smooth).

Approximately half of a transverse section is illustrated. The mucosa consists of pseudostratified ciliated columnar epithelium with goblet cells (13), and a lamina propria (11, 14) of fine connective tissue with diffuse lymphatic tissue and occasional solitary nodules. In the deep part of the lamina propria, elastic fibers become concentrated to form a longitudinal elastic membrane (15). In the submucosa (16) of loose connective tissue are tubuloalveolar mixed glands (4, 5) whose ducts (10, 17) pass through the lamina propria to open into the lumen of the trachea.

The plate of hyaline cartilage (3) is surrounded by its perichondrium (2) of dense fibrous tissue, which merges internally with the submucosa and externally with the adventitia (1). Numerous blood vessels and nerves (6) course in the adventitia and supply smaller branches to the other layers.

The mucosa is folded (12) along the posterior wall of the trachea where cartilage is absent. The trachealis muscle (9) lies deep to the elastic membrane of the mucosa, embedded in the fibroelastic tissue that occupies the area between the ends of the cartilages. Most muscle fibers insert into the perichondrium of the cartilage (2, upper leader). Mixed glands continue to be present, sometimes intermingled with muscle fibers and extending into the adventitia (8).

PLATE 77 (Fig. 2)

TRACHEA (SECTIONAL VIEW)

A small section of trachea at a higher magnification shows detailed structure of the components making up the wall, as seen with hematoxylin-eosin. In the surface epithelium are seen ciliated cells (5) and goblet cells (10), the typical irregular arrangement of nuclei, and the characteristic thickened basement membrane (6). In the deep lamina propria, a longitudinal elastic membrane (7) is visible. A duct (8) and a group of mucous alveoli (9) represent tracheal glands. Adjacent is the perichondrium (1) of the cartilage. The usual relationship of cartilage to perichondrium is seen, with the larger lacunae and chondrocytes in the interior of the plate becoming progressively flattened (3) toward the perichondrium, and the matrix (2) gradually blending with the connective tissue.

PLATE 77 (Fig. 3)

TRACHEA (SECTIONAL VIEW): ELASTIC FIBER STAIN

The section is similar to Figure 2 but has been stained with Gallego's method for selectively demonstrating elastic fibers, which stain red with carbol-fuchsin. The elastic fibers making up the elastic membrane (8) are now seen prominently. Collagenous fibers stain blue with aniline blue, providing a striking contrast where they intermingle with the elastic fibers. Collagenous fibers are also demonstrated in the perichondrium (1, lower leader), submucosa (3) and in the superficial lamina propria (9).

PLATE 77

TRACHEA

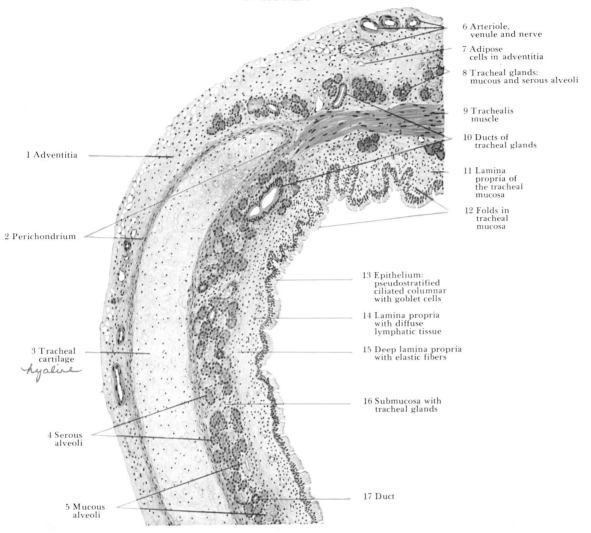

1 Adventitia

2 Perichondrium

3 Tracheal
cartilage
hyaline

4 Serous
alveoli

5 Mucous
alveoli

6 Arteriole,
venule and nerve

7 Adipose
cells in adventitia

8 Tracheal glands:
mucous and serous alveoli

9 Trachealis
muscle

10 Ducts of
tracheal glands

11 Lamina
propria of
the tracheal
mucosa

12 Folds in
tracheal
mucosa

13 Epithelium:
pseudostratified
ciliated columnar
with goblet cells

14 Lamina propria
with diffuse
lymphatic tissue

15 Deep lamina propria
with elastic fibers

16 Submucosa with
tracheal glands

17 Duct

Fig. 1. *Trachea (panoramic view, transverse section).*
Stain: hematoxylin-eosin. 50×.

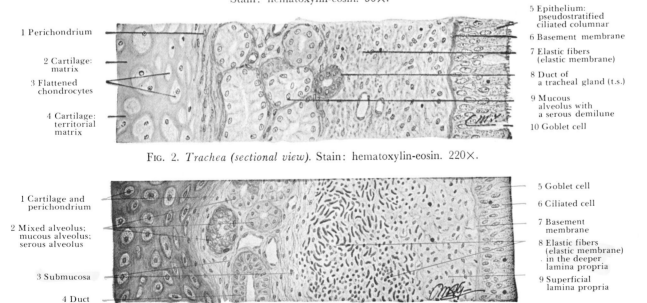

1 Perichondrium

2 Cartilage:
matrix

3 Flattened
chondrocytes

4 Cartilage:
territorial
matrix

5 Epithelium:
pseudostratified
ciliated columnar

6 Basement membrane

7 Elastic fibers
(elastic membrane)

8 Duct of
a tracheal gland (t.s.)

9 Mucous
alveolus with
a serous demilune

10 Goblet cell

Fig. 2. *Trachea (sectional view).* Stain: hematoxylin-eosin. 220×.

1 Cartilage and
perichondrium

2 Mixed alveolus;
mucous alveolus;
serous alveolus

3 Submucosa

4 Duct

5 Goblet cell

6 Ciliated cell

7 Basement
membrane

8 Elastic fibers
(elastic membrane)
in the deeper
lamina propria

9 Superficial
lamina propria

Fig. 3. *Trachea (sectional view).* Stain: Gallego's method for elastic fibers. 220×.

PLATE 78

LUNG (PANORAMIC VIEW)

Terminology has varied for the different divisions of the respiratory tract. The terminology employed here is that in current use, based on the concept of bronchopulmonary segments. From the exterior to the alveolus, the divisions are: primary bronchi, secondary or lobar bronchi, segmental (small or tertiary) bronchi, bronchioles, terminal bronchioles, respiratory bronchioles, alveolar ducts, alveolar sacs, alveoli. The histological characteristics of several of these divisions are shown on Plate 79. The distinguishing features are indicated on this panoramic view of lung tissue.

Structure of the primary bronchi is at first like that of the trachea. When they enter the lung, the C-shaped cartilage is replaced by separate plates of cartilage which encircle the bronchus, and the smooth muscle spreads out from the trachealis muscle to form an incomplete layer around the lumen.

A secondary or lobar bronchus is identified by the closeness of its several cartilage plates (33, and Plate 79, Fig. 1). The lining epithelium is pseudostratified columnar ciliated with goblet cells (32). Making up the wall, one sees, in succession, a thin lamina propria, a narrow layer of smooth muscle (31), a submucosa in which are scattered bronchial glands, hyaline cartilage plates (30), and the adventitia.

Segmental bronchi retain a similar structure, but the epithelium becomes lower, and each of the other elements decreases in amount.

In bronchioles (16), the epithelium is low pseudostratified columnar ciliated with occasional goblet cells. The mucosa is typically folded, producing a stellate lumen in cross section. The band of smooth muscle is prominent. Adventitia surrounds this, since glands and cartilage are no longer present.

Each terminal bronchiole (6, 12) has a spacious, irregular lumen, with a wavy epithelial lining when seen in cross-section. The epithelium is ciliated columnar; goblet cells are lacking. Still present are a thin lamina propria, the layer of smooth muscle, and an adventitia.

The respiratory bronchioles (5, 8, 17, 23, 26, 27) are the tubules in direct connection with alveolar ducts and alveoli. The epithelium is low columnar or cuboidal (5, 8); it may be ciliated in the proximal portion. Minimal connective tissue supports the band of intermingled smooth muscle and elastic fibers of the lamina propria and the accompanying blood vessels. Alveoli appear in the wall, on the side opposite the pulmonary artery (5; 26, left side). These increase in number going distally (5; 26, 23); here epithelium and muscle of the distal respiratory bronchiole are seen as small, intermittent areas between the openings of the numerous alveoli (5, upper leader; 17; 23, 24, 25).

Each distal respiratory bronchiole opens into two or more alveolar ducts, although in sections only one such alveolar duct may be seen (5 and 2, lower leader; 23, upper leader and 22, middle leader). Walls of alveolar ducts are formed by a series of alveoli lying adjacent to each other (2, 15, 22). A group or cluster of alveoli opening into an alveolar duct is an alveolar sac (14, 20).

The alveoli (4, 21, 25) form the mass of the parenchyma of the lung, giving the appearance of fine lace. (See Fig. 4, Plate 79, for details.)

A fortuitous plane of section shows a continuous passageway from terminal bronchiole into alveolar ducts (6, 5, lowest leader of 2; 26, 23, middle leader of 22).

The pulmonary artery (an elastic artery) branches repeatedly to accompany the divisions of the bronchial tree (7, 10, 28). Larger pulmonary vein branches accompany the bronchi and bronchioles; numerous small branches are seen in the trabeculae of the lung (3).

Very small bronchial arteries supply the walls of the various bronchi and bronchioles and included structures (and other areas). Small bronchial veins (29) may be seen in the larger bronchi.

The visceral pleura (1) is composed of a thin layer of connective tissue (19) and a layer of mesothelium (18).

PLATE 78

LUNG (PANORAMIC VIEW)

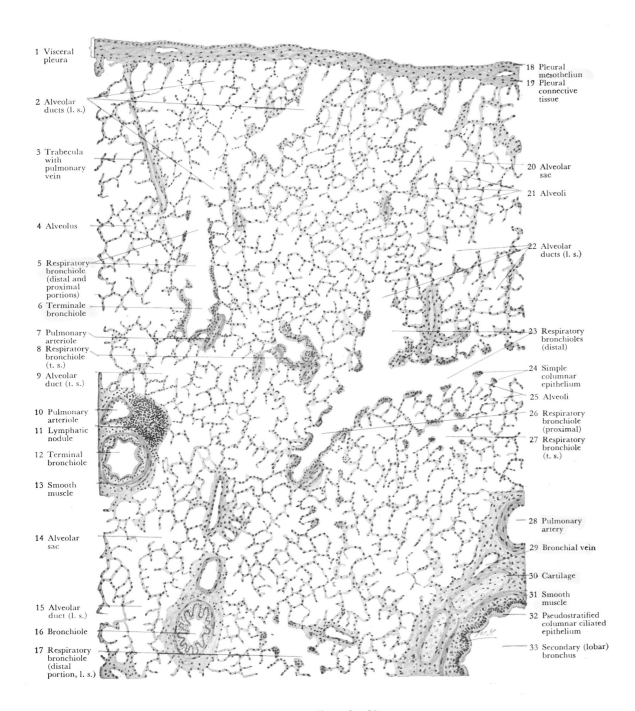

1 Visceral
   pleura

2 Alveolar
   ducts (l. s.)

3 Trabecula
   with
   pulmonary
   vein

4 Alveolus

5 Respiratory
   bronchiole
   (distal and
   proximal
   portions)

6 Terminale
   bronchiole

7 Pulmonary
   arteriole

8 Respiratory
   bronchiole
   (t. s.)

9 Alveolar
   duct (t. s.)

10 Pulmonary
   arteriole

11 Lymphatic
   nodule

12 Terminal
   bronchiole

13 Smooth
   muscle

14 Alveolar
   sac

15 Alveolar
   duct (l. s.)

16 Bronchiole

17 Respiratory
   bronchiole
   (distal
   portion, l. s.)

18 Pleural
   mesotheliun

19 Pleural
   connective
   tissue

20 Alveolar
   sac

21 Alveoli

22 Alveolar
   ducts (l. s.)

23 Respiratory
   bronchioles
   (distal)

24 Simple
   columnar
   epithelium

25 Alveoli

26 Respiratory
   bronchiole
   (proximal)

27 Respiratory
   bronchiole
   (t. s.)

28 Pulmonary
   artery

29 Bronchial vein

30 Cartilage

31 Smooth
   muscle

32 Pseudostratified
   columnar ciliated
   epithelium

33 Secondary (lobar)
   bronchus

Stain: hematoxylin-eosin. 30×.

Plate 79 (Fig. 1)

SECONDARY (LOBAR) BRONCHUS

The secondary (lobar) bronchus is lined with pseudostratified columnar ciliated epithelium (12). This is surrounded by a thin lamina propria (13) of fine fibered connective tissue with many elastic fibers (not illustrated) and scanty lymphocytes. Ducts (2) of submucosal glands pass through it to open into the lumen. A thin layer of smooth muscle (6) surrounds the lamina propria.

In the submucosa are glands, which may consist of groups of serous alveoli only (5, 8), or groups of serous and mucous alveoli intermingled (10); demilunes may be present.

The several cartilage plates (4) are close together. They will become smaller and farther apart as division of bronchi continues. Between them, connective tissue of the submucosa blends with that of the adventitia (3), which is a well developed layer.

The accompanying branch of the pulmonary artery (15) may be seen in the outer adventitia or adjacent to it. A small branch of the pulmonary artery (7) probably accompanies a small bronchus or bronchiole which is in another plane of section.

Bronchial vessels are seen in the connective tissue of the bronchus: an arteriole (16), a venule (11), and capillaries (9).

Plate 79 (Fig. 2)

BRONCHIOLE

A bronchiole is of small diameter, about 1 mm. Mucosal folds are prominent (4). The epithelium is low pseudostratified columnar ciliated, with fewer goblet cells. It becomes columnar ciliated in terminal bronchioles; usually goblet cells are absent. A well developed smooth muscle layer (3) surrounds a thin lamina propria, and is in turn surrounded by the adventitia (2). Cartilage and glands are lacking.

Adjacent to the bronchiole is a branch of the pulmonary artery (6). The bronchiole is surrounded by parenchyma (alveoli) of the lung (1).

Plate 79 (Fig. 3)

RESPIRATORY BRONCHIOLE

A respiratory bronchiole and associated structures are illustrated. The wall of the bronchiole is lined with cuboidal epithelium (4); cilia and goblet cells are lacking. Smooth muscle forms a layer close to the epithelium (3). A branch of the pulmonary artery (5) accompanies the respiratory bronchiole.

Also seen is an alveolar duct (2), arising from this respiratory bronchiole, and pulmonary alveoli (1) which open into it.

Plate 79 (Fig. 4)

ALVEOLAR WALLS (INTERALVEOLAR SEPTA)

The rounded or oval alveoli (5) are lined with squamous epithelium, not distinctly discernible at this magnification. Adjacent alveoli have a common wall (interalveolar septum) (4). Within this thin wall are capillary plexuses (1, 3) supported by a minimal amount of fine connective tissue in which are fibroblasts and a few other cells. The capillaries, therefore, are close to the squamous lining cells of adjacent alveoli, separated from the epithelium only by the sparse connective tissue. In a routine section of lung tissue, it is difficult to distinguish between nuclei of squamous cells, endothelial cells and fibroblasts (6).

At the free ends of the interalveolar septa, around the open ends of the alveoli, is a narrow band of smooth muscle (2), continued down from the muscle layer of the respiratory bronchiole.

PLATE 79

LUNG

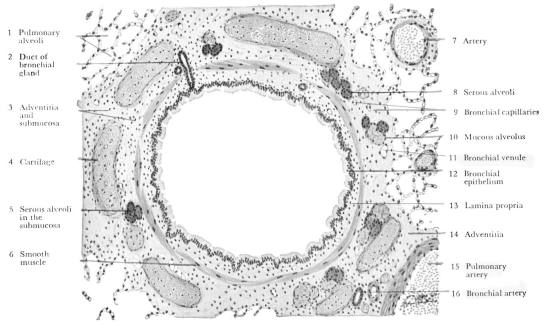

1 Pulmonary alveoli

2 Duct of bronchial gland

3 Adventitia and submucosa

4 Cartilage

5 Serous alveoli in the submucosa

6 Smooth muscle

7 Artery

8 Serous alveoli

9 Bronchial capillaries

10 Mucous alveolus

11 Bronchial venule

12 Bronchial epithelium

13 Lamina propria

14 Adventitia

15 Pulmonary artery

16 Bronchial artery

FIG. 1. *Secondary (lobar) bronchus.* 50×.

intrapulmonary bronchus

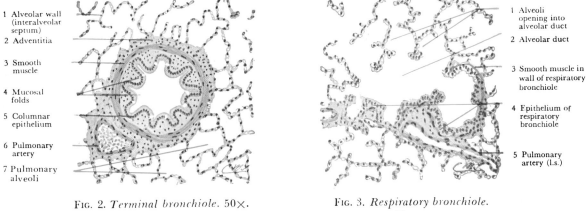

1 Alveolar wall (interalveolar septum)

2 Adventitia

3 Smooth muscle

4 Mucosal folds

5 Columnar epithelium

6 Pulmonary artery

7 Pulmonary alveoli

1 Alveoli opening into alveolar duct

2 Alveolar duct

3 Smooth muscle in wall of respiratory bronchiole

4 Epithelium of respiratory bronchiole

5 Pulmonary artery (l.s.)

FIG. 2. *Terminal bronchiole.* 50×.

FIG. 3. *Respiratory bronchiole.* 80×.

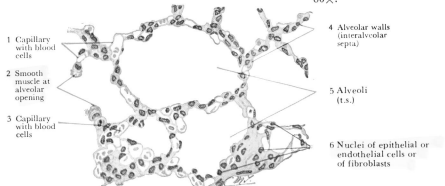

1 Capillary with blood cells

2 Smooth muscle at alveolar opening

3 Capillary with blood cells

4 Alveolar walls (interalveolar septa)

5 Alveoli (t.s.)

6 Nuclei of epithelial or endothelial cells or of fibroblasts

FIG. 4. *Alveolar walls (interalveolar septa).* 700X. Stain: hematoxylin-eosin.

PLATE 80

KIDNEY: CORTEX AND ONE PYRAMID
(PANORAMIC VIEW)

The substance of the kidney is divided into cortex (20) and medulla (21). The cortex is covered by a capsule (19) and perirenal connective and adipose tissues (18).

In the cortex are seen alternating areas of convoluted tubules (3) and glomeruli (2, 8), and areas of straight tubules (4); the regions are called pars convoluta or cortical labyrinths and medullary rays (5) respectively. The pars convoluta is made up of renal corpuscles (glomerular capsules and glomeruli) and adjacent proximal and distal convolutions (3) of nephrons, together with interlobular arteries and veins (6, 7) which course through this area. The medullary rays (5) contain straight portions of nephrons and collecting tubules. Medullary rays do not reach the capsule of the kidney; a narrow zone of convoluted tubules separates them (1).

The medulla is composed of a number of renal pyramids. Each pyramid lies with its base adjacent to cortex (11) and its apex directed inward. The apices of two or three renal pyramids coalesce to form a papilla (16) which projects into a minor calyx (14).

The medulla contains loops of the nephrons, the medullary loops of Henle (descending straight proximal tubules, thin segments, and ascending straight segments), and collecting tubules. Collecting tubules coalesce as they pass through the medulla to form large papillary ducts (Plate 82).

The papilla is usually covered with simple columnar epithelium (12) which also forms the lining of the inner wall of the calyx. As this epithelium reflects to the outer wall of the calyx, it becomes transitional epithelium (13). A thin layer of connective tissue and smooth muscle (not indicated) underlies the epithelium (14). This merges with the connective tissue of the renal sinus (17).

In the renal sinus are branches of the renal artery and vein (15). Branches of these penetrate into the parenchyma of the kidney as interlobar vessels, which then arch over the base of the pyramid as arcuate vessels (9). From arcuate vessels arise small interlobular arteries and veins (6, 7, 10) which pass into the pars convoluta areas of the cortex, giving off afferent glomerular arteries along their course.

PLATE 80

KIDNEY: CORTEX AND ONE PYRAMID (PANORAMIC VIEW)

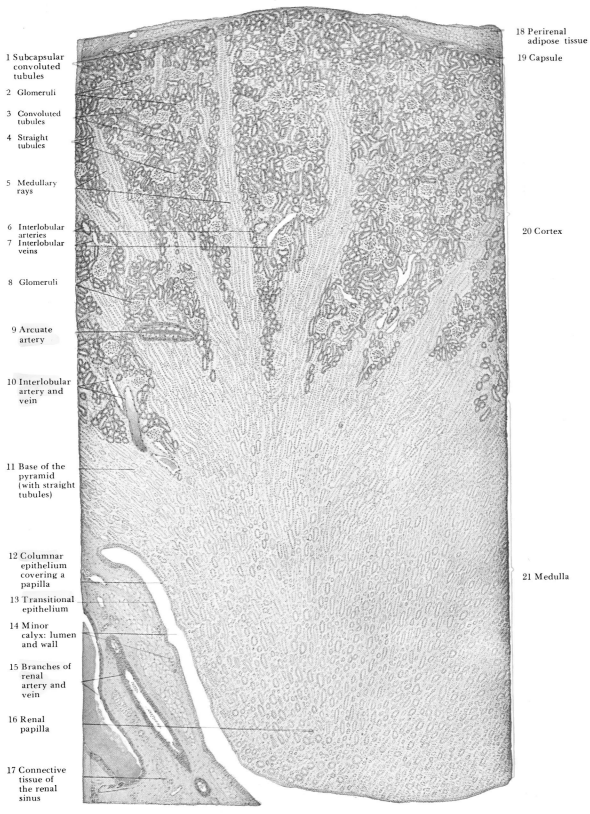

1 Subcapsular convoluted tubules

2 Glomeruli

3 Convoluted tubules

4 Straight tubules

5 Medullary rays

6 Interlobular arteries
7 Interlobular veins

8 Glomeruli

9 Arcuate artery

10 Interlobular artery and vein

11 Base of the pyramid (with straight tubules)

12 Columnar epithelium covering a papilla

13 Transitional epithelium

14 Minor calyx: lumen and wall

15 Branches of renal artery and vein

16 Renal papilla

17 Connective tissue of the renal sinus

18 Perirenal adipose tissue

19 Capsule

20 Cortex

21 Medulla

Stain: hematoxylin-eosin. 25×.

PLATE 81 (Fig. 1)

KIDNEY: DEEP CORTICAL AREA AND OUTER MEDULLA

At a higher magnification, renal corpuscles are more distinguishable, each corpuscle consisting of a glomerulus (3) and a glomerular capsule (Bowman's capsule) (2, 17). The glomerulus (3) is a mass of branching capillaries, supported by scant connective tissue, formed by the division of the afferent glomerular arteriole.

The visceral layer of the glomerular capsule (Bowman's capsule) is a layer of squamous cells, the glomerular epithelium (17), which follows closely the contours of the glomerulus. It then reflects at the vascular pole to become the parietal layer or capsular epithelium (17), leaving the capsular space (Bowman's space) between them. The capsular space opens into the neck of the proximal convoluted tubule; the squamous epithelium of the parietal layer changes quickly to the cuboidal cells of the neck of the proximal tubule (9).

Numerous tubules, sectioned in various planes, lie adjacent to the renal corpuscles. These are of two types, proximal convoluted (4, 10, 15, 21) and distal convoluted (1, 14, 21) which are actually the initial and terminal segments, respectively, of the nephron. The proximal convoluted tubules are numerous, have a relatively small, often uneven, lumen and are composed of large broad cuboidal cells whose granular cytoplasm stains deeply with eosin. Brush borders (15) are present but are not always well preserved in sections.

Distal convoluted tubules (14) are fewer in number, have a larger regular lumen, the cells are smaller and more distinctly cuboidal, their cytoplasm stains less deeply, and brush borders are not present (14, compare with 15).

Renal corpuscles and their associated tubules constitute the cortical labyrinths (pars convoluta) of the cortex. Cortical labyrinths surround medullary rays (pars radiata) which are made up of straight portions of the nephrons and collecting tubules.

The medullary rays include three types of tubules. The straight segments of proximal tubules (proximal or thick descending segments of nephrons or of Henle's loops) (6) are generally similar in structure to the convoluted parts of proximal tubules. The ascending thick segments (distal segments of nephrons or of Henle's loops) (11, 20) are generally similar in structure to distal convoluted tubules with which they are continuous. Collecting tubules (5, 19) are distinct because of their lightly stained cuboidal cells with visible cell membranes.

The medulla contains only straight portions of tubules and loops of nephrons (Henle's loops). In the small area of outer medulla illustrated here are seen thin segments of nephrons or of Henle's loops (13, 23) lined with a very low epithelium, thick ascending segments (20), and collecting tubules (12, 22).

PLATE 81 (Fig. 2)

KIDNEY CORTEX: JUXTAGLOMERULAR COMPLEX

The section is stained with PASH (periodic acid-Schiff and hematoxylin) to demonstrate basement membranes and brush borders, which take a red color. Nuclei are stained with hematoxylin.

A small area of cortex illustrates a renal corpuscle and its adjacent structures, which include a juxtaglomerular apparatus and a macula densa.

In the renal corpuscle are seen glomerular capillaries (3), the parietal and visceral layers of the glomerular capsule (Bowman's capsule) (2) and the capsular space. Brush borders on proximal convoluted tubules (1) distinguish these readily from distal convoluted tubules (8) which lack brush borders. Basement membranes (9) are distinct.

In favorable sections, the juxtaglomerular apparatus may be seen as a collar of epithelioid cells (6) replacing some of the smooth muscle of the afferent glomerular arteriole (5) as it nears the renal corpuscle. In the adjacent segment of the distal convoluted tubule, the cells which border the juxtaglomerular area are more columnar than elsewhere in the tubule and form a palisade arrangement, the macula densa (7).

PLATE 81

FIG. 1. KIDNEY: DEEP CORTICAL AREA AND OUTER MEDULLA

1 Distal convoluted tubules

2 Glomerular capsule (Bowman's capsule)

3 Glomerulus

4 Proximal convoluted tubules

5 Collecting tubules

6 Straight segment of a proximal convoluted tubule

7 Interlobular vein

8 Glomerular arteriole (t.s.)

9 Junction of glomerular capsule with proximal tubule

10 Proximal convoluted tubules

11 Ascending thick segments of Henle's loops

12 Collecting tubules

13 Thin segments of Henle's loops

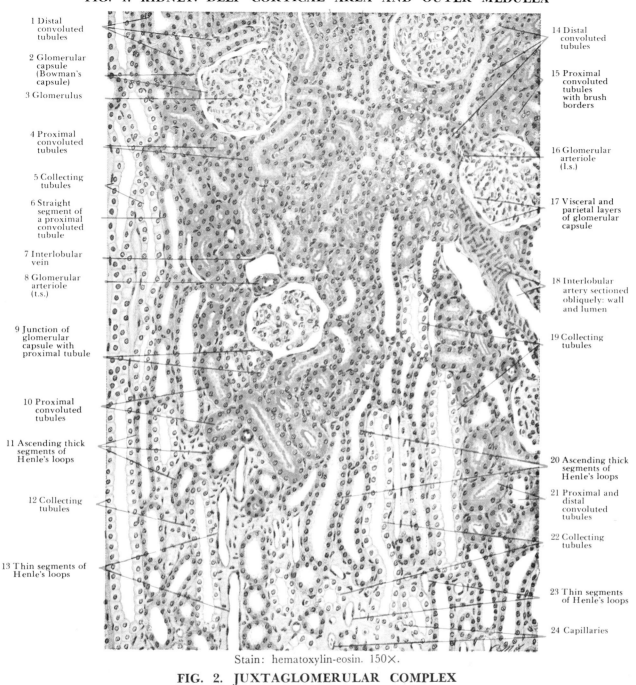

14 Distal convoluted tubules

15 Proximal convoluted tubules with brush borders

16 Glomerular arteriole (l.s.)

17 Visceral and parietal layers of glomerular capsule

18 Interlobular artery sectioned obliquely: wall and lumen

19 Collecting tubules

20 Ascending thick segments of Henle's loops

21 Proximal and distal convoluted tubules

22 Collecting tubules

23 Thin segments of Henle's loops

24 Capillaries

Stain: hematoxylin-eosin. 150×.

FIG. 2. JUXTAGLOMERULAR COMPLEX

1 Brush borders on proximal convoluted tubule cells

2 Glomerular capsule: parietal and visceral layers

3 Glomerular capillaries

4 Distal convoluted tubule

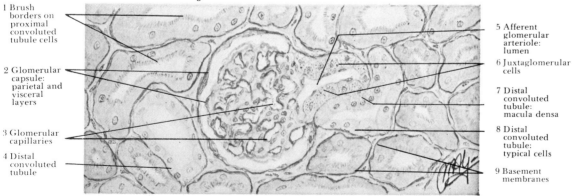

5 Afferent glomerular arteriole: lumen

6 Juxtaglomerular cells

7 Distal convoluted tubule: macula densa

8 Distal convoluted tubule: typical cells

9 Basement membranes

Stain: periodic acid-Schiff and hematoxylin. 280×.

PLATE 82 (Fig. 1)

KIDNEY MEDULLA: PAPILLA (TRANSVERSE SECTION)

In the papilla are seen the terminal collecting tubules, the papillary ducts (2, 6). These are of large diameter, have wide lumens, and are lined with tall, clear columnar cells. Also present are cross sections of thin segments of medullary loops of nephrons (Henle's loops) (3, 8) and thick ascending segments (1, 7). Connective tissue (10) is more abundant than elsewhere in the kidney; the tubules are not as close together. Numerous capillaries (4, 9) are present.

PLATE 82 (Fig. 2)

KIDNEY MEDULLA: PAPILLA ADJACENT TO A CALYX (LONGITUDINAL SECTION)

Terminal collecting tubules, the papillary ducts (5), are seen near their openings at the tip of the papilla. In this illustration, the papilla is covered with a stratified cuboidal epithelium (8). However, at the actual area cribrosa, the covering epithelium is usually a simple columnar epithelium, a continuation of that lining the papillary ducts. Also present are thin segments of medullary loops (of Henle) (3, 4, 6) and thick ascending segments (1). Abundant connective tissue (7) and many capillaries (2) are seen.

—176—

PLATE 82

KIDNEY MEDULLA: PAPILLA

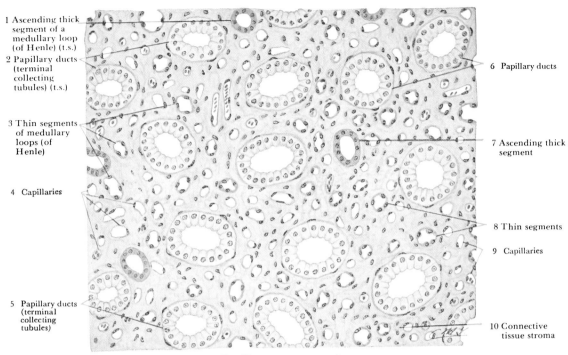

1 Ascending thick segment of a medullary loop (of Henle) (t.s.)

2 Papillary ducts (terminal collecting tubules) (t.s.)

3 Thin segments of medullary loops (of Henle)

4 Capillaries

5 Papillary ducts (terminal collecting tubules)

6 Papillary ducts

7 Ascending thick segment

8 Thin segments

9 Capillaries

10 Connective tissue stroma

FIG. 1. *Papilla, transverse section.*
Stain: hematoxylin-eosin.   170x

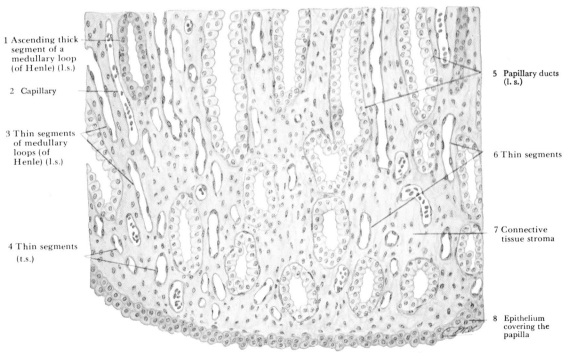

1 Ascending thick segment of a medullary loop (of Henle) (l.s.)

2 Capillary

3 Thin segments of medullary loops (of Henle) (l.s.)

4 Thin segments (t.s.)

5 Papillary ducts (l. s.)

6 Thin segments

7 Connective tissue stroma

8 Epithelium covering the papilla

FIG. 2. *Papilla, longitudinal section through an area adjacent to a calyx.*
Stain: hematoxylin-eosin. 120×.

PLATE 83 (Fig. 1)

URETER (TRANSVERSE SECTION)

The undistended ureter has a convoluted lumen, the convolutions being due to longitudinal mucosal folds. Its wall consists of a mucosa, muscularis and adventitia.

The mucosa consists of transitional epithelium (9, 10) and a wide lamina propria (5). The epithelium has several layers of cells, the outermost of which are large cuboidal or rounded (9) and sometimes show a narrow acidophilic band. The intermediate cells are pear-shaped or irregularly polyhedral. In the basal row, the cells are low columnar or cuboidal (10) but may be somewhat rounded. The basal surface of the epithelium is smooth; there are no connective tissue papillae indenting it.

The wide lamina propria (5) is fibroelastic connective tissue, more dense and with more fibroblasts under the epithelium, and usually loose near the muscularis. Scanty diffuse lymphatic tissue and occasional small lymphatic nodules may be present.

The muscularis consists of an inner longitudinal layer (3) and an outer circular layer of smooth muscle (2) which are not always clearly defined as two layers. An outer longitudinal layer is also present in the lower ureter.

The adventitia (6) is continuous with surrounding fibroelastic connective tissue and adipose tissue (subserous fascia) (1, 12) in which are numerous blood vessels (8, 11) and small nerves (7).

PLATE 83 (Fig. 2)

URETER: WALL (TRANSVERSE SECTION)

Higher magnification shows the structure of the different coats in more detail. The transitional epithelium (8, 9, 10) shows the arrangement of cell layers as described in Fig. 1. The outermost cells often stain more deeply than cells in the remaining layers. The surface membrane, seen as a narrow acidophilic band (9), renders the cells impermeable to urine.

In the lamina propria (12), fibroblasts are somewhat more numerous in the connective tissue under the epithelium than in the deeper area.

The muscle of the muscularis is often loosely arranged bundles with abundant connective tissue between them, as seen here in the inner longitudinal layer (11).

The adventitia (5) merges with the vascular subserous connective tissue (6) in which the abdominal part of the ureter is embedded.

PLATE 83

URETER

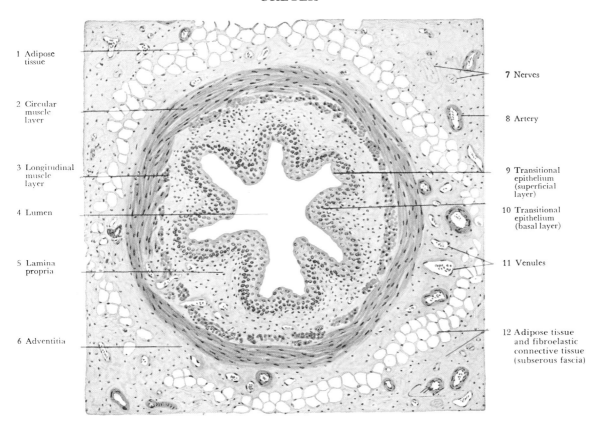

1 Adipose
  tissue

2 Circular
  muscle
  layer

3 Longitudinal
  muscle
  layer

4 Lumen

5 Lamina
  propria

6 Adventitia

7 Nerves

8 Artery

9 Transitional
  epithelium
  (superficial
  layer)

10 Transitional
   epithelium
   (basal layer)

11 Venules

12 Adipose tissue
   and fibroelastic
   connective tissue
   (subserous fascia)

FIG. 1. *Transverse section.*
Stain: hematoxylin-eosin. 50×.

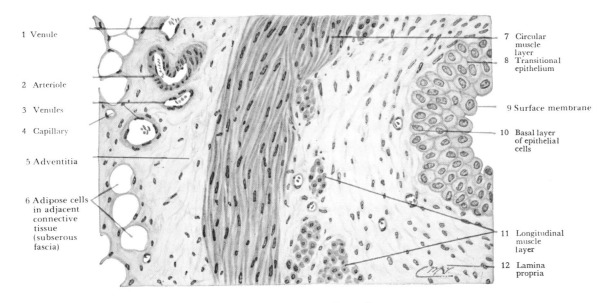

1 Venule

2 Arteriole

3 Venules

4 Capillary

5 Adventitia

6 Adipose cells
  in adjacent
  connective
  tissue
  (subserous
  fascia)

7 Circular
  muscle
  layer

8 Transitional
  epithelium

9 Surface membrane

10 Basal layer
   of epithelial
   cells

11 Longitudinal
   muscle
   layer

12 Lamina
   propria

FIG. 2. *A sector of the wall.*
Stain: hematoxylin-eosin. 150×.

PLATE 84 (Fig. 1)

URINARY BLADDER, UPPER PART: WALL
(TRANSVERSE SECTION)

The layers of the wall of the bladder are similar to those of the ureter but the thick muscular coat (1) of the bladder is distinctive.

The wall consists of a mucosa (6–9), a muscularis (1, 10) and a serosa (4, 5) in the upper bladder. The lower part has an adventitia which merges with connective tissue of adjacent structures.

The mucosa in the empty bladder is thrown into numerous folds (6) but these are obliterated when it is distended. The transitional epithelium (7, 8) and lamina propria (9) are as in the ureter but the epithelium has more cell layers, the lamina propria is wider and the loose connective tissue in its deeper zone contains many elastic fibers.

The muscularis (1, 10) is a thick coat. It is more or less in three layers; the middle layer is the widest. Actually, the muscle fibers are arranged in anastomosing bundles (1) between which is loose connective tissue (2). In a section, the groups of muscle fibers are seen in various planes (1) and three layers are difficult to distinguish. The interstitial connective tissue merges with the connective tissue of the serosa (4). Mesothelium (5) covers this.

PLATE 84 (Fig. 2)

URINARY BLADDER: MUCOSA

The mucosa of the bladder is shown at a higher magnification.

In transitional epithelium (5) in a relaxed state, the outermost or superficial cells are low broad cuboidal or columnar (6) or somewhat convex. Where the epithelium is stretched over the top of a fold (or in a distended state) the cells may be broad squamous (8). The acidophilic surface membrane (6) of the superficial cells may be quite prominent. The deeper layers of cells are rounded or oval; the basal cells are more columnar.

In the lamina propria (2) are seen two zones as in the ureter but more pronounced here. The subepithelial region is more dense but fine-fibered with numerous fibroblasts (2, upper leader); the deeper zone (2, lower leader) is typical loose or moderately dense irregular connective tissue. The latter extends between bundles of muscle as interstitial connective tissue.

PLATE 84

URINARY BLADDER (UPPER PART)

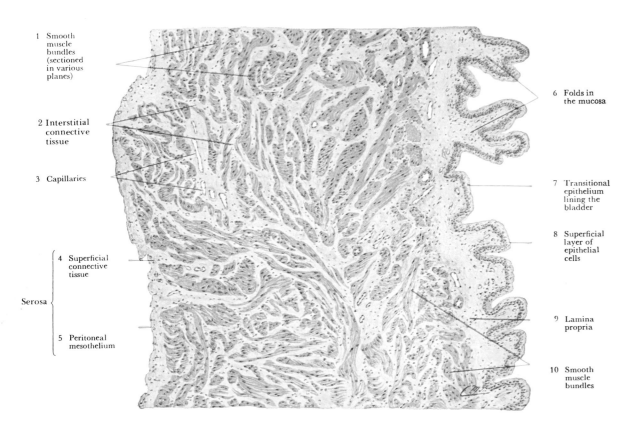

1 Smooth
muscle
bundles
(sectioned
in various
planes)

2 Interstitial
connective
tissue

3 Capillaries

4 Superficial
connective
tissue

Serosa

5 Peritoneal
mesothelium

6 Folds in
the mucosa

7 Transitional
epithelium
lining the
bladder

8 Superficial
layer of
epithelial
cells

9 Lamina
propria

10 Smooth
muscle
bundles

FIG. 1. *Wall (transverse section).*
Stain: hematoxylin-eosin. 40×.

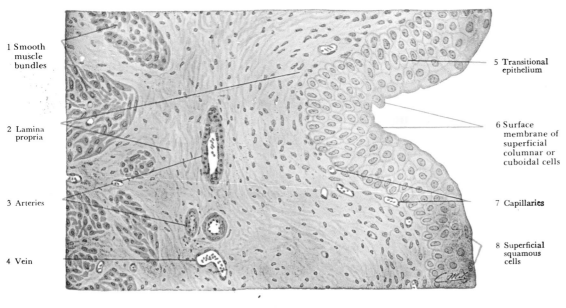

1 Smooth
muscle
bundles

2 Lamina
propria

3 Arteries

4 Vein

5 Transitional
epithelium

6 Surface
membrane of
superficial
columnar or
cuboidal cells

7 Capillaries

8 Superficial
squamous
cells

FIG. 2. *Mucosa (transverse section).*
Stain: hematoxylin-eosin. 160×.

PLATE 85 (Fig. 1)

HYPOPHYSIS (PITUITARY GLAND): PANORAMIC VIEW, SAGITTAL SECTION

There are four divisions of the hypophysis: pars anterior or pars distalis (anterior lobe) (5); pars nervosa or infundibular process (11); pars intermedia (10); and pars tuberalis (9) which enfolds the infundibular stalk (stem, peduncle) like a sheath and is therefore seen above and below the stalk in a sagittal section.

The pars anterior or distalis (5) is the largest of the four divisions. Its glandular substance is composed of two main types of cells, chromophobe cells (1) and chromophil cells (3, 4). Chromophobes are also called reserve or chief cells. Chromophils are further classified as alpha (acidophilic) cells (3) and beta (basophilic) cells (4). (See Fig. 2 below.)

The pars nervosa or infundibular process (11) is the second largest of the four divisions. Together with the pars intermedia it forms the posterior lobe of the hypophysis. It is predominantly fibrillar in structure (nerve fibers and processes of neuroglia cells). Numerous small connective septa (12), arising from the capsule, penetrate into its substance.

The pars intermedia (10) lies between the pars anterior and the pars nervosa. In it are vesicles filled with colloid. Basophilic types of cells predominate.

The pars tuberalis (9) surrounds the infundibular peduncle (stalk) (8), rising higher on the anterior than on the posterior aspect. The infundibular peduncle (8) connects the hypophysis to the base of the brain.

The pars nervosa or infundibular process is part of the larger unit, the neurohypophysis, which includes also the tuber cinereum of the median eminence and the infundibular stalk. The adenohypophysis includes the cellular portions derived from oral ectoderm: the pars distalis (5), pars intermedia (10) and pars tuberalis (9).

PLATE 85 (Fig. 2)

HYPOPHYSIS (PITUITARY GLAND): SECTIONAL VIEW

Under higher magnification, cells of the pars anterior or distalis may be distinguished. Chromophobe cells (4) have a homogeneous cytoplasm and stain lightly. Typically they are smaller than chromophil cells, thus in groups their nuclei are closer together. Chromophils stain well, as red, acidophilic or alpha cells (3), and blue basophils or beta cells (5).

Numerous sinusoidal capillaries (6) are seen in the pars anterior.

The vesicles (7) of the pars intermedia are lined with low columnar epithelial cells, with or without basophilic granules in their cytoplasm. Their lumens are filled with colloid. Follicles lined with basophilic cells (8) are often present. Some of the cells contain secretory granules (8, lower leader).

The pars nervosa or infundibular process is recognized by the presence of nerve fibers (9) among which are numerous nuclei of modified neuroglial cells, the pituicytes (10).

PLATE 85

HYPOPHYSIS (PITUITARY GLAND)

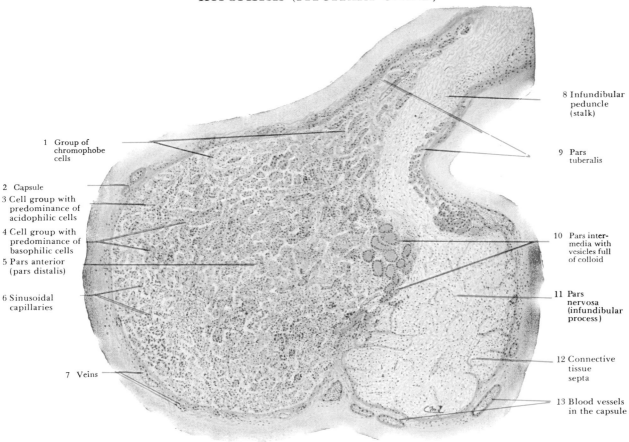

1 Group of chromophobe cells

2 Capsule

3 Cell group with predominance of acidophilic cells

4 Cell group with predominance of basophilic cells

5 Pars anterior (pars distalis)

6 Sinusoidal capillaries

7 Veins

8 Infundibular peduncle (stalk)

9 Pars tuberalis

10 Pars intermedia with vesicles full of colloid

11 Pars nervosa (infundibular process)

12 Connective tissue septa

13 Blood vessels in the capsule

FIG. 1. *Panoramic view (sagittal section).*
Stain: hematoxylin-eosin. 22×.

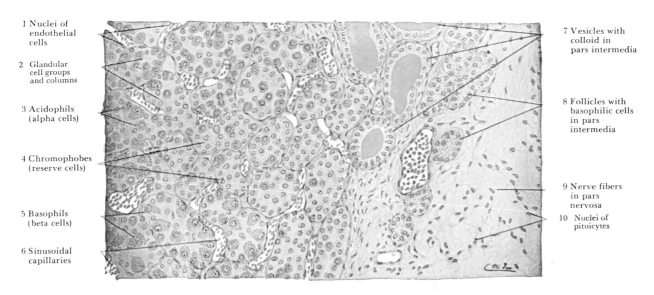

1 Nuclei of endothelial cells

2 Glandular cell groups and columns

3 Acidophils (alpha cells)

4 Chromophobes (reserve cells)

5 Basophils (beta cells)

6 Sinusoidal capillaries

7 Vesicles with colloid in pars intermedia

8 Follicles with basophilic cells in pars intermedia

9 Nerve fibers in pars nervosa

10 Nuclei of pituicytes

FIG. 2. *Sectional view.*
Stain: hematoxylin-eosin. 200×.

Plate 86 (Fig. 1)

HYPOPHYSIS: PARS ANTERIOR (PARS DISTALIS); AZAN STAIN

Cell types in the pars anterior (pars distalis) are readily identified by the use of special fixatives and/or special stains. In this preparation, a corrosive sublimate mixture was used as fixative. The section was then stained with azocarmine and differentiated with aniline oil. Phosphotungstic acid was then used to destain connective tissue, followed by aniline blue and orange G as cytoplasmic stains. Cytoplasmic granules stain red, orange or blue, according to their respective affinities. Nuclei of all cells stain orange.

Chromophobes (3) stain lightly, as after any other stain. Nuclei are pale, cytoplasm is pale orange, cell outlines are poorly defined. The frequent arrangement of chromophobes in groups or clumps is apparent.

Two types of acidophils can be distinguished (although not as clearly as after certain other specific stains) by their staining reaction, those whose coarse granules stain red with azocarmine (1), and those whose smaller granules stain with orange G (6).

Basophils are readily recognized by the blue staining of their granules (2, 5). The different types of basophils are not distinguishable, but it can be seen that the degree of granularity, and therefore the density of the stain, varies in different cells.

Plate 86 (Fig. 2)

HYPOPHYSIS: CELL GROUPS (AZAN STAIN)

Typical cells of the hypophysis, stained with azan as in Fig. 1, are shown here at a higher magnification. Nuclei of all cells are stained orange-red.

In chromophobes (a), the light orange stain of the cytoplasm emphasizes its non-granular character and the vagueness of cell boundaries.

In the rounded or oval acidophils (b), the heavy granules in the cytoplasm take an intense red stain. Cell outlines are clearly defined. A sinusoidal capillary is seen in close proximity to the acidophils.

The basophils (c) shown here illustrate varying shapes of these cells, round, polyhedral or angular. The blue granules vary in size, and are not as compactly arranged as are acidophilic granules.

At (d) are pituicytes from the pars nervosa. Cells and their nuclei are of different shapes and sizes (1). The small amount of cytoplasm, stained orange, sends out diffuse processes (2) for varying distances.

FIG. 1. HYPOPHYSIS: PARS DISTALIS (AZAN STAIN)

1 Acidophils
(alpha cells)
with red
granules

2 Basophils
(beta cells)

3 Chromophobes

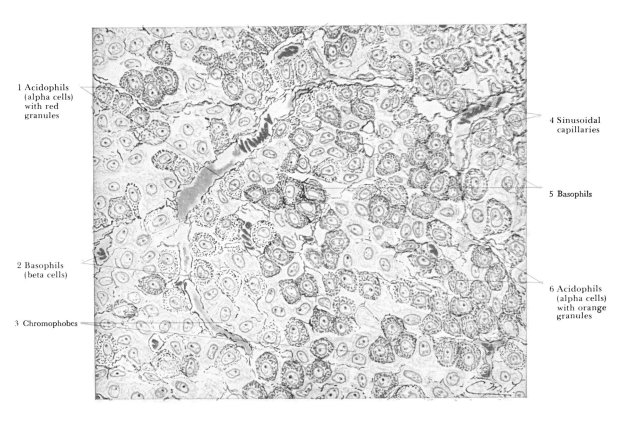

4 Sinusoidal
capillaries

5 Basophils

6 Acidophils
(alpha cells)
with orange
granules

Sectional view. Nuclei: orange; cytoplasmic granules of alpha cells: red or orange; cytoplasmic granules of beta cells: deep blue; collagenous and reticular fibers: blue; erythrocytes: bright red; hemolyzed blood: deep yellow. About 500×.

FIG. 2. HYPOPHYSIS: CELL GROUPS (AZAN STAIN) 800×

1 Connective
tissue

2 Nucleus
and
cytoplasm

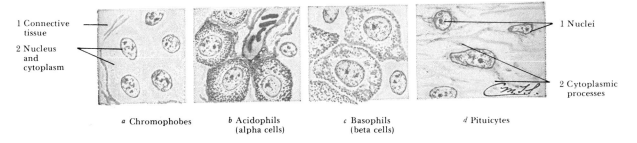

1 Nuclei

2 Cytoplasmic
processes

a Chromophobes   *b* Acidophils   *c* Basophils   *d* Pituicytes
                (alpha cells)   (beta cells)

PLATE 87 (Fig. 1)

THYROID GLAND (GENERAL VIEW)

The thyroid gland is composed of follicles (3, 6) which have a large lumen and are lined with a simple columnar or cuboidal epithelium (6). The epithelium is made up chiefly of follicle cells (principal thyroid cells) which have large rounded nuclei. The follicles vary in size. They are usually filled with colloid (3) which takes an acidophilic stain. Often the colloid shrinks away from the follicular wall (1) because of the reagents used in section preparation. Between follicles may be seen groups of cells not showing a lumen; these are tangential sections through the follicular wall (4).

Connective tissue septa (5), arising from the capsule which encloses the thyroid gland, penetrate into the body of the gland, dividing it into groups of follicles or lobules. Relatively little connective tissue is found between the follicles of a group (interfollicular connective tissue). It supports numerous sinusoidal capillaries (2) which are in close association with the follicular epithelium.

PLATE 87 (Fig. 2)

THYROID GLAND: FOLLICLES (SECTIONAL VIEW)

At a higher magnification, variations may be seen in the epithelium of different follicles. In some, the follicle cells are somewhat flattened (1, upper leader); in others, they are cuboidal (2) or low columnar. Nuclei are vesicular (1). The epithelium, as well as colloid and size of follicles, may vary considerably in different functional states.

As in Fig. 1, most follicles are filled with acidophilic colloid (5). In some follicles, colloid is retracted (4); in others, the colloid may have vacuoles (7). Tangential sections through the walls of follicles (8) are seen as discrete clumps of cells within the interfollicular connective tissue. Sinusoidal capillaries (3) are prominent.

PLATE 87

THYROID GLAND

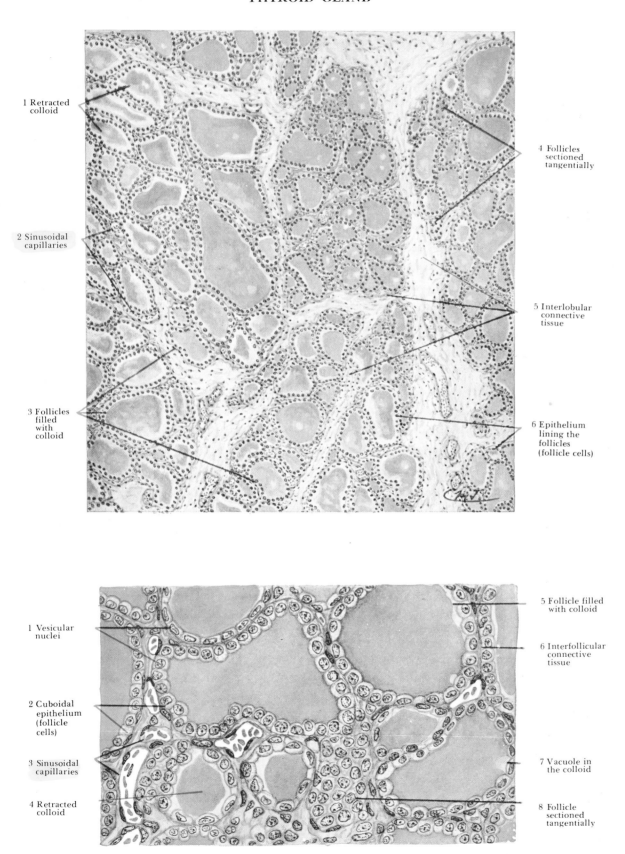

1 Retracted
colloid

2 Sinusoidal
capillaries

3 Follicles
filled
with
colloid

4 Follicles
sectioned
tangentially

5 Interlobular
connective
tissue

6 Epithelium
lining the
follicles
(follicle cells)

1 Vesicular
nuclei

2 Cuboidal
epithelium
(follicle
cells)

3 Sinusoidal
capillaries

4 Retracted
colloid

5 Follicle filled
with colloid

6 Interfollicular
connective
tissue

7 Vacuole in
the colloid

8 Follicle
sectioned
tangentially

PLATE 88 (Fig. 1)

THYROID AND ADJACENT PARATHYROID GLAND

The anatomical proximity of these two glands makes it possible to examine them in the same histological section and to note their relationships and structural differences.

A section of thyroid gland (7) is seen in the upper field. Its follicles of various sizes (1) contain colloid, and the interfollicular connective tissue is rich in capillaries.

The thin capsule (8, 2) of the thyroid gland separates the thyroid (7) from the parathyroid (9) and at the same time binds them together. From the capsule, trabeculae extend into the parathyroid (5, 6) bringing in larger blood vessels (6) which distribute capillaries among the parathyroid cells. Nerves accompany the vessels. The trabeculae may contain adipose cells (5).

The parathyroid cells are single cells, not arranged into follicles as in the thyroid gland. The cells are very close together. The majority, occurring mainly in groups of various sizes, are principal or chief cells (3). Occasional larger cells, sometimes in small groups, are oxyphils or acidophils (4).

PLATE 88 (Fig. 2)

PARATHYROID GLAND

Features of the parathyroid gland, as illustrated in Fig. 1, are seen here at a higher magnification.

Principal or chief cells (1, 7) are by far the most numerous, are close together arranged in masses or columns, with capillaries coursing among groups of cells (5). Principal cells are rounded, are pale with lightly acidophilic cytoplasm, and have vesicular nuclei. Oxyphils or acidophils (3, 6) occur singly or in groups. They are larger than the principal cells, cytoplasm is granular and distinctly acidophilic, nuclei are smaller and more darkly stained. In man, transitional forms between oxyphils and principal cells are common. Oxyphils are not normally present in children.

Spaces filled with colloid (2) occur occasionally (colloid vesicles).

Trabeculae are present (4, 8) but do not form distinct lobules as in the thyroid gland.

PLATE 88

THYROID AND PARATHYROID GLANDS

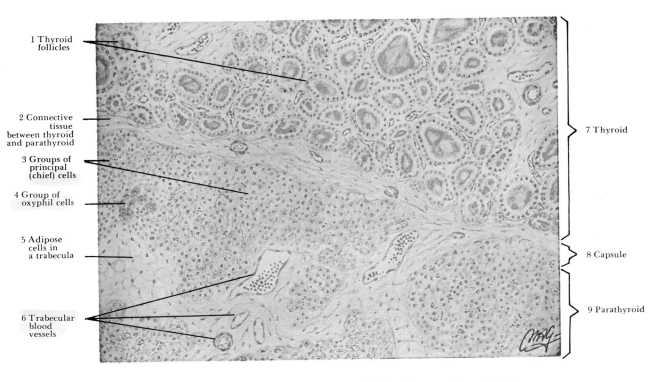

1 Thyroid follicles

2 Connective tissue between thyroid and parathyroid

3 Groups of principal (chief) cells

4 Group of oxyphil cells

5 Adipose cells in a trabecula

6 Trabecular blood vessels

7 Thyroid

8 Capsule

9 Parathyroid

FIG. 1. *Thyroid and adjacent parathyroid gland.* Stain: hematoxylin-eosin. 90×.

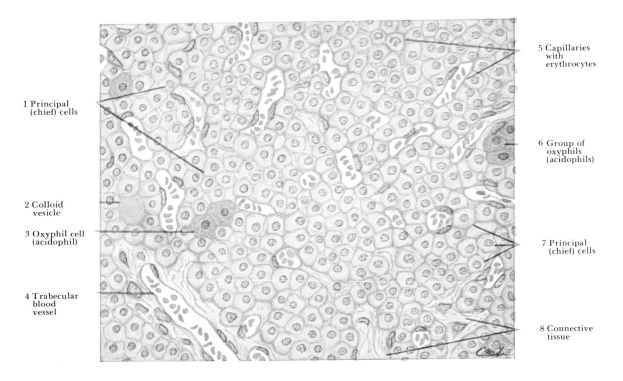

1 Principal (chief) cells

2 Colloid vesicle

3 Oxyphil cell (acidophil)

4 Trabecular blood vessel

5 Capillaries with erythrocytes

6 Group of oxyphils (acidophils)

7 Principal (chief) cells

8 Connective tissue

FIG. 2. *Parathyroid gland.* Stain: hematoxylin-eosin. 550×.

PLATE 89

ADRENAL (SUPRARENAL) GLAND

Each adrenal gland is encased in a thick capsule of connective tissue in which are branches of the main arteries that supply the gland, nerves whose fibers are largely unmyelinated (5), venules and lymphatics. Septa (trabeculae) penetrate the cortex. The larger ones carry arteries (4) to the medulla. Sinusoidal capillaries are present throughout the cortex and medulla.

Each adrenal gland has a cortex (2) and medulla (3).

In the cortex are three zones which are not sharply separated from each other. The zona glomerulosa (2a) is the outer zone. The cells are arranged in ovoid groups. Cytoplasm of the cells (6) contains sparse lipid droplets which appear as vacuoles in hematoxylin-eosin preparations; nuclei stain relatively darkly. Sinusoidal capillaries (7) course between cell groups. Cells of the zona fasciculata (2b) are arranged into columns or plates oriented in a radial direction. Abundant lipid droplets in the cytoplasm give the cells a greatly vacuolated appearance, thus they are often called spongiocytes (8). Nuclei are vesicular. Sinusoidal capillaries (9) between the columns of cells follow a similar radial course. Cells of the zona reticularis (2c) form anastomosing cords which run in various directions. The cells are frequently filled with yellow pigment (11). The intervening capillaries are irregularly arranged.

Cells which make up the major portion of the medulla (3, 14) are arranged in groups. Cytoplasm is relatively clear (14), but following fixation in potassium bichromate, fine brown granules are present. This is the chromaffin reaction and indicates the presence of epinephrine. The medulla also contains sympathetic ganglion cells (13) seen singly or in groups. They have the characteristic vesicular nucleus and prominent nucleolus and a small amount of peripherally placed chromatin. Sinusoidal capillaries are present in the medulla. These drain into medullary veins (12).

PLATE 89

ADRENAL (SUPRARENAL) GLAND

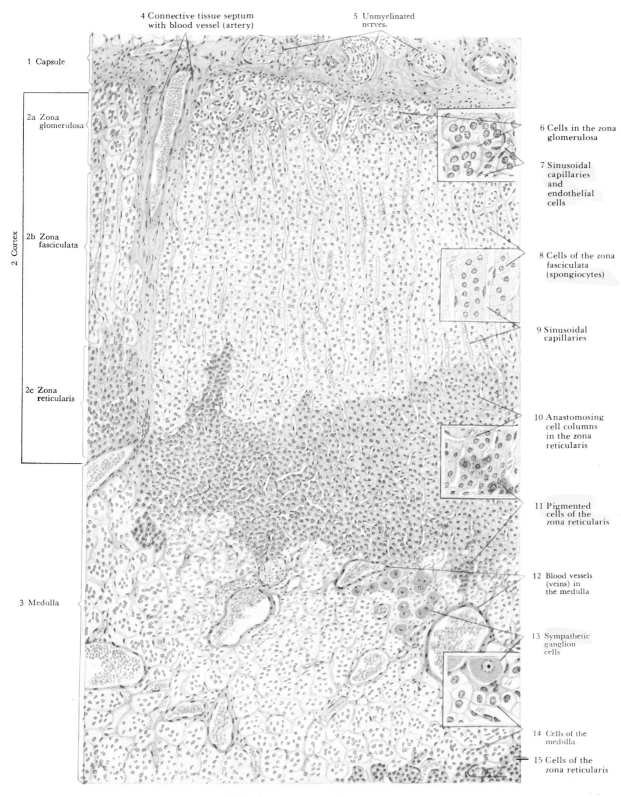

4 Connective tissue septum
with blood vessel (artery)

5 Unmyelinated
nerves.

1 Capsule

2 Cortex

2a Zona
glomerulosa

2b Zona
fasciculata

2c Zona
reticularis

3 Medulla

6 Cells in the zona
glomerulosa

7 Sinusoidal
capillaries
and
endothelial
cells

8 Cells of the zona
fasciculata
(spongiocytes)

9 Sinusoidal
capillaries

10 Anastomosing
cell columns
in the zona
reticularis

11 Pigmented
cells of the
zona reticularis

12 Blood vessels
(veins) in
the medulla

13 Sympathetic
ganglion
cells

14 Cells of the
medulla

15 Cells of the
zona reticularis

Stain: hematoxylin-eosin. 200×.

PLATE 90 (Fig. 1)

TESTIS

The testis is enclosed in a thick fibrous capsule, the tunica albuginea (1). A layer of loose vascular connective tissue beneath this is the tunica vasculosa (2). This merges with the stroma of the testis, the intertubular or interstitial connective tissue (7) which is rich in blood vessels (10). It supports the seminiferous tubules (3, 4, 9).

Seminiferous tubules are long, extremely convoluted tubules, thus they are seen sectioned in various planes (3, 4, 9). They are lined with several rows of highly specialized epithelium (spermatogenic cells and supporting cells of Sertoli) which rests on a thin basement membrane (5). (See Plate 91 for detailed structure.)

In the interstitial connective tissue are groups of epithelioid cells, the interstitial cells (of Leydig) (8).

PLATE 90 (Fig. 2)

SEMINIFEROUS TUBULES, STRAIGHT TUBULES, RETE TESTIS AND DUCTULI EFFERENTES

Illustrated is a section which passes through the mediastinum of the testis, and includes a small area of testis proper and the beginning of the ductuli efferentes.

Seminiferous tubules (1) are seen at the left, lined with spermatogenic cells and supporting cells of Sertoli. The interstitial connective tissue becomes continuous with the connective tissue of the mediastinum (3). At the junction of the testis and mediastinum, the seminiferous tubules of each lobule converge to form a narrow straight tubule (2), a short duct lined with cuboidal or low columnar epithelium.

Straight tubules pass into a series of rete testis tubules (4) which lie in the connective tissue of the mediastinum (3). These are irregular anastomosing channels with broad lumens and thin walls of cuboidal or low columnar epithelium (6); they become wider as they approach the efferent ductules (ductuli efferentes) (5) into which they empty. The efferent ductules (ductuli efferentes) are straight tubules at their origin, but become highly convoluted as they pass toward and into the head of the epididymis (see Plate 92, Fig. 1).

PLATE 90

FIG. 1. TESTIS

1 Tunica albuginea

2 Tunica vasculosa

3 Seminiferous tubules (o.s.)

6 Spermatozoa

7 Interstitial connective tissue

4 Seminiferous tubules (t.s.)

8 Interstitial cells (of Leydig)

9 Seminiferous tubule (tg. s.)

5 Basement membrane of seminiferous tubules

10 Blood vessels

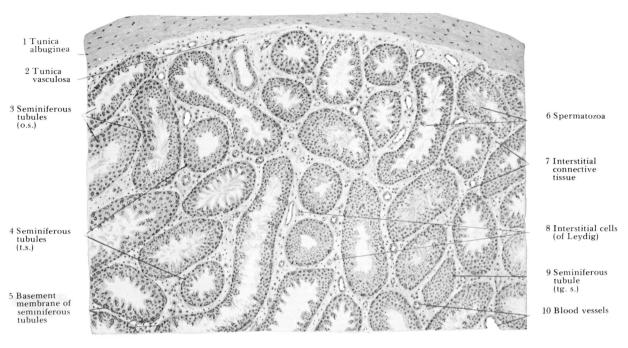

Stain: hematoxylin-eosin. 70×.

FIG. 2. SEMINIFEROUS TUBULES, STRAIGHT TUBULES, RETE TESTIS AND DUCTULI EFFERENTES

1 Seminiferous tubules

3 Connective tissue of mediastinum

4 Rete testis tubules

5 Ductuli efferentes (efferent ductules)

2 Straight tubules

6 Rete testis tubules

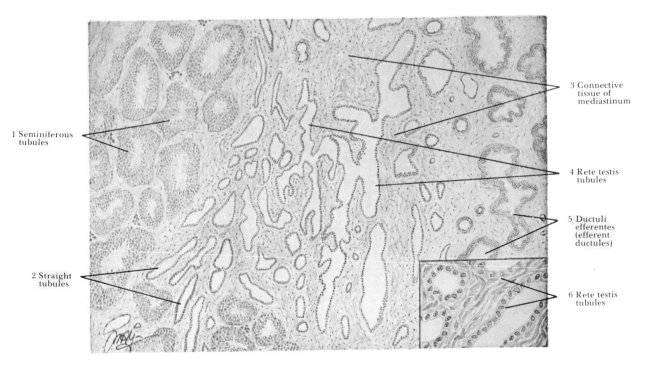

Stain: hematoxylin-eosin. 60× and 400×.

PLATE 91

TESTIS: SEMINIFEROUS TUBULES (TRANSVERSE SECTION)

Sections of several seminiferous tubules are shown. Between the tubules is the interstitial (intertubular) connective tissue which contains fibroblasts (2) and other characteristic cells, blood vessels (4, 12, 25), nerves, and lymphatics. Also present are the specific interstitial cells (of Leydig) which occur typically in groups (3) but may also be seen singly. They are large, rounded or polygonal cells with granular cytoplasm and a distinct ovoid or wrinkled nucleus (3). They constitute the endocrine gland of the testis and produce testosterone.

Each seminiferous tubule is surrounded by an outer lamina propria of compact connective tissue with flattened fibroblasts and an inner, thin, basement membrane (6). Enclosed by the membrane is the complex seminiferous epithelium consisting of two kinds of cells, the supporting cells of Sertoli and the spermatogenic cells. The characteristic arrangement of these cells is seen best in a transverse section of a seminiferous tubule (5).

The supporting cells of Sertoli are slender, elongated cells with irregular outlines extending from the basement membrane to the lumen (19, 32). The cytoplasm often exhibits faint longitudinal striations. The distinctive nucleus is ovoid or somewhat triangular in shape, clearly outlined, pale-staining with fine, sparse chromatin, and contains one or more prominent nucleoli. Nuclei may vary in position in different cells. In tangential sections of seminiferous tubules (15), supporting cells are seen as ovoid rounded cross sections (16).

Spermatogenic cells are arranged in rows between and around supporting cells of Sertoli; in sections, they often appear superimposed on supporting cells, obscuring their cytoplasm in varying degrees (8, 13). The most primitive spermatogenic cells, the spermatogonia (17, 18), lie beneath the basement membrane of the seminiferous tubule. Many divide by mitosis (1, 21) to produce several generations of spermatogonia. After proper fixation and when viewed under high magnification, two types of spermatogonia can be distinguished. Type A (27) shows lightly stained cytoplasm and a rounded or ovoid nucleus with small chromatin granules. One or two nucleoli may be present lying against the nuclear membrane. In a later type B spermatogonium (28), the chromatin granules in the rounded nucleus are of various sizes, and a concentration occurs along the nuclear membrane. A nucleolus is centrally located (not illustrated).

By division and differentiation of type B spermatogonia, primary spermatocytes (11, 22) are formed, which lie adjacent to spermatogonia but nearer the lumen. Their nuclei have variable appearances (11, 22) due to different states of activity of the chromatin. Meiotic figures are prevalent (7), representing stages of the first maturation division (meiosis). The formation of thin chromosomes in the nucleus indicates the leptotene stage (29). An increase in cell size and thickening of the chromosomes (and darker staining) indicates the zygotene stage (30). The pachytene stage (31) is characterized by further increase in cell size and shorter, much thicker chromosomes. By meiotic division, each primary spermatocyte gives rise to two secondary spermatocytes.

Secondary spermatocytes are smaller than primary spermatocytes and the nuclear chromatin is less dense (23, 33). They divide soon after formation and therefore are not seen frequently in stained testicular tissue. This second maturation division gives rise to two spermatids.

Spermatids are much smaller cells (24) with small nuclei containing fine as well as larger chromatin granules, lying usually in groups close to the lumen of the seminiferous tubule (24). They become closely associated with supporting cells of Sertoli and here undergo metamorphosis to form spermatozoa (26; 34 a, b, c).

The small, deeply-staining heads of spermatozoa appear to be embedded in the cytoplasm of supporting cells (20), their tails extending into the lumen of the seminiferous tubule. A mature spermatozoan in profile and frontal view is illustrated (35 a and b).

PLATE 91

TESTIS: SEMINIFEROUS TUBULES (TRANSVERSE SECTION)

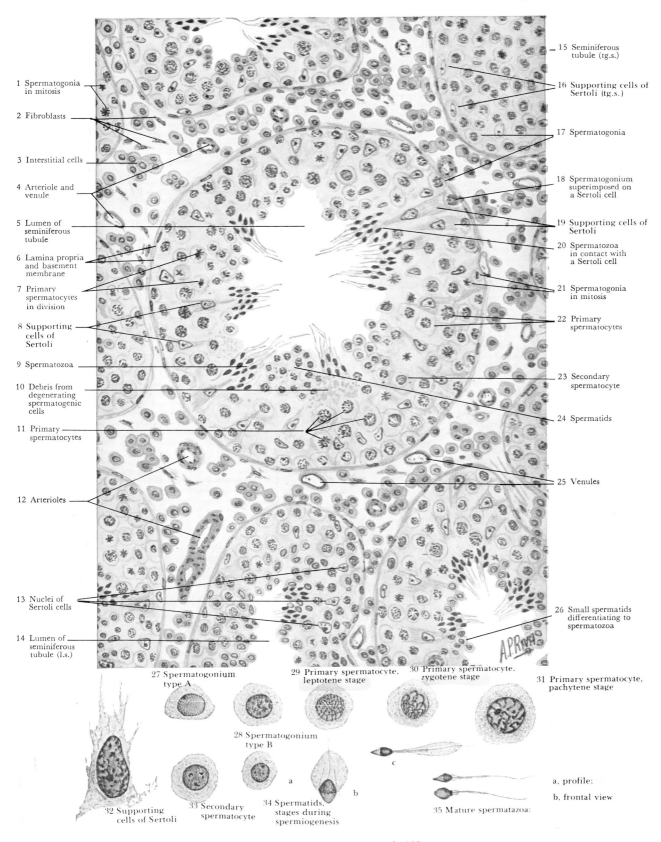

1 Spermatogonia in mitosis

2 Fibroblasts

3 Interstitial cells

4 Arteriole and venule

5 Lumen of seminiferous tubule

6 Lamina propria and basement membrane

7 Primary spermatocytes in division

8 Supporting cells of Sertoli

9 Spermatozoa

10 Debris from degenerating spermatogenic cells

11 Primary spermatocytes

12 Arterioles

13 Nuclei of Sertoli cells

14 Lumen of seminiferous tubule (l.s.)

15 Seminiferous tubule (tg.s.)

16 Supporting cells of Sertoli (tg.s.)

17 Spermatogonia

18 Spermatogonium superimposed on a Sertoli cell

19 Supporting cells of Sertoli

20 Spermatozoa in contact with a Sertoli cell

21 Spermatogonia in mitosis

22 Primary spermatocytes

23 Secondary spermatocyte

24 Spermatids

25 Venules

26 Small spermatids differentiating to spermatozoa

27 Spermatogonium type A

28 Spermatogonium type B

29 Primary spermatocyte, leptotene stage

30 Primary spermatocyte, zygotene stage

31 Primary spermatocyte, pachytene stage

32 Supporting cells of Sertoli

33 Secondary spermatocyte

34 Spermatids, stages during spermiogenesis

35 Mature spermatazoa:

a, profile;

b, frontal view

Stain: hematoxylin-eosin. 300× and 1000×.

PLATE 92 (Fig. 1)

DUCTULI EFFERENTES AND TRANSITION
TO DUCTUS EPIDIDYMIDIS

The ductuli efferentes or efferent ductules (1, 5), after arising from the rete testis, are embedded in the connective tissue of the epididymis (2) and form part of the head of the latter. Because of the tortuous, winding course of the tubules, they appear in sections as isolated tubules cut in various planes (1, 5).

The lumens of the ductuli have a characteristic, wavy appearance (4). The lining epithelium is basically simple, consisting of alternating groups of columnar cells, usually ciliated, and groups of cuboidal cells (4) which are apparently absorptive. Occasional basal cells may be present, thus the epithelium may be pseudostratified in part. The basal surface of the tubules is smooth in contour. Beneath the basement membrane is a thin layer of dense connective tissue (lamina propria) with smooth muscle fibers (3).

The distal ends of the ductuli, as they approach the epididymis, are lined with columnar cells only (6), thus the lumens have an even contour. As the ductuli enter the ductus epididymidis, there is an abrupt transition to the tall pseudostratified columnar epithelium of the ductus epididymidis.

PLATE 92 (Fig. 2)

DUCTUS EPIDIDYMIDIS (DUCT OF THE EPIDIDYMIS)

The ductus epididymidis is a long, greatly convoluted tubule embedded in the connective tissue of the epididymis. A transverse section through this shows the convolutions of the tubule as varied individual sections (2, 5, 6) surrounded by connective tissue (1). Both internal and external surfaces of the epithelium are smooth in contour.

The lining of the tubule is pseudostratified epithelium (4), consisting of very tall columnar cells (9) with long stereocilia (8) and small basal cells (10). The columnar cells (9) apparently function primarily as absorptive (resorptive) cells; other suggested functions have not been clarified. The stereocilia (8) are long, branching microvilli. Function of the basal cells (10) is unknown. The basement membrane (3) is distinct. The lamina propria, with circularly arranged smooth muscle fibers (7) is thin but more pronounced than that of the ductuli efferentes.

Clumps of spermatozoa may be seen in the lumens of some of the tubules.

PLATE 92

FIG. 1. DUCTULI EFFERENTES AND TRANSITION TO DUCTUS EPIDIDYMIDIS

1 Ductuli efferentes

2 Connective tissue of the epididymis

3 Smooth muscle fibers

4 Undulating epithelium of ductuli efferentes

5 Ductuli efferentes: typical tubules

6 Ductuli efferentes: distal transition tubules

7 Ductus epididymidis

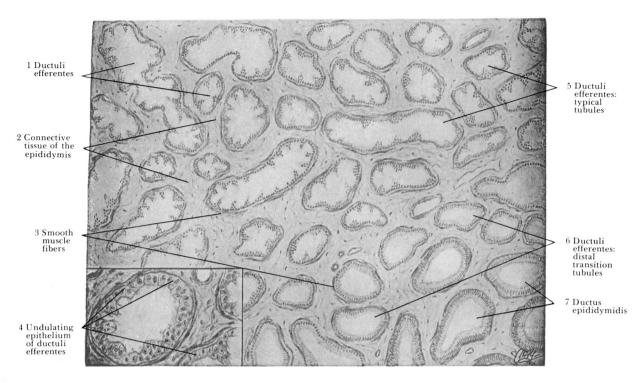

Stain: hematoxylin-eosin. 60× and 240×.

FIG. 2. DUCTUS EPIDIDYMIDIS (DUCT OF THE EPIDIDYMIS)

1 Connective tissue

2 Cross sections of the ductus epididymidis

3 Basement membrane

4 Pseudo-stratified columnar epithelium with stereocilia

5 Section through a U-bend of the ductus epididymidis

6 Epididymal wall cut tangentially

7 Smooth muscle fibers

8 Stereocilia

9 Columnar cells

10 Basal cell

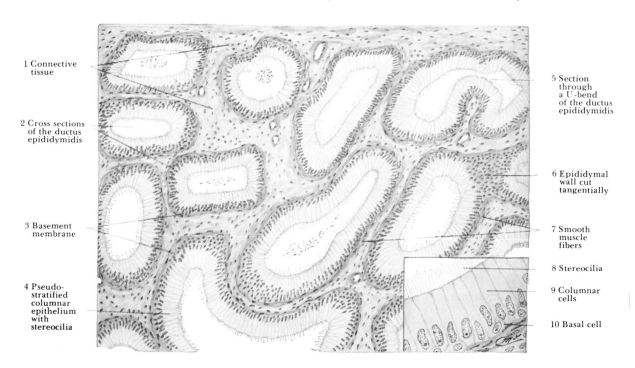

Stain: hematoxylin-eosin. 90×.

PLATE 93 (Fig. 1)

DUCTUS DEFERENS (TRANSVERSE SECTION)

The ductus deferens (vas deferens) has a narrow, irregular lumen, a thin mucosa, and a thick muscularis surrounded by adventitia. The irregularity of the lumen is caused by longitudinal folds of the lamina propria (5, 6), which in transverse sections have the appearance of crests or papillae (6).

The epithelium is pseudostratified columnar (7), lower than that in the ductus epididymidis, resting on a thin basement membrane. Stereocilia are usually present but their distribution varies. The thin lamina propria (5, 6) is compact collagenous fibers with fine elastic networks.

The muscularis consists of a thin inner longitudinal layer (3), a thick middle circular layer (2) and a thinner but well developed outer longitudinal layer (1). The adventitia (4) contains abundant blood vessels and nerves. It merges with the surrounding connective tissue of the spermatic cord.

PLATE 93 (Fig. 2)

SEMINAL VESICLE

Each seminal vesicle is an elongated sac with a highly convoluted, irregular lumen. A section through the wall shows complex primary folds (5) and innumerable thinner secondary folds (6), frequently joined by anastomoses, forming many crypts and cavities (1). Extensions of lamina propria form the core of the larger folds (5) and the thin stroma of the smaller ones (6).

The epithelium (4) is usually a low pseudostratified with some basal cells, and short columnar or cuboidal cells which are secretory but not ciliated. The epithelium may appear simple. The thin lamina propria (7) extends around the bases of the folds and sends projections into them.

The muscularis (2) is more or less in the form of an inner circular and an outer longitudinal layer. This is often difficult to discern in sections because of the convolutions of the vesicles. An adventitia (3) surrounds the muscularis.

PLATE 93

FIG. 1. DUCTUS DEFERENS (TRANSVERSE SECTION)

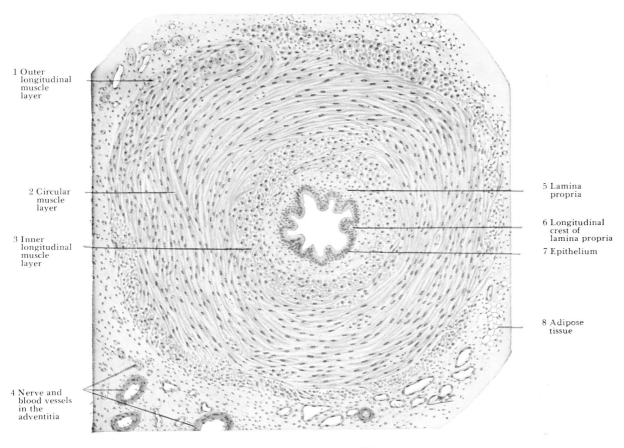

1 Outer
   longitudinal
   muscle
   layer

2 Circular
   muscle
   layer

3 Inner
   longitudinal
   muscle
   layer

4 Nerve and
   blood vessels
   in the
   adventitia

5 Lamina
   propria

6 Longitudinal
   crest of
   lamina propria

7 Epithelium

8 Adipose
   tissue

Stain: hematoxylin-eosin. 40×.

FIG. 2. SEMINAL VESICLE

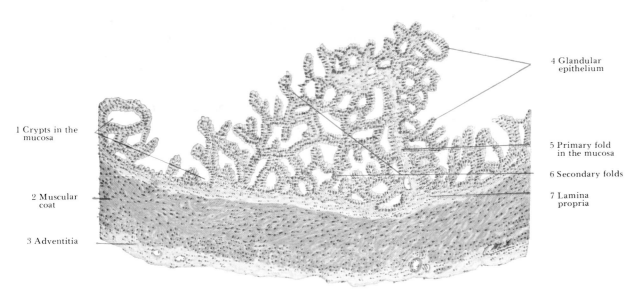

1 Crypts in the
   mucosa

2 Muscular
   coat

3 Adventitia

4 Glandular
   epithelium

5 Primary fold
   in the mucosa

6 Secondary folds

7 Lamina
   propria

Stain: hematoxylin-eosin. 60×.

PLATE 94 (Fig. 1)

PROSTATE GLAND WITH PROSTATIC URETHRA

Illustrated is a section of the prostate gland which includes the prostatic urethra, the colliculus seminalis and the utriculus.

In the prostatic tissue, the glandular alveoli (4, 5) seen are the terminal tubules of many small, irregularly branching tubuloalveolar glands. The alveoli vary in size (4, 5). Lumens are wide and markedly irregular in the larger alveoli (4). Epithelium is variable (see Fig. 2).

The glands are embedded in a distinctive fibromuscular stroma (3, 6). Strands of smooth muscle (6) course in various directions, together with collagenous fibers and fine elastic networks.

The prostatic urethra (1) is seen as a crescent-shaped structure with small diverticula along its lumen (8), especially prominent in the urethral recesses. The epithelium is usually transitional. Fibromuscular stroma of the prostate surrounds the urethra, but a thin lamina propria may be present.

The colliculus seminalis (2), a ridge of dense fibromuscular stroma without glands, protrudes into the urethral lumen, giving it the crescent shape. The prostatic utriculus (9) lies in the mass of the colliculus; frequently it is dilated at its distal end (7) before it opens into the urethra. Its thin mucous membrane is typically folded. The epithelium is usually secretory simple or pseudo-stratified columnar.

Ejaculatory ducts (10) penetrate the prostate, course alongside the utriculus and open finally into the urethra.

PLATE 94 (Fig. 2)

PROSTATE GLAND (SECTIONAL VIEW)

Illustrated is a small section of prostate gland at a high magnification. In this specimen, glands are closer together than in Fig. 1; the stroma between them is more concentrated.

As in Fig. 1, alveoli (2) vary in size, lumens are wide, and frequently uneven in contour. The epithelium (4) is secretory, is usually columnar or pseudostratified, and the cells stain lightly in their superficial portions. There is considerable variation, however; the epithelium may be squamous or cuboidal. The alveoli may contain prostatic concretions (1), formed by concentric layers of coagulated secretions which may become calcified.

Ducts (3) of the glands may be quite similar to alveoli and difficult to distinguish. Terminally, the epithelium usually becomes columnar and stains more darkly (5) prior to becoming transitional as the ducts open into the urethra.

The abundance of smooth muscle (6) in the stroma is emphasized.

PLATE 94

FIG. 1. PROSTATE GLAND WITH PROSTATIC URETHRA

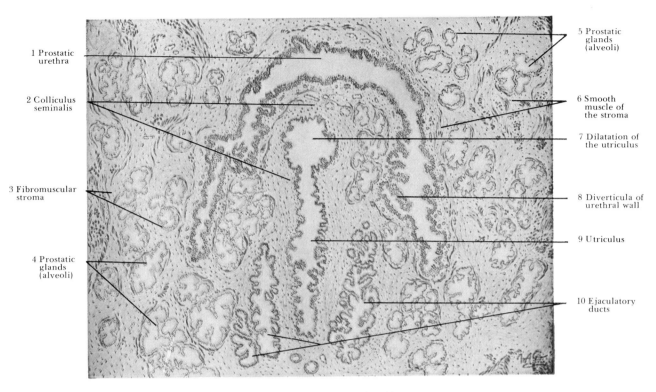

1 Prostatic urethra

2 Colliculus seminalis

3 Fibromuscular stroma

4 Prostatic glands (alveoli)

5 Prostatic glands (alveoli)

6 Smooth muscle of the stroma

7 Dilatation of the utriculus

8 Diverticula of urethral wall

9 Utriculus

10 Ejaculatory ducts

Stain: hematoxylin-eosin. 80×.

FIG. 2. PROSTATE GLAND (SECTIONAL VIEW)

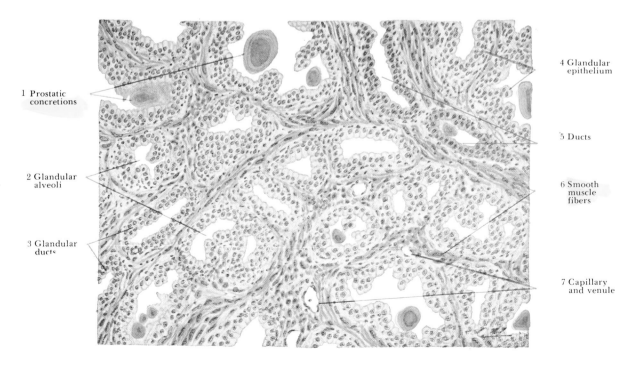

1 Prostatic concretions

2 Glandular alveoli

3 Glandular ducts

4 Glandular epithelium

5 Ducts

6 Smooth muscle fibers

7 Capillary and venule

Stain: hematoxylin-eosin. 180×.

PLATE 95

PENIS (TRANSVERSE SECTION)

A cross-section of the penis reveals sections through the three cavernous bodies: two dorso-lateral corpora cavernosa (9) and a single mid-ventral corpus spongiosum (16) which surrounds the urethra (15). A tunic of collagenous fibers lies at the periphery of each. Surrounding the two larger corpora cavernosa is their tunica albuginea (5) which extends between them as the medial septum (10). This septum is better developed at the base of the penis than at the tip. Surrounding the corpus spongiosum is the tunica albuginea of the corpus spongiosum (6).

All three cavernous bodies are bound together by loose connective tissue, the deep penile fascia (Buck's fascia) (4). This fascia in turn is surrounded by the connective tissue of the dermis (2) underlying the epidermis (1). Strands of smooth muscle, the dartos tunic (3), and an abundance of peripheral blood vessels are embedded in the dermis. Sebaceous glands (7) are present in the dermis on the ventral side of the penis.

The core of each corpus cavernosum is occupied by numerous trabeculae (14), consisting of collagenous fibers, elastic fibers and smooth muscle, which surround the cavities or lacunae (cavernous veins) (12) of the corpora cavernosa. Nerves and blood vessels also lie in the trabeculae. The cavities of the corpora cavernosa (12) are lined with endothelium. They receive blood from two sources, the dorsal arterial system (8) and the central deep arteries (11). Arterial branches of the latter open directly into the cavities. The corpus spongiosum (corpus cavernosa urethrae) receives its blood supply largely from the bulbo-urethral artery. From its cavities blood exits mainly by way of the superficial veins (13) in the vascularized dermis (2) and the deep dorsal vein.

The urethra in the shaft of the penis is designated as the spongiosa part (15) or the cavernous urethra. Toward the base of the shaft of the penis, the urethra is lined with pseudostratified or stratified columnar epithelium, but toward the external orifice, the epithelium grades into stratified squamous epithelium.

Not apparent at this magnification are numerous small but deep invaginations of the mucous membrane, the urethral lacunae (of Morgagni) which contain single or groups of mucous cells. Branched tubular urethral glands (of Littré) open into these.

PLATE 95

PENIS (TRANSVERSE SECTION)

1 Epidermis

2 Dermis

3 Dartos tunic

4 Deep penile
fascia

5 Tunica
albuginea of
corpus
cavernosum

6 Tunica
albuginea of
corpus
spongiosum

7 Sebaceous
gland in
dermis

8 Dorsal artery

9 Corpus
cavernosum

10 Medial septum

11 Central (deep)
artery

12 Cavities (cavernous
veins) of corpus
cavernosum

13 Superficial vein

14 Trabeculae

15 Urethra

16 Corpus
spongiosum

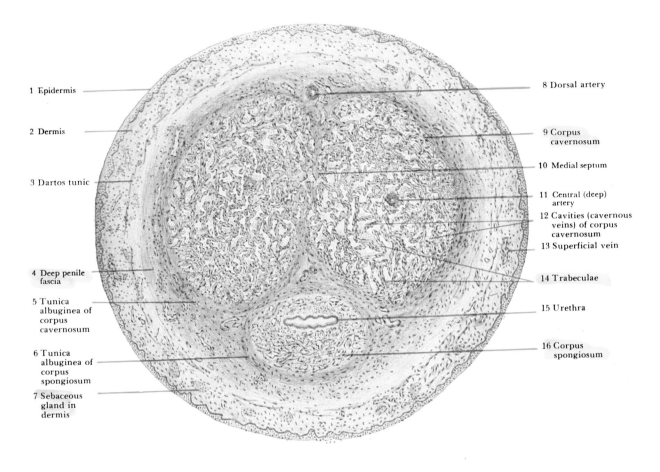

Stain: Hematoxylin-eosin. 12×.

PLATE 96

OVARY (PANORAMIC VIEW)

The surface of the ovary is covered with surface epithelium (germinal epithelium) (1), the modified mesothelium of the visceral peritoneum. In young women, this is a cuboidal epithelium; it usually becomes flattened in later life. Beneath the epithelium is the tunica albuginea (2), a thin zone of collagenous connective tissue (modified stroma).

The cortex occupies the greater part of the ovary. Its stroma (8) is a primitive type of connective tissue, in which large, spindle-shaped fibroblasts predominate (see Plate 97, Fig. 1: 8). Coursing in all directions between them are compactly arranged fine collagenous and reticular fibers.

The stroma of the medulla (24) is typical dense irregular connective tissue continuous with that of the mesovarium (13). Numerous blood vessels course in the medulla (10). From these, smaller vessels are distributed to all parts of the cortex. The mesovarium is covered in part by ovarian surface epithelium (12) and in part by peritoneal mesothelium (14).

Numerous follicles in various stages of development are embedded in the stroma of the cortex (3, 4, 7, 9, 16–20, 22, 27, 28); detailed structure of some of these is shown on Plate 97. The most numerous are primary follicles (3, 28), found in the peripheral zone of the cortex just under the tunica albuginea; they are the smallest and simplest in structure. The largest of the follicles (16–20) is an almost mature follicle. Its various parts can be identified: the thecae (16) surrounding the follicle, the stratum granulosum or membrana granulosa (17), the large antrum (18) filled with follicular fluid (liquor folliculi), and the cumulus oophorus (19) in which is embedded the ovum (20). Smaller follicles with stratified follicular cells surrounding the ovum are growing follicles (4, 22). Larger follicles with cavities of various sizes are termed vesicular follicles (7, 9, 27). They are situated deeper in the cortex and are surrounded by connective tissue capsules, the thecae folliculi (6) derived from the stroma. Most of the follicles illustrated contain an ovum (such as 20, 27) with its nucleus or germinal vesicle. The ovum is small in primary follicles, then increases gradually in size in growing follicles.

Many follicles never attain maturity, but undergo degeneration (atresia) at various stages of growth, thus becoming atretic follicles (11, 21, 26; see also Plate 98). As atresia progresses, the degenerating follicles are gradually replaced by stroma.

Following ovulation, a corpus luteum is formed. Stages in regression of a corpus luteum are indicated (5, 15, 23) and Plates 98, 99 illustrate these at a higher magnification.

PLATE 96

OVARY (PANORAMIC VIEW)

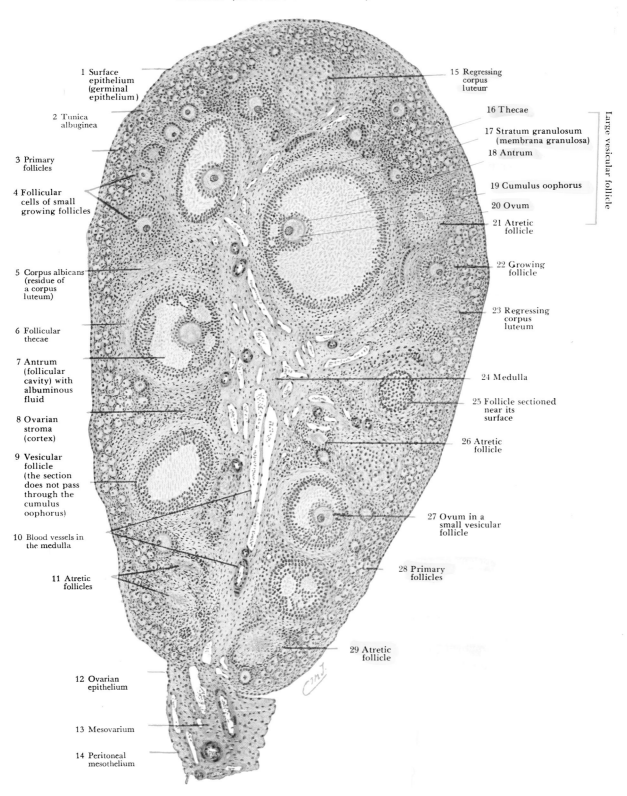

1 Surface epithelium (germinal epithelium)

2 Tunica albuginea

3 Primary follicles

4 Follicular cells of small growing follicles

5 Corpus albicans (residue of a corpus luteum)

6 Follicular thecae

7 Antrum (follicular cavity) with albuminous fluid

8 Ovarian stroma (cortex)

9 Vesicular follicle (the section does not pass through the cumulus oophorus)

10 Blood vessels in the medulla

11 Atretic follicles

12 Ovarian epithelium

13 Mesovarium

14 Peritoneal mesothelium

15 Regressing corpus luteum

16 Thecae

17 Stratum granulosum (membrana granulosa)

18 Antrum

19 Cumulus oophorus

20 Ovum

21 Atretic follicle

Large vesicular follicle

22 Growing follicle

23 Regressing corpus luteum

24 Medulla

25 Follicle sectioned near its surface

26 Atretic follicle

27 Ovum in a small vesicular follicle

28 Primary follicles

29 Atretic follicle

Stain: hematoxylin-eosin. 60×.

—205—

PLATE 97 (Fig. 1)

OVARY: CORTEX, PRIMARY AND GROWING FOLLICLES

The surface epithelium (germinal epithelium) (1), composed of cuboidal cells, covers the ovary. Beneath it lies the tunica albuginea (2), a layer of dense connective tissue (modified stroma).

Numerous primary follicles (5, 6) lie in the outer zone of the ovarian stroma, immediately beneath the tunica albuginea (2). Each follicle consists of an ovum (5) surrounded by a single layer of follicular cells (6).

Intermediate follicles at later stages of development are seen at (7) and (4). In the former (7), the developing ovum is surrounded by a single layer of follicular cells which have become low columnar. In the latter (4), the follicular cells (10) have divided by mitosis (3) to form a a stratified epithelium of large cuboidal or columnar cells around the developing ovum; this epithelium will become the stratum granulosum (membrana granulosa). The innermost layer of the follicular cells is beginning to differentiate to the corona radiata (13); they are more columnar than the other follicular cells. Between the corona radiata and the ovum is the non-cellular zona pellucida (12). Stromal cells have concentrated around the follicular cells to form the follicular theca (9) which will later differentiate into two layers, the theca interna and theca externa. Within the ovum (4) is a large eccentrically placed nucleus (germinal vesicle) (11) with a conspicuous nucleolus (germinal spot).

An atretic follicle (15) is seen, containing the remnants of a disintegrating ovum.

PLATE 97 (Fig. 2)

OVARY: WALL OF A MATURE VESICULAR FOLLICLE

This figure illustrates that part of a mature vesicular follicle which contains the ovum. It is comparable to that area in Plate 96 which contains the ovum in the cumulus oophorus (19, 20) and the wall of the follicle to the left.

The stratum granulosum (membrana granulosa) (6), formed by hypertrophied follicular cells, surrounds and encloses the central cavity or antrum (8) of the follicle. The central cavity (8) is filled with follicular fluid secreted by the follicular and granulosa cells. Smaller isolated intercellular accumulations of follicular fluid may occur (14); these may form rounded vacuoles which stain deeply (Call-Exner vacuoles) (3, 7).

The mass of granulosa cells enclosing the mature ovum (11) projects into the antrum, forming a hillock, the cumulus oophorus (12). The ovum is surrounded by the prominent zona pellucida (10). The corona radiata (9) is now a well-defined, radially arranged layer of columnar cells.

The basal row of granulosa cells rests on a thin basement membrane (5). Surrounding this are the theca interna (4), which is a layer of modified stroma with hypertrophied stromal cells, and the theca externa (2), a layer of concentrated stroma forming an indistinct capsule.

PLATE 97

OVARY

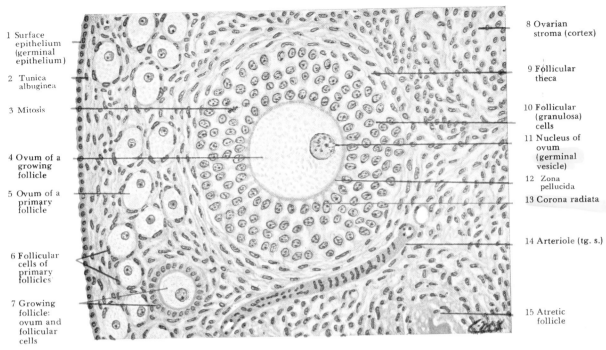

1 Surface epithelium (germinal epithelium)

2 Tunica albuginea

3 Mitosis

4 Ovum of a growing follicle

5 Ovum of a primary follicle

6 Follicular cells of primary follicles

7 Growing follicle: ovum and follicular cells

8 Ovarian stroma (cortex)

9 Follicular theca

10 Follicular (granulosa) cells

11 Nucleus of ovum (germinal vesicle)

12 Zona pellucida

13 Corona radiata

14 Arteriole (tg. s.)

15 Atretic follicle

FIG. 1. *Cortex, primary and growing follicles.*
Stain: hematoxylin-eosin. 320×.

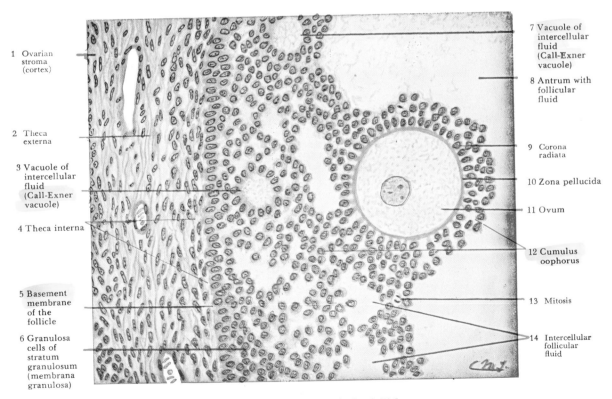

1 Ovarian stroma (cortex)

2 Theca externa

3 Vacuole of intercellular fluid (Call-Exner vacuole)

4 Theca interna

5 Basement membrane of the follicle

6 Granulosa cells of stratum granulosum (membrana granulosa)

7 Vacuole of intercellular fluid (Call-Exner vacuole)

8 Antrum with follicular fluid

9 Corona radiata

10 Zona pellucida

11 Ovum

12 Cumulus oophorus

13 Mitosis

14 Intercellular follicular fluid

FIG. 2. *Wall of a mature vesicular follicle.*
Stain: hematoxylin-eosin. 320×.

PLATE 98

OVARY: CORPORA LUTEA AND ATRETIC FOLLICLES

This plate illustrates a newly formed corpus luteum, corpora lutea in various stages of regression, and several stages of atresia of large follicles.

As in Plate 96, surface epithelium (1) covers the external surface of the ovary; the thin tunica albuginea underlies this. The cortex (2, 18) constitutes the greater part of the ovary; it contains follicles and corpora lutea. The medulla (7) occupies the interior. It contains the larger blood vessels which will distribute to all parts of the cortex.

A few primary follicles (12) are present in the peripheral zone of the cortex. Two small growing follicles (one at 8) without an antrum are seen, and a large vesicular follicle (17) shows its various component parts.

The newly formed corpus luteum (3), resulting from the rupture of the mature follicle and collapse of its wall, is a large structure. Its wall is folded. The thin zone of theca lutein cells (4), formed from the theca interna cells of the follicle, are on the periphery of the corpus luteum and follow along the indentations between the folds. (See Plate 99 for details.) The mass of the wall is granulosa lutein cells (5) formed by hypertrophy of the granulosa cells of the follicle. Connective tissue (fine collagenous fibers and fibroblasts) has proliferated from the theca externa, forming the stroma for abundant capillaries in the wall of the corpus luteum, and is also filling in the former follicular cavity (6).

At (10) is seen a small part of a corpus luteum in moderate regression; the section passes through its wall. The granulosa lutein cells are smaller, nuclei are pyknotic (10a) and larger blood vessels are growing in from the stroma (10b). Theca lutein cells have lost their identity.

A later stage of regression at (16) shows further shrinkage of lutein cells and pyknosis of nuclei (16b), and a fibrous central core (16a). Connective tissue is intermingled with the regressing luteal cells and replaces them as they degenerate. The stroma forms somewhat of a capsule (16c) around this regressing corpus luteum, but this is not a constant feature. When connective tissue has replaced completely all lutein cells, a fibrous or hyalinized scar, the corpus albicans (15) remains.

Vesicular follicles may undergo regressive changes (atresia) at any time before reaching maturity. At (17) is a large normal follicle showing its theca interna (17a) and the thick stratum granulosum (membrana granulosa) (17b), with a thin basement membrane between these two layers. In the cumulus oophorus (17d) is a normal ovum (17e). The antrum (follicular cavity) is filled with follicular fluid (17c).

Atresia of such large follicles is gradual but the series of changes can be followed by noting follicles at different stages in the atretic processes. The follicle at (14) shows very early atretic changes. The theca interna (14a) and membrana granulosa (14b) are intact but some cells of the latter are beginning to slough into the antrum (14e) which still contains follicular fluid (14d). Disruption of the cumulus oophorus has already taken place and degeneration of the ovum is advanced. A remnant of ovum, surrounded by swollen zona pellucida (14c) is seen free in the antrum.

At (13) is a follicle with more advanced, but still early, atresia. The theca interna (13a) is present; its cells are somewhat hypertrophied. The membrana granulosa is no longer present; all of its cells have sloughed off and have been resorbed. The basement membrane between these two layers has thickened and become folded, and is now called the hypertrophied glassy membrane (13b). Loose connective tissue is growing in from the stroma (13e) and has partially filled the reduced cavity (13d) in which follicular fluid (13c) is still present.

With further atresia, stroma replaces the theca interna cells (9a), the hypertrophied glassy membrane (9b) becomes thicker and more folded, and loose connective tissue with small blood vessels completely fills the former antrum (9c). Finally, this, too, is replaced by stroma, but the hypertrophied and folded glassy membrane (11) remains for some time as the only indication of the former follicle.

PLATE 98

OVARY: CORPORA LUTEA AND ATRETIC FOLLICLES

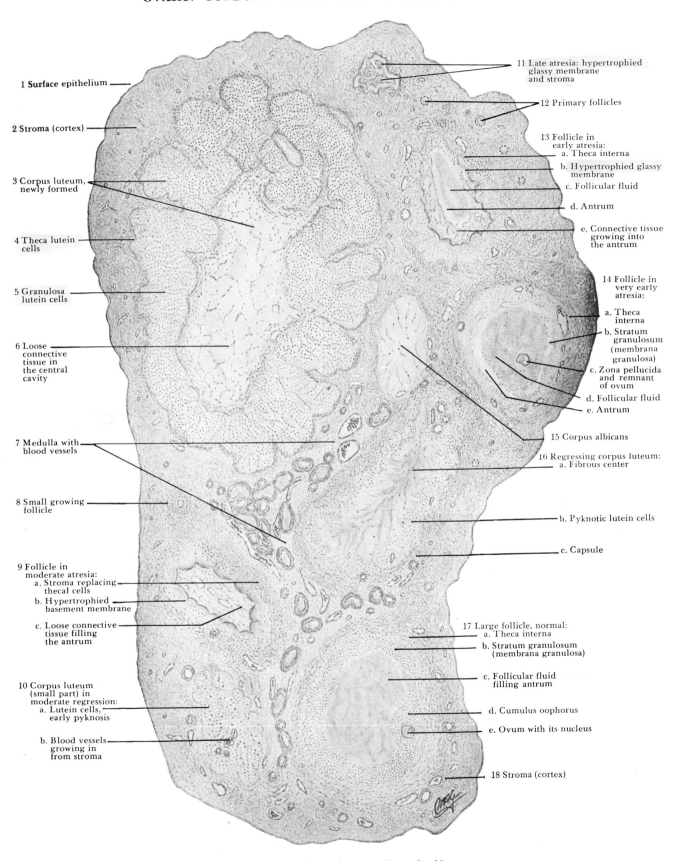

1 **Surface** epithelium

2 Stroma (cortex)

3 Corpus luteum,
newly formed

4 Theca lutein
cells

5 Granulosa
lutein cells

6 Loose
connective
tissue in
the central
cavity

7 Medulla with
blood vessels

8 Small growing
follicle

9 Follicle in
moderate atresia:
a. Stroma replacing
thecal cells
b. Hypertrophied
basement membrane

c. Loose connective
tissue filling
the antrum

10 Corpus luteum
(small part) in
moderate regression:
a. Lutein cells,
early pyknosis

b. Blood vessels
growing in
from stroma

11 Late atresia: hypertrophied
glassy membrane
and stroma

12 Primary follicles

13 Follicle in
early atresia:
a. Theca interna

b. Hypertrophied glassy
membrane

c. Follicular fluid

d. Antrum

e. Connective tissue
growing into
the antrum

14 Follicle in
very early
atresia:

a. Theca
interna

b. Stratum
granulosum
(membrana
granulosa)

c. Zona pellucida
and remnant
of ovum

d. Follicular fluid

e. Antrum

15 Corpus albicans

16 Regressing corpus luteum:
a. Fibrous center

b. Pyknotic lutein cells

c. Capsule

17 Large follicle, normal:
a. Theca interna

b. Stratum granulosum
(membrana granulosa)

c. Follicular fluid
filling antrum

d. Cumulus oophorus

e. Ovum with its nucleus

18 Stroma (cortex)

Human ovary. Stain: hematoxylin-eosin. 80×.

PLATE 99 (Fig. 1)

CORPUS LUTEUM (PANORAMIC VIEW)

In cross-section, the corpus luteum appears as a highly folded thick mass of glandular tissue (3) with a central core consisting of remains of follicular fluid, serum, sometimes a little blood, and loose connective tissue (7–9).

The glandular tissue is made up of anastomosing columns or cords of epithelioid cells (3) consisting principally of granulosa lutein cells (3, upper leader) and peripherally of theca lutein cells (3, lower leader). Theca lutein cells also extend into the depressions between folds of the wall.

Theca externa forms a poorly defined capsule (1) around the developing corpus luteum. From it, or from stroma, thin septa of connective tissue may extend into the depressions between folds (2, 6).

The core of the corpus luteum (the former follicular cavity) is filling in with loose connective tissue which has proliferated from the theca externa and penetrated through the layers of glandular tissue, first forming a covering over the inner surface of the glandular layer (7), then gradually spreading throughout the cavity (8).

The stroma (4) surrounding the corpus luteum is highly vascular (5).

PLATE 99 (Fig. 2)

CORPUS LUTEUM (PERIPHERAL WALL)

Granulosa lutein cells (7) make up the mass of the corpus luteum. These are hypertrophied former granulosa cells of the mature follicle. They are large, lightly stained in part because of lipid inclusions, and have large vesicular nuclei. Theca lutein cells (2), the former theca interna cells, are limited to the periphery of the corpus luteum and the depressions between folds, retaining their position external to the granulosa lutein cells. The cells (2) are smaller than granulosa lutein cells, the granular cytoplasm stains more deeply, nuclei are smaller and darker.

Between the anastomosing columns of lutein cells are numerous capillaries (8), which, together with fine connective tissue, have proliferated inward from the theca externa.

The capsule (5) is poorly defined. The stroma surrounding the corpus luteum is very vascular (1, 3, 4).

PLATE 99

CORPUS LUTEUM

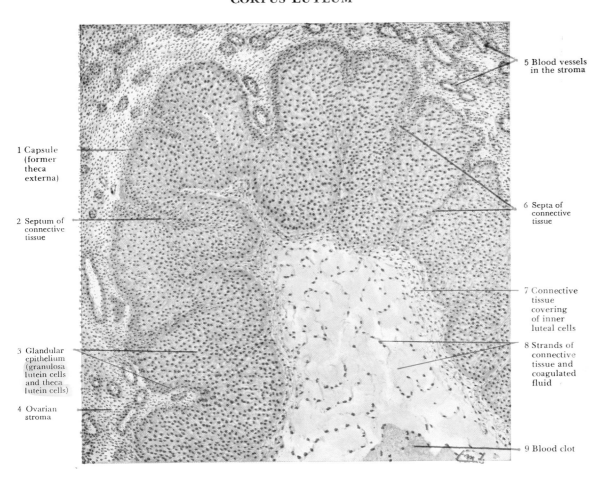

1 Capsule
(former
theca
externa)

2 Septum of
connective
tissue

3 Glandular
epithelium
(granulosa
lutein cells
and theca
lutein cells)

4 Ovarian
stroma

5 Blood vessels
in the stroma

6 Septa of
connective
tissue

7 Connective
tissue
covering
of inner
luteal cells

8 Strands of
connective
tissue and
coagulated
fluid

9 Blood clot

FIG. 1. *Panoramic view.*
Stain: hematoxylin-eosin. 80×.

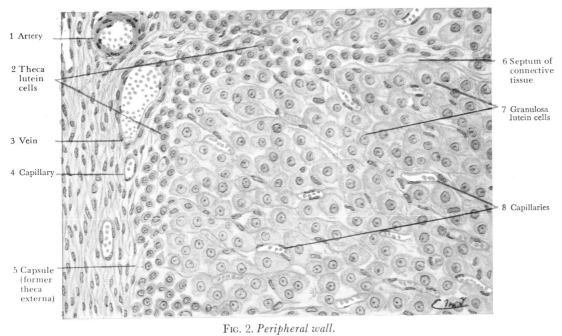

1 Artery

2 Theca
lutein
cells

3 Vein

4 Capillary

5 Capsule
(former
theca
externa)

6 Septum of
connective
tissue

7 Granulosa
lutein cells

8 Capillaries

FIG. 2. *Peripheral wall.*
Stain: hematoxylin-eosin. 250×.

PLATE 100 (Fig. 1)

UTERINE TUBE: AMPULLA (PANORAMIC VIEW, TRANSVERSE SECTION)

Numerous tall, ramified mucosal folds (9) give a highly irregular contour to the lumen of the uterine tube (Fallopian tube). Extensions of the lumen form deep grooves between the folds. The lining epithelium (10) is simple columnar. The lamina propria (8) is well-vascularized loose connective tissue. The muscularis is in two layers, an inner circular layer (1) and an outer longitudinal layer (6). However, interstitial connective tissue (2) is abundant, so that the layering of muscle is not too distinct, especially in the outer layer. Serosa (7) forms the external coat.

PLATE 100 (Fig. 2)

UTERINE TUBE: MUCOSA

The epithelium (1) is composed of ciliated columnar cells (3) and peg-shaped non-ciliated secretory cells (4). The cilia beat toward the uterus. The proportion of these two cell types varies with stages of the menstrual cycle.

The lamina propria (2) is a loose connective tissue, with thin fibers and numerous fibroblasts, many of which have processes and are apparently less differentiated than ordinary fibroblasts. This connective tissue is capable of reacting like the stroma of the uterine endometrium if an incipient embryo becomes inadvertently planted in the wall of the tube; many of the fibroblasts become decidual cells.

—212—

PLATE 100

UTERINE TUBE: AMPULLA

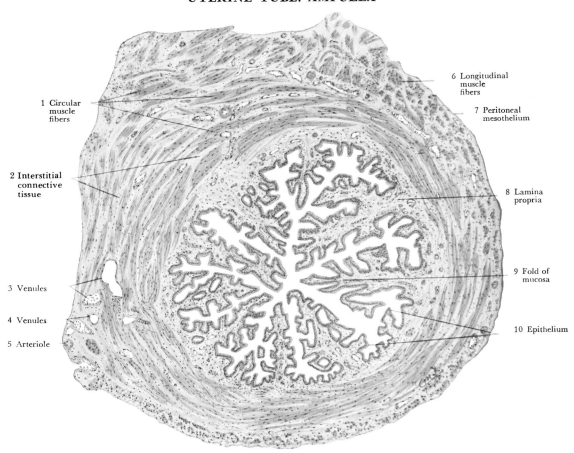

6 Longitudinal muscle fibers

7 Peritoneal mesothelium

1 Circular muscle fibers

2 Interstitial connective tissue

8 Lamina propria

9 Fold of mucosa

3 Venules

4 Venules

5 Arteriole

10 Epithelium

FIG. 1. *Panoramic view.*
Stain: hematoxylin-eosin. 40×.

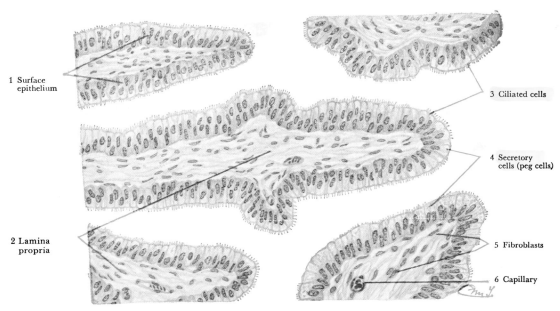

1 Surface epithelium

3 Ciliated cells

4 Secretory cells (peg cells)

2 Lamina propria

5 Fibroblasts

6 Capillary

FIG. 2. *Mucosal folds.*
Stain: hematoxylin-eosin. 320×.

Plate 101

UTERUS: FOLLICULAR (PROLIFERATIVE) PHASE

Cyclic activity of the uterus in non-pregnancy may be divided into three phases: a follicular phase, a progravid or secretory phase and a menstrual phase. The uterine wall, as seen typically during each of these phases, is shown respectively in Plates 101, 102, 103.

The uterine wall consists of three layers: the inner endometrium or mucous membrane (1–4), the middle myometrium or muscularis (5, 6, 12, 13), and the perimetrium or outer serous membrane.

In the endometrium can be distinguished two zones or layers: a narrow, deep layer, the basal stratum or basalis (4, 15), and a wide superficial layer above this, the functional stratum or functionalis (1, 2, 3, 14). The endometrium is composed of a simple columnar secretory epithelium (1) overlying a broad lamina propria (2, 3, 4). Long, tubular glands, the uterine glands (8) are present in the lamina propria. These glands are usually straight in the superficial portion of the endometrium (8), but forked or coiled in the deep portion so that they are seen in cross sections (10). Interglandular stroma (3) is abundant. Cross sections of coiled arteries (9) are seen in the deep layers of the endometrium, but not yet in the superficial layers which contain only veins and capillaries.

The connective tissue or stroma of the endometrium is a "cellular" type, with masses of branching fibroblasts held in a meshwork of reticular fibers and fine collagenous fibers. It is more compact in the basalis (not indicated in this illustration).

The endometrium is firmly attached to the underlying myometrium, which consists of compactly arranged smooth muscle bundles (5, 6, 13), separated by thin partitions of connective tissue (12) and arranged into three poorly defined layers. The myometrium is well supplied with blood vessels (7).

PLATE 101

UTERUS: FOLLICULAR (PROLIFERATIVE) PHASE

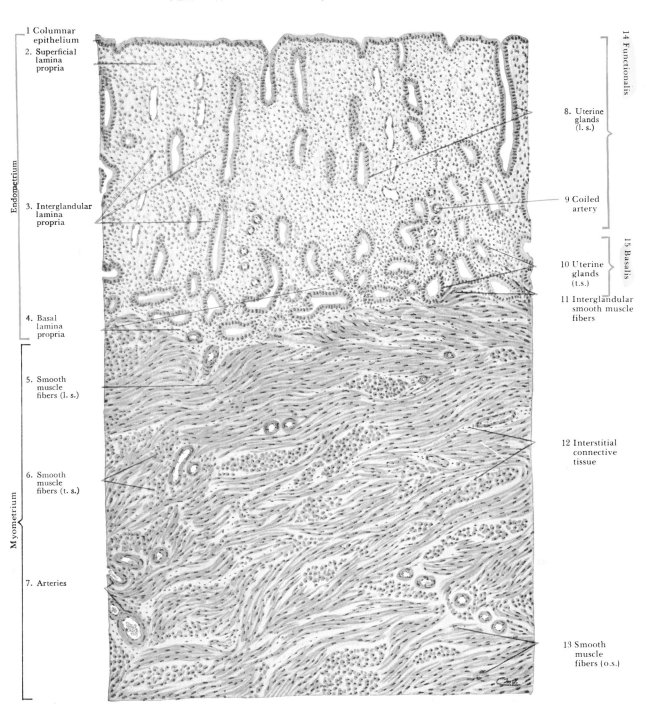

1 Columnar epithelium

2. Superficial lamina propria

Endometrium

3. Interglandular lamina propria

4. Basal lamina propria

5. Smooth muscle fibers (l. s.)

Myometrium

6. Smooth muscle fibers (t. s.)

7. Arteries

14 Functionalis

8. Uterine glands (l. s.)

9 Coiled artery

15 Basalis

10 Uterine glands (t.s.)

11 Interglandular smooth muscle fibers

12 Interstitial connective tissue

13 Smooth muscle fibers (o.s.)

Stain: hematoxylin-eosin. 45×.

PLATE 102

UTERUS: PROGRAVID (SECRETORY) PHASE

During the progravid phase, the endometrium becomes much thicker due largely to the increase in secretory activity of the glands and to edema fluid in the stroma. Cells of the glands have hypertrophied (4) because of the accumulation of large quantities of secretory products. The glands have become tortuous (3, 4, 9), lumens are dilated, and are often filled with secretion (5, 10). In the stroma (8), tissue fluid has increased greatly, causing edema. The coiled arteries (7) have extended throughout the endometrium into its superficial part.

These changes in the glands and stroma take place throughout the greater part of the functionalis layer of the endometrium. Two zones can now be distinguished in the functionalis: a narrow compact stratum or compacta (12) beneath the epithelium, where there is little edema and where the glands are constricted and straight (2), and the wide spongy stratum or spongiosa (13) with changes as described above. In the basal stratum or basalis (11, 14), neither glands nor stroma show much change during the different phases of the menstrual cycle.

PLATE 102

UTERUS: PROGRAVID (SECRETORY) PHASE

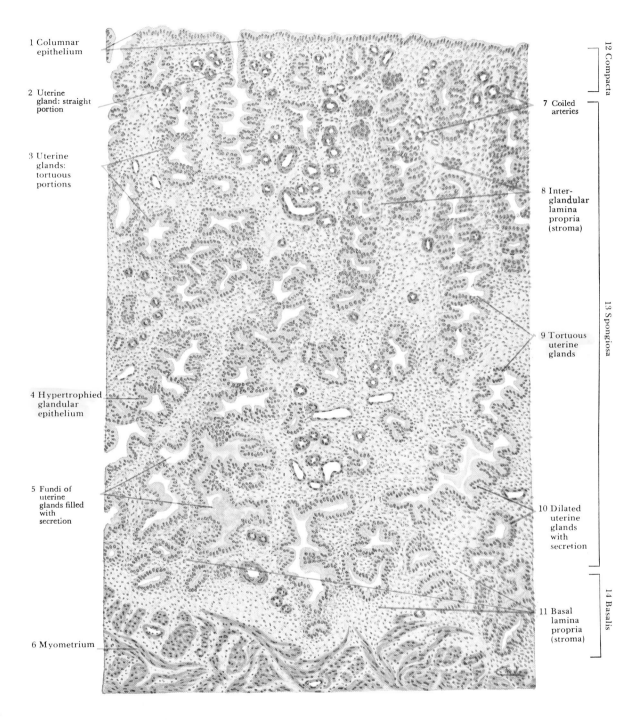

1 Columnar epithelium

2 Uterine gland: straight portion

3 Uterine glands: tortuous portions

4 Hypertrophied glandular epithelium

5 Fundi of uterine glands filled with secretion

6 Myometrium

7 Coiled arteries

8 Inter-glandular lamina propria (stroma)

9 Tortuous uterine glands

10 Dilated uterine glands with secretion

11 Basal lamina propria (stroma)

12 Compacta

13 Spongiosa

14 Basalis

Stain: hematoxylin-eosin. 45×.

PLATE 103

UTERUS: MENSTRUAL PHASE

During the menstrual phase, the surface of the endometrium loses its epithelium (1) and much of the underlying tissue; the eroded surface is covered with blood clots (7) together with fragments of disintegrated stroma (6) and glands. Some of the intact uterine glands are filled with blood (2). In the deeper lamina propria, the fundi of the glands are intact (9).

In the lamina propria of most of the spongiosa region are aggregations of free erythrocytes (8) which have been extruded from the disintegrating blood vessels. There is a moderate infiltration of lymphocytes and neutrophils. The basilar part of the lamina propria remains generally unaffected (4).

Distal portions of the coiled arteries undergo necrosis and only the deeper parts remain (3).

PLATE 103

UTERUS: MENSTRUAL PHASE

1 Superficial endometrium without epithelium

2 Glandular lumen filled with blood

3 Coiled arteries

4 Interglandular lamina propria of basal region

5 Smooth muscle fibers (myometrium)

6 Fragments of disintegrated mucosa

7 Blood clots

8 Erythrocytes in lamina propria

9 Intact fundi of uterine glands

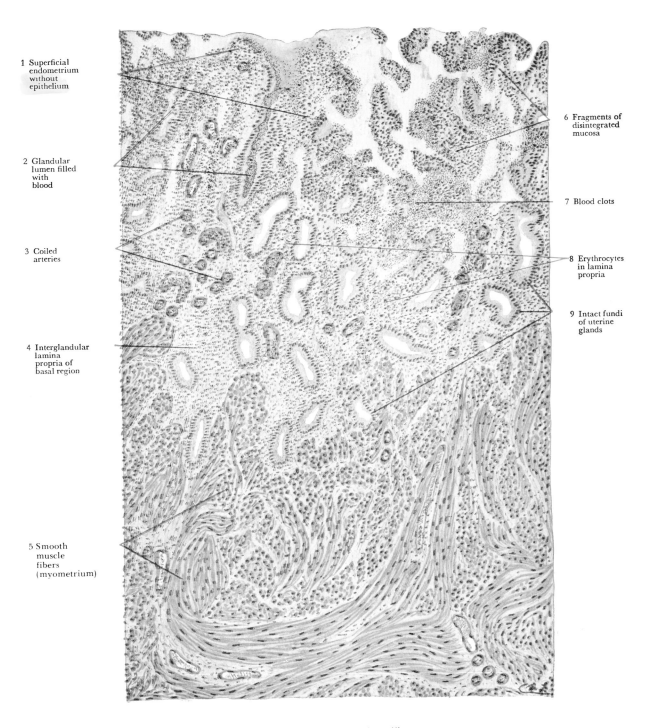

Stain: hematoxylin-eosin. 45X.

PLATE 104

Fig. 1. PLACENTA: FIVE MONTHS' PREGNANCY

The upper part of the plate corresponds to the fetal portion of the placenta (10, 11). The maternal placenta includes the functionalis of the endometrium (12–14) which lies beneath the fetal placenta. Below this is the basal portion of the endometrium, containing the deep parts of the uterine glands (15), which is not sloughed off during parturition. A small area of myometrium (17) is seen in the lower field.

On the upper surface of the section is seen the squamous epithelium of the amnion (1). The layer of connective tissue (2) represents merged connective tissue of the amnion and chorion. Below this is the chorionic plate (3, 10). Details of the trophoblast are not distinguishable at this magnification.

Anchoring villi arising from the chorionic plate (4, upper leaders) extend to the uterine wall and embed in the decidua basalis (7). This continuity is not seen in this plate, but larger units in the fetal placenta probably represent sections of anchoring villi (4, lower leader). These will increase in size and complexity.

Innumerable floating villi are seen (chorion frondosum), sectioned in various planes (5, 11) because of their outgrowth in all directions from the anchoring villi. They "float" in the intervillous spaces (6) which are filled with maternal blood. The structure of these villi is shown in Fig. 2.

The maternal portion of the placenta, or decidua basalis, shows anchoring villi embedded in it (7), groups of large decidual cells (8) as well as typical stroma, distal portions of uterine glands which are in various stages of regression (14) and which usually disappear entirely later, and maternal blood vessels, recognized by their size or by red blood corpuscles in their lumens (9). A maternal blood vessel is seen opening into an intervillous space (13).

Coiled arteries (16) and basal portions of uterine glands (15) are present in the deep zone of the endometrium. Fibrin deposits are seen on the surface of the decidua basalis (12). These will increase in volume and extent.

Fig. 2. CHORIONIC VILLI (PLACENTA AT FIVE MONTHS)

The plate shows several chorionic villi, from the above placenta of a fetus of five months, at a higher magnification. It is seen that the trophoblastic epithelium is composed of an external layer of syncytial cells, the syncytial trophoblast (1) and another deeper layer of well outlined cells, the cytotrophoblast or layer of Langhans (2). In the interior of the villus, which is embryonic connective tissue (3), one finds fetal blood vessels (5) which are branches of umbilical arteries and veins; both nucleated and non-nucleated erythrocytes may be present. Intervillous spaces (4) contain maternal blood, erythrocytes are non-nucleated. One of the villi shown is attached to the endometrium (6). Several decidual cells (7) are seen in the stroma.

Fig. 3. CHORIONIC VILLI (PLACENTA AT TERM)

This plate shows several chorionic villi from a placenta of a fetus at term. In contrast to the villi in Fig. 2, the chorionic epithelium here is present only as syncytial trophoblast (1), whose syncytial character is more pronounced than in Fig. 2. The connective tissue (2) is more differentiated, showing more fibers, fewer typical fibroblasts, and many large, rounded macrophages (Hofbauer cells) (4). Fetal blood vessels are numerous (3), having increased in complexity of branching as pregnancy progressed.

—220—

PLATE 104 . PLACENTA

FIG. 1. PLACENTA: FIVE MONTHS' PREGNANCY
(PANORAMIC VIEW)

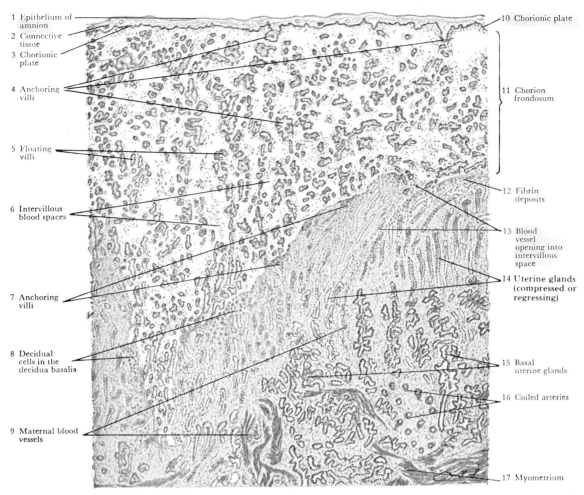

1 Epithelium of amnion
2 Connective tissue
3 Chorionic plate
4 Anchoring villi
5 Floating villi
6 Intervillous blood spaces
7 Anchoring villi
8 Decidual cells in the decidua basalis
9 Maternal blood vessels
10 Chorionic plate
11 Chorion frondosum
12 Fibrin deposits
13 Blood vessel opening into intervillous space
14 Uterine glands (compressed or regressing)
15 Basal uterine glands
16 Coiled arteries
17 Myometrium

Stain: hematoxylin-eosin. 10×.

FIG. 2. CHORIONIC VILLI
(Placenta at Five Months)

FIG. 3. CHORIONIC VILLI
(Placenta at Term)

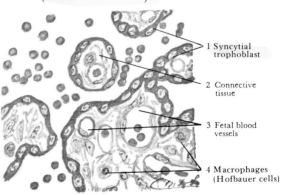

1 Syncytial trophoblast
2 Cytotrophoblast
3 Embryonic connective tissue
4 Intervillous space
5 Fetal blood vessels
6 Attached villus
7 Decidual cell

1 Syncytial trophoblast
2 Connective tissue
3 Fetal blood vessels
4 Macrophages (Hofbauer cells)

Stain: hematoxylin-eosin. 350×.   Stain: hematoxylin-eosin. 350×.

PLATE 105

CERVIX: LONGITUDINAL SECTION

The mucosa of the endocervix (cervix uteri) is lined with tall, mucus-secreting columnar epithelium (1), differing from that lining the body of the uterus with which it is continuous. This type of epithelium also lines the numerous highly branched tubular cervical glands (2) which extend deep into the wide lamina propria (4). The lamina propria is still a "cellular" type of connective tissue as in the body of the uterus, but is becoming more fibrous.

In the lower part of the cervix, at the os cervix (5) or opening of the cervical canal into the vaginal canal, the columnar epithelium changes abruptly to stratified squamous. This continues over the vaginal portion of the cervix, the portio vaginalis (6) and its external wall (8), which lies in the fornix of the vagina. At the base of the fornix (7), the epithelium reflects to continue over the vaginal wall proper.

The muscularis (3, 10) is not as compact as in the body of the uterus and more connective tissue is interspersed. Both muscularis and lamina propria are well vascularized.

PLATE 105

CERVIX (LONGITUDINAL SECTION)

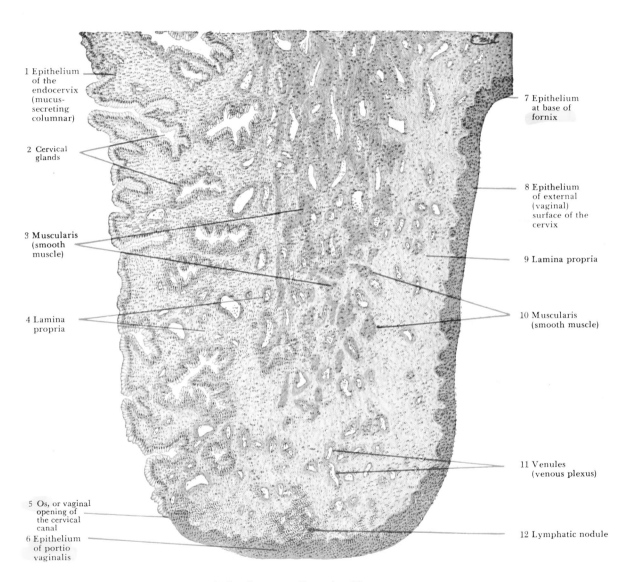

1 Epithelium
of the
endocervix
(mucus-
secreting
columnar)

2 Cervical
glands

3 Muscularis
(smooth
muscle)

4 Lamina
propria

5 Os, or vaginal
opening of
the cervical
canal

6 Epithelium
of portio
vaginalis

7 Epithelium
at base of
fornix

8 Epithelium
of external
(vaginal)
surface of the
cervix

9 Lamina propria

10 Muscularis
(smooth muscle)

11 Venules
(venous plexus)

12 Lymphatic nodule

Stain: hematoxylin-eosin. 20X.

PLATE 106 (Fig. 1)

VAGINA (LONGITUDINAL SECTION)

The mucosa has numerous transverse folds (5). The lining epithelium is non-cornified stratified squamous (1) whose cells are rich in glycogen (see Fig. 2). Connective tissue papillae vary from small ones (2) to tall ones in the posterior wall of the vagina.

The broad lamina propria (4) is moderately dense irregular connective tissue with excessive elastic fibers; however, it is looser in the deeper area and extensions from it pass into the muscularis. Diffuse lymphatic tissue is usually present under the epithelium, and lymphatic nodules (3) may occur. Small blood vessels are numerous throughout the lamina propria.

The muscularis is made up predominantly of longitudinal (6) and obliquely (8) arranged bundles of muscle fibers. Circular fibers (10) are less numerous and more frequently found in the inner layers. Interstitial connective tissue is rich in elastic fibers.

In the adventitia (7) are numerous veins (9) (part of a large venous plexus), as well as other blood vessels.

PLATE 106 (Fig. 2)

GLYCOGEN IN HUMAN VAGINAL EPITHELIUM

Glycogen is a prominent component of the cells in the vaginal epithelium, except in the deepest layers, where normally there is little or none. It accumulates during the follicular phase, reaching its maximum just before ovulation. It can be demonstrated by the use of iodine vapor, or iodine solution in mineral oil (Mancini's method). Glycogen stains a reddish-purple.

Figures (a) and (b) were similarly prepared by fixation in absolute alcohol and formaldehyde. In (a), one sees the amount of glycogen present during the interfollicular phase of the cycle. In (b), during the follicular phase, the amount of glycogen is increased, especially in the intermediate layers, but extending also into the more superficial cells.

Figure (c), from the same specimen as (b), but fixed by the Altmann-Gersch method (freezing and drying in a vacuum) with less shrinkage of tissue, shows that glycogen is abundant during the follicular phase, and that it is distributed diffusely throughout the cytoplasm.

PLATE 106
Fig. 1. VAGINA (LONGITUDINAL SECTION)

1 Stratified
  squamous
  epithelium

2 Papillae in the
  superficial layer
  of the lamina
  propria

3 Lymphatic
  nodule

4 Lamina
  propria

5 Folds of
  the mucosa

6 Longitudinal
  bundles
  of smooth
  muscle
  fibers

7 Adventitia

8 Oblique
  bundles of
  smooth
  muscle
  fibers

9 Veins and
  artery

10 Transverse
   bundles of
   muscle
   fibers

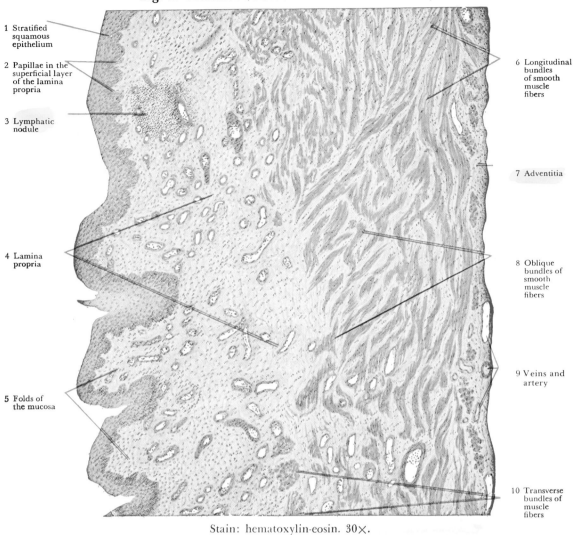

Stain: hematoxylin-eosin. 30×.

Fig. 2. GLYCOGEN IN HUMAN VAGINAL EPITHELIUM

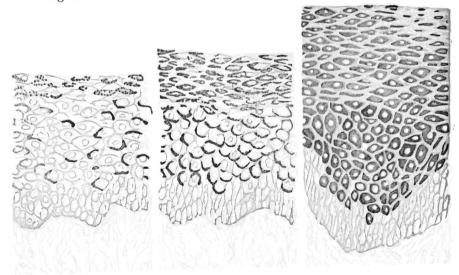

a. Interfollicular phase.   b. Follicular phase.   c. Follicular phase.

Stain: Mancini's iodine technique.

PLATE 107

VAGINA: EXFOLIATE CYTOLOGY

This plate shows smears, from vaginal material obtained by suction, on different days of the menstrual cycle of a normal woman, and also smears obtained during the early months of pregnancy and during menopause. The Shorr trichrome stain employed (Biebrich scarlet, Orange G and Fast Green) plus Harris hematoxylin, facilitates recognition of the different cellular types.

Fig. 7 presents individual cell types. At (a) is a superficial acidophil of the vaginal mucosa. It is flat, somewhat irregular in outline, is from 35 to 65 μ in diameter, has a small pyknotic nucleus, and ample cytoplasm tinted an orange color. At (b) is a similar superficial basophil with bluish-green cytoplasm. At (c) is an intermediate cell from the intermediate stratum of the vaginal epithelium. It is flattened like the superficial cells, but smaller (20 to 40 μ), and has a basophilic blue green-cytoplasm. Its nucleus is somewhat larger and often vesicular. Cells at (d) are intermediate cells in profile (navicular cells), characterized by their elongated form with folded borders and an elongated nucleus placed eccentrically. At (e) are represented cells of the deep layers of the vaginal epithelium, the basal cells. The larger ones, considered to be the more superficial cells, are called parabasal cells. All are rounded or oval, from 12 to 15 μ in diameter, and have a relatively large nucleus with a more prominent chromatin network. Most of them are basophilic.

Fig. 1 represents a vaginal smear from the 5th day of the menstrual cycle (post menstrual phase). In predominance are intermediate cells (1) from the outer layers of the intermediate stratum (transitions to the deeper superficial cells). A few superficial acidophils and basophils (2) and a few leucocytes are also present.

Fig. 2, a smear from the 14th day of the cycle (ovulatory stage), is characterized by predominance of large superficial acidophils (8), the scarcity of superficial basophils (10) and intermediate cells (9), and the absence of leucocytes. It is the expression of the high estrogenic level achieved by the time of ovulation, and is therefore called the "follicular type" smear. The superficial cells "mature" with increase in estrogen and become acidophilic. This same type of smear can be obtained from a menopausic patient when she is under intensive estrogenic treatment.

Fig. 3, from the 21st day of the cycle, represents the luteal stage (progestational stage), under the influence of high levels of progesterone and diminished estrogens. In predominance are large intermediate cells (precornified superficial cells) with folded borders (3) which aggregate into groups. Superficial acidophils (4), superficial basophils (5) and leucocytes are scarce.

Fig. 4 represents the premenstrual stage on the 28th day of the cycle, characterized by the great predominance of intermediate cells with folded borders (13, 14) which tend to form groups (14), by an increase in neutrophils (12), a scarcity of superficial cells (11), and by an abundance of mucus which gives a blurred aspect to these preparations.

Fig. 5, from a 3 months' pregnancy, shows predominantly intermediate cells of the navicular type, many with folded borders (6). Typically these form dense groups or conglomerations (7). Superficial cells and neutrophils are very scarce.

Fig. 6. The smear during menopause is quite different from all others. In a typical "atrophic" smear, the dominant cells are the rounded or oval basal cells of varied diameters (17). Intermediate cells are scarce (15), neutrophils are abundant (16). However, menopausal smears will vary, depending on the stage of menopause and the estrogen levels present.

Vaginal exfoliate cytology is correlated with the ovarian cycle. Its study permits recognition of the degree of follicular activity, whether normally or after estrogenic or other therapy, and provides information (together with cells from the endocervix) for the recognition of regional malignant processes.

PLATE 107

VAGINA: EXFOLIATE CYTOLOGY (VAGINAL SMEARS)

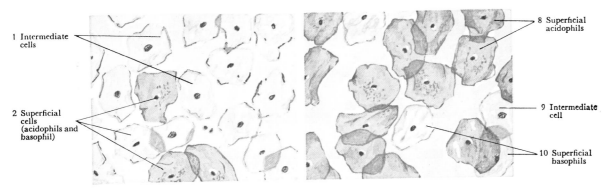

1 Intermediate cells

2 Superficial cells (acidophils and basophil)

8 Superficial acidophils

9 Intermediate cell

10 Superficial basophils

FIG. 1. *Post-menstrual phase, 5th day of normal cycle.*

FIG. 2. *Ovulatory phase, 14th day.*

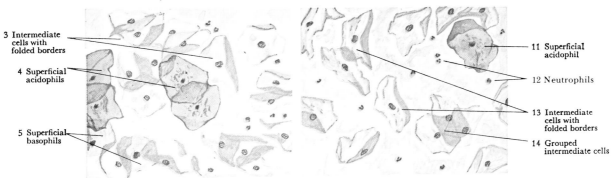

3 Intermediate cells with folded borders

4 Superficial acidophils

5 Superficial basophils

11 Superficial acidophil

12 Neutrophils

13 Intermediate cells with folded borders

14 Grouped intermediate cells

FIG. 3. *Luteal phase, 21st day.*

FIG. 4. *Premenstrual phase, 28th day.*

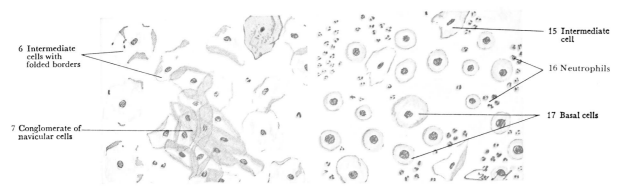

6 Intermediate cells with folded borders

7 Conglomerate of navicular cells

15 Intermediate cell

16 Neutrophils

17 Basal cells

FIG. 5. *Three months' pregnancy.*

FIG. 6. *Menopause, atrophic phase.*

a Superficial acidophil b Superficial basophil c Intermediate cell d Intermediate (navicular) cell in profile e Basal and parabasal cells: basophils and an acidophil

FIG. 7. *Types of cells found in vaginal smears of a normal cycle.*

Stain: Shorr's trichrome. 250 × and 450 ×.

PLATE 108 (Fig. 1)

MAMMARY GLAND, INACTIVE

In the inactive mammary gland, connective tissue is abundant and glandular elements are minimal. Lobes and lobules are not well defined.

The glandular elements consist of groups of potential secretory tubules (3, 10) lined with cuboidal or low columnar epithelium. These are intralobular ducts with perhaps inactive alveoli at their terminal ends. Rarely is it possible to distinguish between ducts and alveoli. An occasional tubule lined with smaller cells may indicate a duct (6), or a tubule may be seen emerging from a lobule (8) to join an interlobular duct. Tubules may be present in an indifferentiated form as solid cords of cells (5).

The tubules are surrounded by a loose, fine-fibered, vascular connective tissue with numerous fibroblasts, the intralobular connective tissue (4). Between the lobules are masses of dense collagenous fibers, the interlobular connective tissue (2) in which adipose tissue is usually present (11).

PLATE 108 (Fig. 2)

MAMMARY GLAND DURING THE FIRST HALF OF PREGNANCY

Growth of secretory tubules with continued branchings of their terminal ends continues throughout the first half of pregnancy. Alveoli differentiate at the ends of the ducts but it is still difficult to distinguish intralobular ducts from alveoli (9, 6). Most of the alveoli are empty (6) but secretion is present in some (5).

The loose intralobular connective tissue (7) enables the continued expansion of the ducts and alveoli. In addition to numerous fibroblasts, other cells appear in increasing numbers, mainly lymphocytes, plasma cells and eosinophils.

The lobules become more apparent (1) and stand out distinctly in contrast to their indistinctness in the inactive gland. The dense interlobular connective tissue (3) now appears as septa between the lobules of glandular tissue. Interlobular ducts (4), lined with columnar cells, course in these septa. These empty into large lactiferous ducts (8), lined usually with low pseudostratified columnar epithelium. Each lactiferous duct collects the secretions of a lobe.

PLATE 108

MAMMARY GLAND

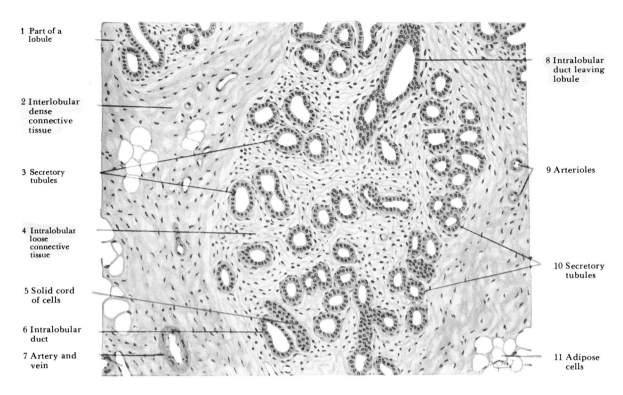

1 Part of a
lobule

2 Interlobular
dense
connective
tissue

3 Secretory
tubules

4 Intralobular
loose
connective
tissue

5 Solid cord
of cells

6 Intralobular
duct

7 Artery and
vein

8 Intralobular
duct leaving
lobule

9 Arterioles

10 Secretory
tubules

11 Adipose
cells

Fig. 1. *Mammary gland, inactive.*
Stain: hematoxylin-eosin. 90×.

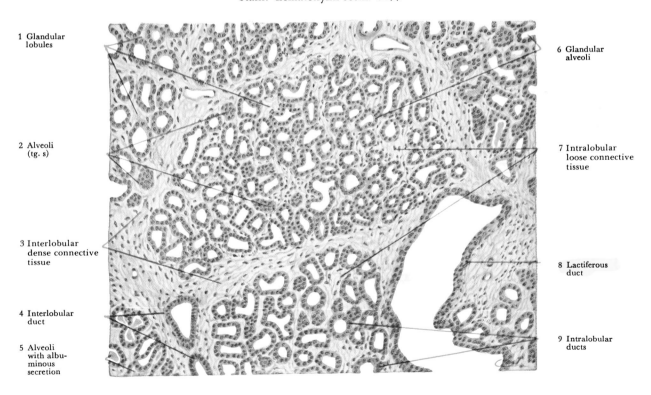

1 Glandular
lobules

2 Alveoli
(tg. s)

3 Interlobular
dense connective
tissue

4 Interlobular
duct

5 Alveoli
with albu-
minous
secretion

6 Glandular
alveoli

7 Intralobular
loose connective
tissue

8 Lactiferous
duct

9 Intralobular
ducts

Fig. 2. *Mammary gland during the first half of pregnancy.*
Stain: hematoxylin-eosin. 90×.

PLATE 109 (Fig. 1)

MAMMARY GLAND, SEVENTH MONTH OF PREGNANCY

The general features of a mammary gland of pregnancy are similar to those illustrated on Plate 108, Fig. 2.

At seven months, alveoli are expanding and cells are becoming secretory (1), so secretion is often seen in the alveolar lumens. Intralobular ducts also secrete (6) so distinction between alveoli and ducts continues to be difficult. Occasionally a fortuitous section shows rounded alveoli (7) opening into an elongated duct (6).

Further relative reduction is seen in the amount of intralobular connective tissue (3) within the lobules and interlobular connective tissue (5). In the latter are seen interlobular ducts (2) and a lactiferous duct (4) with secretion in its lumen.

PLATE 109 (Fig. 2)

MAMMARY GLAND DURING LACTATION

General structures illustrated are as in Fig. 1.

The principal differences here are the various sizes and irregular shapes of the alveoli (1, 3) and the presence of secretion in most of the lumens. All alveoli are not in the same state of activity at the same time. Some are storing secretion in their cells (8); the cells are large, broad and contain vacuoles due to removal of fat droplets during section preparation. Others may be in a resting state (7); the epithelium is low cuboidal, the cells having been reduced in size when the secretory products in their apical portions were released into the lumen of the alveolus.

PLATE 109

MAMMARY GLAND

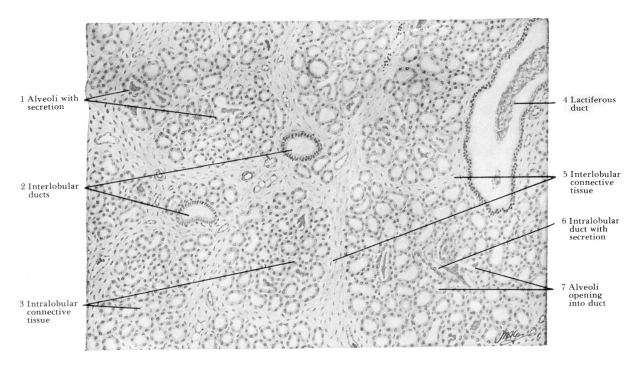

1 Alveoli with secretion

4 Lactiferous duct

2 Interlobular ducts

5 Interlobular connective tissue

6 Intralobular duct with secretion

3 Intralobular connective tissue

7 Alveoli opening into duct

FIG. 1. *Mammary gland, seventh month of pregnancy.* Stain: hematoxylin-eosin. 90×.

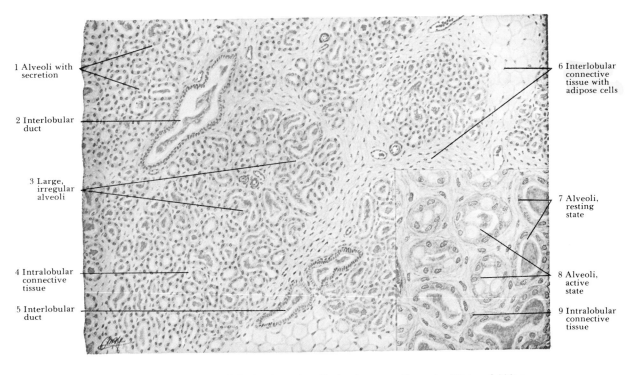

1 Alveoli with secretion

6 Interlobular connective tissue with adipose cells

2 Interlobular duct

3 Large, irregular alveoli

7 Alveoli, resting state

4 Intralobular connective tissue

8 Alveoli, active state

5 Interlobular duct

9 Intralobular connective tissue

FIG. 2. *Mammary gland during lactation.* Stain: hematoxylin-eosin. 90× and 200×.

PLATE 110

EYELID (SAGITTAL SECTION)

The outer layer of the eyelid is seen at the left; the inner layer, which is adjacent to the eyeball, is at the right.

The outer layer is thin skin, and is therefore covered by stratified squamous epithelium (3) which has some papillae. In the dermis (3) are small hair follicles (1, 4), small sebaceous glands and sweat glands (2).

The inner layer is a mucous membrane, the palpebral conjunctiva (17). The epithelium is a low stratified columnar type (14) with goblet cells scattered among the superficial cells. The stratified squamous epithelium of the skin continues over the margin of the eyelid and a transition is made to the stratified columnar epithelium. The thin lamina propria of the palpebral conjunctiva (17) is fine dense, connective tissue. Beneath this is a plate of dense fibrous tissue, the tarsus (16), in which are embedded tarsal glands (Meibomian glands) (15). These are specialized sebaceous glands; the alveoli open into a long central duct (18) which courses parallel to the conjunctival surface.

At the free end of the lid are the eyelashes, arising from large, long hair follicles (20). Sebaceous glands (of Zeiss) (9) accompany these. Large sweat glands, the ciliary glands (of Moll) (8), are present between the hair follicles.

Three sets of muscle fibers are present in the eyelid: the extensive palpebral part of the orbicularis oculi muscle (5) which is skeletal muscle; the skeletal ciliary muscle (of Riolan) (19) in the region of the hair follicles of the eyelashes and the tarsal glands; and the smooth superior tarsal muscle (of Müller) (10).

The accessory lacrimal gland (of Krause) (12) lies in connective tissue beneath the conjunctiva of the fornix. Diffuse lymphatic tissue (13) is prevalent in this region. Other small accessory tarsal lacrimal glands (of Wolfring) lie in connective tissue above the tarsal plate. They are scattered and vary in number, thus are not necessarily present in every section.

PLATE 110

EYELID (SAGITTAL SECTION)

1 Hair follicles

2 Sweat glands

3 Epidermis
and dermis

4 Rudimentary
hair follicle

5 Palpebral
part of
orbicularis
oculi muscle

6 Connective
tissue

7 Arteriole

8 Ciliary glands:
large sweat
glands
(of Moll)

9 Sebaceous
glands
(of Zeiss)

10 Superior tarsal
muscle (of Müller)

11 Adipose tissue

12 Accessory lac-
crimal gland
(of Krause)

13 Lymphatic tissue

14 Epithelium of
palpebral
conjunctiva

15 Tarsal glands
(Meibomian glands)

16 Tarsus

17 Palpebral
conjunctiva

18 Duct of tarsal
gland
(Meibomian gland)

19 Ciliary muscle
(of Riolan)

20 Hair follicles
of eyelashes

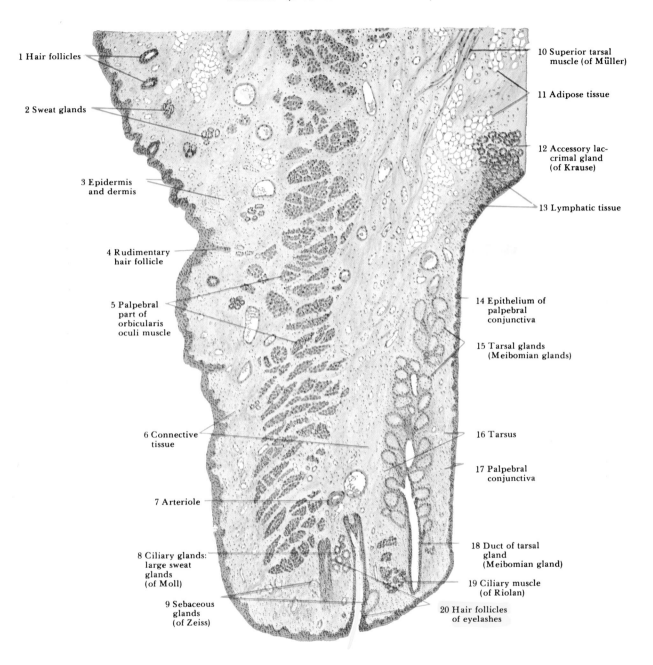

Stain: hematoxylin-eosin. 20×.

PLATE 111 (Fig. 1)

LACRIMAL GLAND

The lacrimal gland is a group of tubuloalveolar glands. The alveoli (1, 8) vary in size and shape. They resemble serous alveoli but their lumens are larger than in typical serous alveoli and there may be irregular outpocketings of cells (5) projecting into them. The cells are more columnar than pyramidal. They contain large secretion granules and lipid droplets and stain lightly. Myoepithelial cells (basal or basket cells) (3) are present.

The smaller intralobular excretory ducts (2, lower leader) are lined with simple cuboidal or columnar epithelium. The larger ones (2, upper leader) and interlobular ducts (7, 11) are lined with two layered low columnar or pseudostratified columnar epithelium.

Interalveolar (intralobular) connective tissue (9) is sparse but interlobular connective tissue (4) is abundant and may contain adipose tissue.

PLATE 111 (Fig. 2)

CORNEA (TRANSVERSE SECTION)

The anterior surface of the cornea is covered with non-papillated stratified squamous epithelium (1, 6, 7). Its lowest layer of columnar cells rests on a typical basement membrane. This is adjacent to a thick, structureless, homogenous anterior limiting membrane (Bowman's membrane) (2) derived from the underlying corneal stroma or substantia propria (3). The corneal stroma forms the body of the cornea. It consists of parallel bundles of collagenous fibrils termed lamellae (9) and rows or layers of flattened, branching corneal cells (8) between the bundles. The corneal cells are modified fibroblasts.

The posterior surface of the cornea is covered with a very low cuboidal epithelium, the posterior epithelium (5, 10). Its basement membrane, the posterior limiting membrane (Descemet's membrane) (4), is unusually wide. It rests on the posterior portion of the corneal stroma.

PLATE 111

FIG. 1. LACRIMAL GLAND

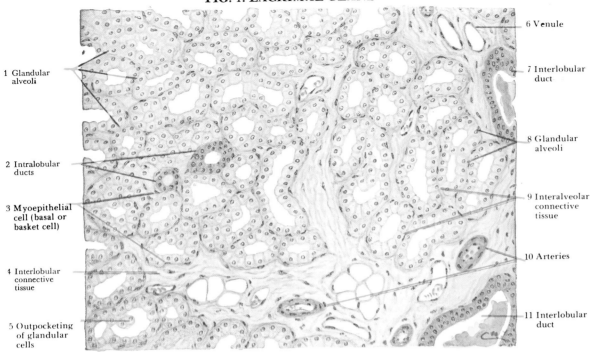

1 Glandular alveoli

2 Intralobular ducts

3 Myoepithelial cell (basal or basket cell)

4 Interlobular connective tissue

5 Outpocketing of glandular cells

6 Venule

7 Interlobular duct

8 Glandular alveoli

9 Interalveolar connective tissue

10 Arteries

11 Interlobular duct

Stain: hematoxylin-eosin. 180×.

FIG. 2. CORNEA (TRANSVERSE SECTION)

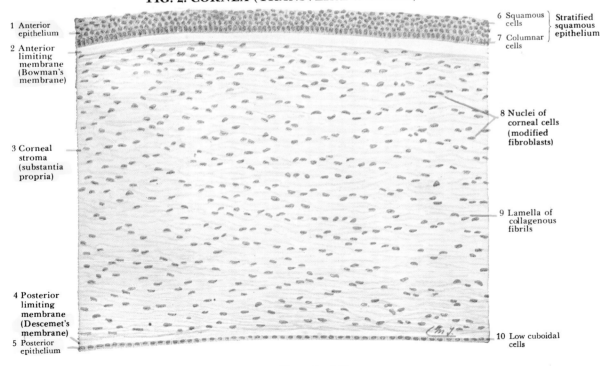

1 Anterior epithelium

2 Anterior limiting membrane (Bowman's membrane)

3 Corneal stroma (substantia propria)

4 Posterior limiting membrane (Descemet's membrane)

5 Posterior epithelium

6 Squamous cells } Stratified squamous epithelium

7 Columnar cells

8 Nuclei of corneal cells (modified fibroblasts)

9 Lamella of collagenous fibrils

10 Low cuboidal cells

Stain: hematoxylin-eosin. 180×.

PLATE 112

EYE (SAGITTAL SECTION)

The capsule of the eye can be divided for descriptive purposes into: a) an outer fibrous tunic, composed of the cornea (1) and the sclera (3, 23); b) a middle vascular layer, the uvea, composed of the choroid (8, 21), the ciliary body (4, 17) and the iris (15); and c) an inner tunic, the retina (7, 18, 20).

The cornea (1) is transparent. Histological details of its structure are shown on Plate 111, Fig. 2.

The sclera (3, 23) is white, opaque, and composed of densely woven collagenous fibers. It is this portion of the capsule which lends rigidity to the eye and appears as the "white" of the eye in situ. The junction of cornea and sclera is the corneal limbus (13). The point at which the optic nerve (27) emerges from the ocular capsule marks the site of continuation of the sclera (9) with the dura mater (11).

The choroid (8, 21) and ciliary body of the uvea lie sub-adjacent to the sclera. When viewed in sagittal section, the ciliary body is triangular in shape. It is composed of the ciliary muscle (4) and the ciliary processes (17). Smooth muscle fibers constitute the ciliary muscle and are disposed in longitudinal, circular, and radial directions. The folded and highly vascularized inward extension of the ciliary body constitutes the ciliary processes (17). To these processes is attached the suspensory ligament of the lens (5), also termed the ciliary zonule (zonule of Zinn). Contraction of the ciliary muscle results in reduction of tension on the suspensory ligament, thus allowing the lens (6) to become more convex.

The iris (15) is the colored portion of the eye as seen in situ. Its circular and radial arrangement of smooth muscle fibers forms the pupil. The anterior chamber (12) lies between the iris and cornea. The posterior chamber (16) lies between the iris and lens. Aqueous humor fills both the anterior and posterior chambers. Behind the lens is the vitreous chamber (22), filled with a gelatinous substance, the vitreous humor.

The inner tunic, or retina (7, 18, 20), is not light receptive throughout. In an anterior hemisection of the eyeball, the posterior rim of the ciliary body appears scalloped. This edge is termed the ora serrata (19). Posterior to the ora serrata is the optic retina (7, 20). It is composed of numerous layers, among which is the layer of light receptive cells, the rods and cones (cf. Plate 113, Fig. 2). Anterior to the ora serrata is the blind retina. As a simplified pigment layer it extends to the tip of the iris. The section of blind retina which is adjacent to the ciliary body is the ciliary retina (18), and that adjacent to the iris is the iridial retina (not labelled).

On the posterior wall of the optic retina lie two landmarks, the macula lutea (25) and the optic papilla (26). In an enucleated eye the macula lutea is a greenish-yellow spot, varying in diameter from 1.05 to 5 mm. A depression in its center marks the fovea centralis, the area of keenest vision. The center of the fovea is devoid of rods and blood vessels but possesses an abundance of cones.

The optic papilla (26) is the site of exit of the optic nerve. This area lacks both rods and cones; hence it constitutes the "blind spot" of the eye.

More extensive histological details of the optic retina are given on Plate 113.

The outer limit of the sclera is contiguous with a spongy mass of orbital fatty tissue (24), composed of loose connective tissue, fat cells, nerves, blood and lymphatic vessels, and glands.

PLATE 112

EYE (SAGITTAL SECTION)

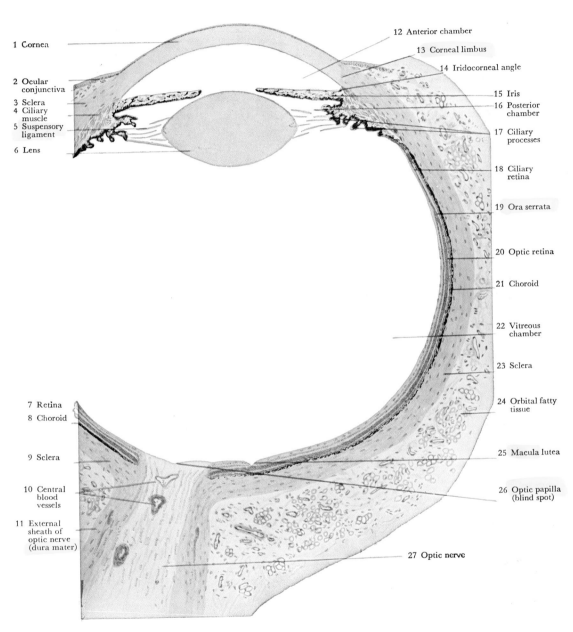

1 Cornea

2 Ocular
conjunctiva

3 Sclera
4 Ciliary
muscle
5 Suspensory
ligament

6 Lens

7 Retina

8 Choroid

9 Sclera

10 Central
blood
vessels

11 External
sheath of
optic nerve
(dura mater)

12 Anterior chamber

13 Corneal limbus

14 Iridocorneal angle

15 Iris

16 Posterior
chamber

17 Ciliary
processes

18 Ciliary
retina

19 Ora serrata

20 Optic retina

21 Choroid

22 Vitreous
chamber

23 Sclera

24 Orbital fatty
tissue

25 Macula lutea

26 Optic papilla
(blind spot)

27 Optic nerve

Stain: hematoxylin-eosin. 15×.

PLATE 113 (Fig. 1)

RETINA, CHOROID AND SCLERA (PANORAMIC VIEW)

For most of its extent, the wall of the eyeball is composed of three coats, the sclera (1), the choroid (2) and the retina (3).

Only the deeper part of the sclera (1) is illustrated. The stroma is composed of dense collagenous fibers (4) coursing in various directions parallel to the surface of the eyeball, and fine elastic networks. Flattened fibroblasts are present throughout and chromatophores (5) are in the deepest layer.

Layers of the choroid are described below.

The human retina has been divided into ten layers except in specialized areas. These are listed in order in the illustration (7–16).

PLATE 113 (Fig. 2)

LAYERS OF THE CHOROID AND RETINA IN DETAIL

The choroid is subdivided into the following layers: the suprachoroid (17), the vessel layer or vascular layer (18), the choriocapillary layer (19) and the transparent limiting membrane, the lamina vitrea or glassy membrane (Bruch's membrane).

The suprachoroid (17) consists of lamellae of fine collagenous fibers with networks of elastic fibers, fibroblasts and numerous large chromatophores. The vessel or vascular layer (18) contains the larger blood vessels (1). In the loose connective tissue stroma between the vessels are numerous large slender chromatophores (2). The choriocapillary layer (19) contains a network of large-lumened capillaries in a stroma of fine collagenous and elastic fibers. The lamina vitrea or glassy membrane, the innermost layer of the choroid, lies adjacent to the pigment epithelium of the retina (3).

The outermost layer of the retina is the pigment epithelium (3). Its basement membrane forms the innermost layer of the glassy membrane of the choroid. Its cuboidal cells contain pigment in the inner apical parts of the cells; processes with pigment granules extend into the layer of rods and cones (20).

Next is a layer of slender rods (4, 22) and thicker cones (5, 21), followed by the outer limiting membrane (6, 23) which is formed by processes of the distinctive neuroglia cells, Müller's cells (30).

The outermost nuclear layer contains nuclei of the rods (8, 25) and cones (7, 24) and the outer processes of Müller's cells (26). In the outer plexiform layer (9), the axons of the rods and cones synapse with dendrites of bipolar cells (28) and horizontal cells (27).

The inner nuclear layer (10) contains the nuclei of bipolar cells (29), horizontal cells and amacrine cells (31) both of which are association cells, and the nuclei of the neuroglial Müller's cells (30). In the inner plexiform layer (11), the axons of bipolar cells (29) synapse (32) with the dendrites of the ganglion cells and amacrine cells.

The ganglion cell layer (12) contains large, multipolar neuron cell bodies (33) and scattered neuroglia cells. Dendrites of the ganglion cells extend into the inner plexiform layer to synapse (32).

The nerve fiber layer (14) contains the vertically and horizontally directed axons of the ganglion cells and the inner fiber network of Müller's cells (37). Axons of the ganglion cells (14, 33) course toward the optic disc where they converge to form the optic nerve. The terminations of the inner fibers of Müller's cells expand to form the inner limiting membrane (15, 36) of the retina.

Blood vessels of the retina course in the nerve fiber layer. They penetrate as deep as the inner nuclear layer (10). Some can be seen (unlabeled) in this layer.

PLATE 113

RETINA, CHOROID AND SCLERA

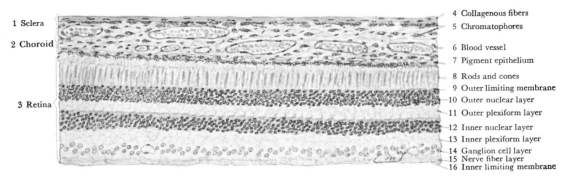

1 Sclera

2 Choroid

3 Retina

4 Collagenous fibers
5 Chromatophores

6 Blood vessel
7 Pigment epithelium

8 Rods and cones
9 Outer limiting membrane
10 Outer nuclear layer
11 Outer plexiform layer
12 Inner nuclear layer
13 Inner plexiform layer
14 Ganglion cell layer
15 Nerve fiber layer
16 Inner limiting membrane

FIG. 1. *Panoramic view.*
Stain: hematoxylin-eosin. 130×.

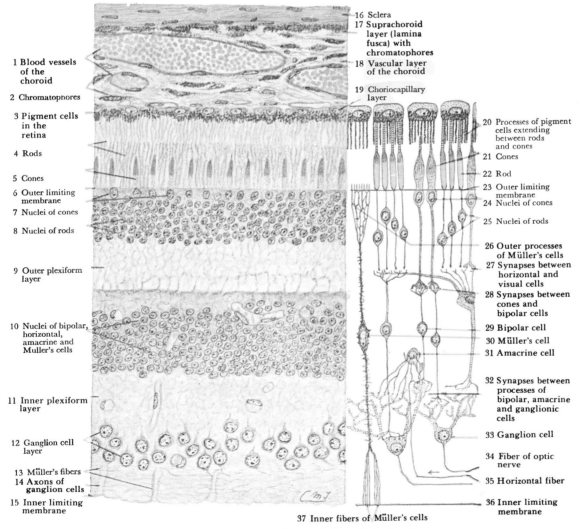

1 Blood vessels
of the
choroid

2 Chromatophores

3 Pigment cells
in the
retina

4 Rods

5 Cones

6 Outer limiting
membrane

7 Nuclei of cones

8 Nuclei of rods

9 Outer plexiform
layer

10 Nuclei of bipolar,
horizontal,
amacrine and
Muller's cells

11 Inner plexiform
layer

12 Ganglion cell
layer

13 Müller's fibers
14 Axons of
ganglion cells

15 Inner limiting
membrane

16 Sclera
17 Suprachoroid
layer (lamina
fusca) with
chromatophores
18 Vascular layer
of the choroid

19 Choriocapillary
layer

20 Processes of pigment
cells extending
between rods
and cones
21 Cones

22 Rod

23 Outer limiting
membrane
24 Nuclei of cones

25 Nuclei of rods

26 Outer processes
of Müller's cells
27 Synapses between
horizontal and
visual cells
28 Synapses between
cones and
bipolar cells

29 Bipolar cell

30 Müller's cell

31 Amacrine cell

32 Synapses between
processes of
bipolar, amacrine
and ganglionic
cells

33 Ganglion cell

34 Fiber of optic
nerve

35 Horizontal fiber

36 Inner limiting
membrane

37 Inner fibers of Müller's cells

FIG. 2. *Layers of the retina and choroid in detail.*

Stain: hematoxylin-eosin. 400×.

PLATE 114 (Fig. 1)

INNER EAR: COCHLEA (VERTICAL SECTION)

A bony tube, the osseous canal of the cochlea, (16, 18) is twisted in a spiral around a central axis of spongy bone, the modiolus (17). The spiral ganglion (14) is embedded in the modiolus. Its bipolar cells give rise to long central processes which become the fibers of the cochlear nerve (9), and short sensory processes to the spiral organ (13).

The osseous canal is divided into two compartments or cavities by the osseous spiral lamina (8) and the basilar membrane (membranous spiral lamina) (7). The osseous spiral lamina (8) projects from the modiolus partway across the spiral canal. The basilar membrane (7) continues from here to the spiral ligament (6) in the outer wall of the cochlea (5). The lower of the two compartments is the tympanic duct (scala tympani) (4). The upper compartment is the vestibular duct (scala vestibuli) (2). Both ducts pursue a spiral course to the apex of the cochlea; here they communicate with each other by a small orifice, the helicotrema (1).

The vestibular membrane (Reissner's membrane) (10) separates the vestibular duct (2) from the cochlear duct (scala media) (3) and forms the roof of the cochlear duct. The specialized cells for receiving sound vibrations and transmitting them as nerve impulses to the brain are in the spiral organ (of Corti) (13) which rests on the basilar membrane (7) on the floor of the cochlear duct. The tectorial membrane (12) overlies the spiral organ.

PLATE 114 (Fig. 2)

INNER EAR: COCHLEAR DUCT

The cochlear duct is shown in detail.

The outer wall of the cochlear duct is formed by the vascular stria (stria vascularis) (16), a stratified columnar epithelium, unusual in that it contains blood vessels and sends processes into the underlying connective tissue. The lamina propria is the spiral ligament (17, 19), consisting of collagenous fibers and fibroblasts with pigment, and supporting many blood vessels.

The roof of the cochlear duct (9) is formed by the vestibular membrane (6) which also separates it from the vestibular duct (7). The vestibular membrane extends from the spiral ligament (17) of the outer wall of the cochlea, at the upper extent of the vascular stria (15), to the thick periosteum of the osseous spiral lamina (4) near the point of origin of the limbus (5).

The spiral limbus (5) forms part of the floor of the cochlear duct (9). The limbus is a thickened mass of connective tissue continued from the periosteum (4) of the osseous spiral lamina (1) which bulges into the cochlear duct. It is supported by a lateral extension of the osseous spiral lamina (1). It is covered by an epithelium that appears columnar. The lateral extension of this epithelium is the tectorial membrane (10) which overlies the inner spiral sulcus (8) and part of the spiral organ (12) including its hair cells (11).

The basilar membrane (13) consists of a plate of vascularized connective tissue underlying a thinner plate of basilar fibers. On these basilar fibers rests the spiral organ (12). This organ extends from the spiral limbus (5) to the spiral ligament (17, 19).

The spiral organ (12) includes the highly specialized sensory cells or hair cells (11), spaces and tunnels, and supporting cells of several types. The deeply staining cells to the left of the hair cells are pillar cells which surround an inner tunnel. Various names are given to the other supporting cells.

From the bipolar cells of the spiral ganglion (3), peripheral (afferent) processes (2) course through channels in the osseous spiral lamina to terminate on the hair cells (11) of the spiral organ (12).

Plate 114

INNER EAR

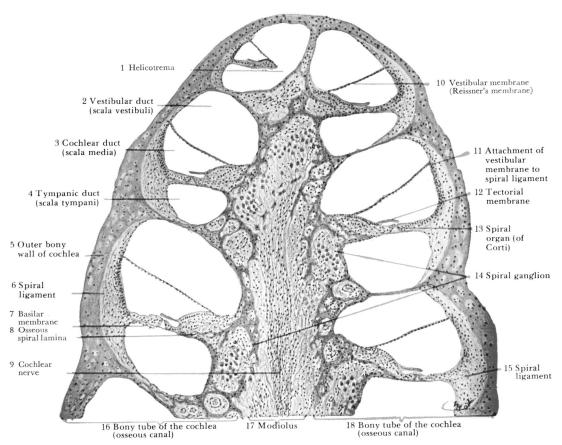

1 Helicotrema

2 Vestibular duct
(scala vestibuli)

3 Cochlear duct
(scala media)

4 Tympanic duct
(scala tympani)

5 Outer bony
wall of cochlea

6 Spiral
ligament

7 Basilar
membrane

8 Osseous
spiral lamina

9 Cochlear
nerve

10 Vestibular membrane
(Reissner's membrane)

11 Attachment of
vestibular
membrane to
spiral ligament

12 Tectorial
membrane

13 Spiral
organ (of
Corti)

14 Spiral ganglion

15 Spiral
ligament

16 Bony tube of the cochlea
(osseous canal)

17 Modiolus

18 Bony tube of the cochlea
(osseous canal)

Fig. 1. *Cochlea (vertical section).*
Stain: hematoxylin-eosin. 55×.

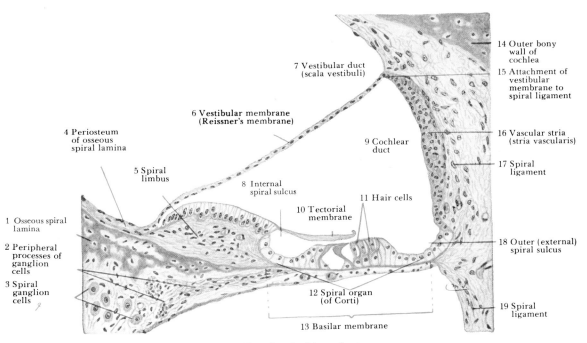

7 Vestibular duct
(scala vestibuli)

6 Vestibular membrane
(Reissner's membrane)

4 Periosteum
of osseous
spiral lamina

5 Spiral
limbus

8 Internal
spiral sulcus

1 Osseous spiral
lamina

2 Peripheral
processes of
ganglion
cells

3 Spiral
ganglion
cells

9 Cochlear
duct

10 Tectorial
membrane

11 Hair cells

12 Spiral organ
(of Corti)

13 Basilar membrane

14 Outer bony
wall of
cochlea

15 Attachment of
vestibular
membrane to
spiral ligament

16 Vascular stria
(stria vascularis)

17 Spiral
ligament

18 Outer (external)
spiral sulcus

19 Spiral
ligament

Fig. 2. *Cochlear duct.*
Stain: hematoxylin-eosin. 200×.

INDEX

A

ACIDOPHILIC cell (alpha cell) of hypophysis, 182–185
— — (oxyphilic cell) of parathyroids, 188, 189
Acinus, pancreatic, 162, 163
—serous, 162, 163
Adipose tissue, 34, 35
Adrenal glands, 190, 191
Adventitia (tunica adventitia)
—of blood vessels, 82–85
—of ductus deferens, 198, 199
—of rectum, 150, 151
—of seminal vesicle, 198, 199
—of ureter, 178, 179
—of vagina, 224, 225
Alpha cell (acidophilic cell) of hypophysis, 182–185
Alveolar ducts of lung, 168–171
—sac, 168, 169
Alveolus of lung, 168–171
—mucous, 118–121
—of mammary gland, 228–231
—of sebaceous glands, 103
—of tooth, 114, 115
—serous, 116–121
Amacrine cell, 238, 239
Ameloblast, 114, 115
Anal canal, 152, 153
Anal valve, 152, 153
Anorectal junction, 152, 153
Anterior chamber of eye, 236, 237
Anterior horn, 62–65, 74–77
— (ventral) median fissure, 74–77
Anterior lateral column of the spinal cord, 74, 75
Aorta, orcein stain, 84, 85
Appendix, 148, 149
Aqueous humor, 236, 237
Arachnoid of spinal cord, 76, 77
Argentaffin cell, 142, 143
Arrector pili muscle, 100–103
Artery, 68, 69, 82–85
—arcuate, 172, 173
—coiled, 214–219
—elastic, 84, 85
—elastic membrane of, 68, 69, 82–85
—endothelium of, 68, 69, 82–85

—hepatic, 154–157
—interlobular of kidney, 172–175
—pulmonary, of heart, 88, 89
— —of lung, 168–171
—renal, 172, 173
—transverse section of, 68, 69, 82–85
—tunica adventitia of, 68, 69, 82–85
—tunica media of, 68, 69, 82–85
Astrocytes (macroglia), 62–67
—perivascular, 66, 67
Auerbach's plexus (myenteric plexus), 130, 131, 140–143, 146–151
Axon, 62, 63, 68, 69–71
—hillock, 62, 63

B

BASEMENT membrane of ductus epididymidis, 196, 197
— —of epithelium, 14–21
— —of seminiferous tubules, 194, 195
— —of villus, 144, 145
Basilar membrane, 240, 241
Basket cell, 116–121, 162, 163
Basophil, 50, 51, 56, 57
Basophilic cell (beta cell) of hypophysis, 182–185
Beta cell (basophilic cell) of hypophysis, 182–185
Bile canaliculi, 156, 157
Bile duct, 154–159
Billroth, cords of (splenic cords), 98
Bipolar cell, 238, 239
Blind spot, 236, 237
Blood cells, Celani's stain of, 52, 53
— —development of, 54–57
— —of bone marrow, 54–57
— —of peripheral blood, 50–53
— —Pappenheim's stain of, 52, 53
— —supravital stain of, 52, 53
Blood platelet, 51–57
Bone, 40–49
—cancellous, 42, 43
—compact, 40, 41
—development of, 42–49
—endochondral, 44–47
—intracartilaginous, 44–47
—intramembranous, 42, 43
—marrow, 54–57

Bowman's capsule, 174, 175
—membrane, 234, 235
Brain, neuroglia of, 66, 67
Bronchiole, 168–171
—respiratory, 168–171
—terminal, 168–171
Bronchus, 168–171
Bruch's membrane, 238
Brunner's glands, 138–141
Brush border of kidney, 174, 175
Buck's fascia, 202

C

CAJAL's stain, 62, 63, 74, 75, 78, 79
Call-Exner vacuole, 206, 207
Calyx, 172, 173
Canaliculi of bone, 40, 41
—bile, of liver, 156, 157
—of teeth, 112, 113
Cardia, 128, 129
Cardiac glands, 128, 129
Cartilage, 36–39
—elastic, 38, 39
—fibrous, 38, 39
—hyaline, 36, 37
—tracheal, 166, 167
Cell, amacrine, 238, 239
—argentaffin, 142, 143
—bipolar, 238, 239
—centroacinar, 162, 163
—Küpffer, 156, 157
—Paneth, 142, 143
—parietal, 128–135
—Sertoli, 194, 195
Cementum of teeth, 112, 113
Centroacinar cell, 162, 163
Cerebellum, 78, 79
—cortical layers of, 78, 79
Cerebral cortex, layers of, 80, 81
Cervical glands, 222, 223
Cervix, 222, 223
Chief cells (principal cells) of para-
    thyroids, 188, 189
— —of stomach, 130–135
Chondrocyte, 36–39, 44, 45
Chorion, of placenta, 220, 221
Chorionic villi, 220, 221
Choroid layer of eye, 236–239
Chromaffin reaction, 190
Chromatophore, 238, 239
Chromophil cell, of hypophysis, 182–
    185

Chromophobe cell, of hypophysis, 182–
    185
Ciliary body of eye, 236
—muscle, 236, 237
—processes, 236, 237
—zonule, 236
Circular furrow, 110, 111
Circumvallate (vallate) papilla, 110,
    111
Cochlea, 240, 241
Cohnheim's fields, 60, 61
Coiled arteries, 214–219
Collagenous fibers, 28–35
Collecting tubules of kidney, 174–175
Column, anterior (ventral), of spinal
    cord, 74, 75
—posterior (dorsal), 74, 75
—of Clarke, 76, 77
—rectal, 150
Cones of retina, 238, 239
Conjunctiva, ocular, 236, 237
—palpebral, 232, 233
Connective tissue, 30–35
— —adipose, 34, 35
— —dense, 30–33
— —embryonic, 34, 35
— —loose, 28–31
Cornea, 234–237
—limbus of, 236, 237
Corona radiata, 206, 207
Corpora cavernosa of penis, 202, 203
Corpus albicans, 208, 209
—cavernosum urethrae, 202
—luteum, 208–211
—spongiosum, 202, 203
Corpuscle, Hassall's, 96, 97
—lamellar, 32, 33, 102, 103, 162, 163
—Meissner's, 100, 101
—Pacinian, 32, 33, 102, 103, 162, 163
—renal, 174, 175
—tactile, 100, 101
—thymic, 96, 97
Corti, organ of, 240, 241
—spiral ganglion of, 240, 241
Cortical labyrinth of kidney, 172, 173
Crypt, tonsillar, 94, 95
Crypts of Lieberkühn, 138–146
Cumulus oophorus, 204–207
Cuticle of hair, 102, 103

D

DARTOS tunic, 202, 203
Decidual cells, 220, 221

Del Rio Hortega's stain, 66, 67, 158, 159
Demilunes, 118–121
Dendrite, 62, 63, 74–77
Dental alveolus, 114, 115
–pulp, 114, 115
–sac, 114, 115
Dentin, 112–115
–tubules, 112, 113
Dermal papillae, 100–103
Dermis, 100–103
Descemet's membrane, 234, 235
Desmosomes, 14, 15, 100
Dorsal (posterior) median sulcus, 74–77
Duct, alveolar, of lung, 168–171
–bile, 154–157
–cochlear, 240, 241
–intercalated, of pancreas, 162, 163
– –of salivary glands, 116–121
–interlobular, of lacrimal gland, 234, 235
– –of mammary gland, 228–231
– –of pancreas, 162, 163
– –of salivary glands, 116–119
–lactiferous, 228–231
–papillary, 176, 177
–striated, 116–121
Ductus deferens, 198, 199
Duodenal (Brunner's) glands, 138–141
Dura mater, 76, 77

E

Ear, inner, 240, 241
Elastic fibers, 28–31
– –in aorta, 84, 85
Eleiden, 100
Enamel, 112–115
–prisms, 114, 115
–pulp, 114, 115
–rods, 112–115
Endocervix, 222, 223
Endometrium, 214–219
Endomysium, 60, 61
Endoneurium, 68–71
Endosteum, 42, 43
Endothelium of blood vessels, 82–84
Eosinophil, 50–57
Ependymal canal, 74–77
Epicardium, 86–89
Epidermis, 100–103
Epididymis, duct of, 196, 197
Epineurium, 70–73

Epithelium, 14–27
–ciliated, 20, 21
–germinal, of ovary, 204–209
–pavement, 14, 15
–peritoneal, 14, 15
–pseudostratified, 20, 21
–simple columnar, 16, 17
–simple squamous, 14, 15
–stratified squamous, 18, 19
–striated-bordered columnar, 16, 17
–transitional, 20, 21
– –of bladder, 180, 181
– –of ureter, 178, 179
Erector muscle, 100–103, 106, 107
Erythroblast, 54–57
Erythrocyte, 50–57
Esophageal glands, 122–125
Esophageal-cardiac junction, 128, 129
Esophagus, 122–127
–Mallory's stain of, 126, 127
–mucosa of, 122–127
–submucosa of, 122–127
–transverse section of, 122–127
–Van Gieson's stain of, 126, 127
Eye, retina of, 236–239
Eyelid, 232, 233

F

Fallopian tube (uterine tube), 212, 213
Fasciculus cuneatus, 74–77
Fasciculus gracilis, 74–77
Fat tissue, 34, 35
Fibroblasts, 28–31
Fibrous connective tissue, 28–33
Filiform papillae, 108, 109
Follicle, hair, 100–103
–ovarian, 204–209
–thyroid, 186, 187
Follicular cells, ovarian, 204–207
–fluid, 204–209
–theca, 204–209
Fornix of cervix, 222, 223
Fovea centralis, 236
Foveolae, 130–139
Fungiform papillae, 108–109

G

Gall bladder, 160, 161
Ganglion, dorsal root, 72, 73
–parasympathetic, 120, 121, 130, 131, 140–143
–spiral, 240, 241

—sympathetic, 72, 73
Gastric glands, 128–135
—pits, 128–137
Germinal center of a lymph node, 92–95
— —of spleen, 98, 99
—epithelium, 204–207
Gland, accessory lacrimal, 232, 233
—adrenal, 190, 191
—anterior lingual, 108, 109
—Brunner's (duodenal), 138–141
—cardiac, 128, 129
—cervical, 222, 223
—compound alveolar, 26, 27
— —tubuloalveolar, 24, 25
—duodenal, 138–141
—esophageal, 122–129
—gastric, 128–135
—intestinal, 138–153
—Krause's, 232, 233
—labial, 106, 107
—lacrimal, 234, 235
—Lieberkühn's (crypts of Lieberkühn), 138–153
—mammary, 228–231
—Meibomian, 232, 233
—Moll's, 232, 233
—of vallate papilla, 110, 111
—parathyroid, 188, 189
—pituitary, 182–185
—posterior lingual, 110–111
—prostate, 200, 201
—pyloric, 136–139
—salivary, 116–121
—sebaceous, 100–103
—simple tubular, 22, 23
—sudoriferous, 100, 105
—sweat, 100–105
—thyroid, 186, 187
—tubular, 22, 23
—uterine, 214–221
—von Ebner's, 110, 111
—Zeiss, 232, 233
Glomerulus of cerebellum, 78, 79
—of kidney, 172–175
Glycogen, liver, 158, 159
—vagina, 224, 225
Goblet cells, 16, 17, 20, 21
— —of large intestine, 146, 147
— —of lung, 168, 170
— —of rectum, 150–153
— —of small intestine, 138–145
Golgi stain of nerve cells, 64, 65
Granulocyte, 50–57

Granulosa lutein cell, 208–211
Gray commissure, 74–76
—matter, 62–65, 74–77

H

HAIR, 100–103
—bulb, 100–103
—follicle, 100–103
Hassall's corpuscle, 96, 97
Haversian canal, 40–43, 48, 49
—systems, 40–43, 48, 49
Heart: atrium, mitral valve, ventricle, 86, 87
—pulmonary artery, valve, ventricle, 88, 89
Helicotrema, 240, 241
Hemocytoblast, 54–57
Hemorrhoidal plexus, 152, 153
Hemorrhoids, 152
Henle's layer, 102, 103
—loop, 174–177
Hepatic artery, 154–157
—triad, 154, 155
Hilus of a lymph node, 90, 91
Histiocytes, 28, 29
Holocrine secretion, 102
Howship's lacuna, 46–49
Huxley's layer, 102, 103
Hypophysis, 182–185

I

ILEUM, 144, 145
Infundibular stalk of hypophysis, 182, 183
Intercalated disc, 60, 61
—duct, 116–121, 162, 163
Intercellular bridges of skin, 100, 101
Interglobular dentin, 112, 113
Interlobular duct of lacrimal gland, 234, 235
— —of mammary gland, 228, 231
— —of pancreas, 162, 163
— —of salivary glands, 116–119
Interstitial cell of testis, 192–195
Intestine, large, 146, 147
—small, 138–145
Involution of corpus luteum, 208, 209
Iris, 236, 237
Islet of Langerhans, 162, 163

J

JEJUNUM, 142, 143
Juxtaglomerular complex, 174, 175

K

KIDNEY, 172–177
Krause, gland of, 232, 233
Küpffer cells, 156, 157

L

LABIAL glands, 106, 107
Lacrimal gland, 234, 235
— —accessory, 232, 233
Lacteal, central, 144, 145
Lactiferous duct, 228–231
Lacunae of bone, 40–42, 46
—Howship's, 46–49
—of cartilage, 36–39
Lamellae of bone, 40
—circumferential, 40, 41
—inner circumferential, 40, 41
—interstitial, 40, 41
—outer circumferential, 40, 41
Lamina fusca (suprachoroid layer), 238, 239
—hepatic (plate), 154–157
—propria of appendix, 148, 149
— —of bladder, 180, 181
— —of cardia, 128, 129
— —of cervix, 222, 223
— —of ductus deferens, 198, 199
— —of esophagus, 122–127
— —of gall bladder, 160, 161
— —of large intestine, 146, 147
— —of lip, 106, 107
— —of rectum, 150, 151
— —of seminal vesicle, 198, 199
— —of small intestine, 140–143
— —of stomach, 130–137
— —of tongue, 108–111
— —of trachea, 166, 167
— —of ureter, 178, 179
— —of uterine tube, 212, 213
— —of uterus, 214–217
— —of vagina, 224, 225
Langerhans, islet of, 162, 163
Large intestine, 146, 147
Larynx, 164, 165
Lens, 236, 237
—suspensory ligament of, 236, 237
Lip, 106, 107
Lieberkühn, crypts (glands) of, 138–153
Lissauer's tract, 74–77
Liver, Altmann's stain of, 158, 159
—Best's carmine stain of, 158, 159
—del Rio Hortega's stain of, 158, 159
—glycogen in, 158, 159
—laminae (plates), 154–157
—lobules of, 154–159
—sinusoids of, 154–159
Lung, 168–171
Lutein cell, granulosa, 208–211
— —theca, 208–211
Lymph node, 90–93
Lymphatic nodules of appendix, 148, 149
— —of ileum, 144, 145
— —of lymph node, 90–93
— —of spleen, 98, 99
— —of tonsil, 94, 95
—vessels, 82, 83, 93
— —afferent, of node, 90, 91
— —efferent, of node, 90, 91
Lymphoblast, 94, 95
Lymphocytes, 50–53, 92–99
—proliferation of, 94–95

M

MACROPHAGES in bone marrow, 54, 55
—in connective tissue, 28, 29
—in liver (Küpffer cells), 156, 157
—in lymphatic tissue, 94, 95, 98, 99
—in placenta (Hofbauer cells), 220, 221
Macula lutea, 236, 237
Mallory-azan stain of heart, 88, 89
— —of nerve, 70, 71
Mammary gland, 228–231
Mast cells, 28, 29
May-Grünwald-Giemsa stain of blood, 50, 51, 56, 57
Medullary cord of a lymph node, 90–93
—ray of kidney, 172, 173
—sinus of a lymph node, 90–93
Megakaryocyte, 46–49, 54–57
Meibomian glands, 232, 233
Meissner's corpuscle, 100, 101
Membrana granulosa, 204–209
Mesenchymal cell, undifferentiated, 30, 31
Mesothelium of the peritoneum, 14, 15, 130, 180, 181
—pleural, 168, 169
—uterine tube, 212, 213
Mesovarium, 204, 205
Metamyelocyte, 54–57

Microglia, 62, 63, 66, 67
Mitochondria in liver cells, 158, 159
Modiolus, 240, 241
Moll, glands of, 232, 233
Monocyte, 51–53, 98, 99
Morgagni, columns of, 150
Mucosa, gastric, 130–137
—of bladder, 180, 181
—of ductus deferens, 198, 199
—of esophagus, 122–127
—of fundus or body, 130–133
—of gall bladder, 160, 161
—of lip, 106, 107
—of rectum, 150–153
—of seminal vesicle, 198, 199
—of trachea, 166, 167
—of uterine tube, 212, 213
—of vagina, 224, 225
Müller, tarsal muscle of, 236, 237
Muscle, cardiac, 60, 61
—ciliary, 236, 237
—orbicularis oculi, 232, 233
—Riolan's, 232, 233
—skeletal, 58–61
—smooth, 58–61
—tarsal, 232, 233
—thyroarytenoid, 164, 165
—trachealis, 166, 167
—vocalis, 164, 165
Muscularis externa of appendix, 148, 149
— —of esophagus, 122, 123, 126, 127
— —of large intestine, 146, 147
— —of small intestine, 140–145
— —of stomach, 130, 131
—mucosae of appendix, 148, 149
— —of esophagus, 122–127
— —of large intestine, 146, 147
— —of pylorus, 136, 137
— —of rectum, 150–153
— —of small intestine, 140–145
— —of stomach, 128–133
Myelinated nerve fibers, 68–71
—sheath, 68–71
Myelocyte, 54–57
Myocardium, 60, 61, 86–89
Myoepithelial cell, 102, 116, 118, 120, 121
Myofibrils, 58–61
Myometrium, 214–219

N

Nerve cell body, 62–65, 74–77
—fibers, 68–73
—transverse section of, 68–71
Nervous tissue, 62–81
Neurofibrils, 62, 63
Neuroglia (neuroglial cells), 66, 67
—of the hypophysis, 182, 183
Neurolemma, 68–71
Neuromotor cell, 74–77
Neurovascular bundle, 84, 85, 122
Neutral red, connective tissue, 28, 29
— —blood cells, 52, 53
Neutrophil, 50–57
Nissl bodies, 62, 63, 76, 77
Normoblast, 54–57
Nucleus dorsalis, 76, 77
—lateral sympathetic, 76–77

O

Odontoblast of teeth, 114, 115
Oligodendrocytes, 62, 63, 66, 67
—type I, 66, 67
—type II, 66, 67
Optic papilla, 236, 237
Ora serrata, 236, 237
Orbicularis oculi muscle, 232, 233
—oris muscle, 106, 107
Os, cervical, 222, 223
Osteoblast, 42–49
Osteoclast, 42, 43, 46–49
Osteon, 40, 41
Osteocyte, 40, 42, 43, 46–49
Ovarian follicle, 204–209
Ovary, 204–211
Ovum, 204–209
Oxyphilic cell (acidophilic cell) of parathyroids, 188, 189

P

Pacinian corpuscle in dermis, 102, 103
— —in pancreas, 162, 163
— —in tendon, 32, 33
Pancreas, 162, 163
—Gomori's stain of, 162, 163
Paneth cells, 142, 143
Papilla, circumvallate, 110, 111
—filiform, 108, 109
—fungiform, 108, 109
—of kidney, 172, 173, 176, 177
—optic, 236, 237
—vallate, 110, 111
Papillary ducts, 176, 177
Parasympathetic ganglion, 130, 131, 140–143, 147–151

Parathyroid glands, 188, 189
Parietal cells of stomach, 130–135
Parotid gland, 116, 117
Pars distalis of hypophysis, 182–185
—intermedia of hypophysis, 182, 183
—nervosa of hypophysis, 182, 183
—tuberalis of hypophysis, 182, 183
Penis, 202, 203
Perichondrium, 36–39, 44–47
Perimysium, 60-61
Perineurium, 68–73
Periosteum, 42–47
Peritoneum, 130, 131, 140–143
Peroxidase reaction, 52, 53
Peyer's patch, 144, 145
Pia mater, 74–77
Pilomotor muscle, 101–103
Pituitary gland (hypophysis), 182–185
— —azan stain of, 184, 185
Placenta, 220, 221
Plasma cell, 98, 99
Platelet, blood, 50–53
Polymorphous cell of cerebral cortex, 80, 81
Portal area of liver, 154, 155
Portal vein, 82, 83
— —of liver, 154–157
Posterior chamber of eye, 236, 237
Predentin, 114, 115
Principal cell (chief cell) of para-thyroids, 188, 189
Prostate gland, 200, 201
Pulmonary artery, heart, 88, 89
— —of lung, 168–171
Pulp cavity, tooth, 112, 113
Purkinje cell of cerebellum, 78, 79
—fibers of heart, 86–89
Pyloric glands of stomach, 136–139
Pyloric sphincter, 138, 139
Pyloric-duodenal junction, 138, 139
Pyramid of kidney, 172, 173
Pyramidal cell of cerebral cortex, 80, 81

R

Ranvier, nodes of, 68–71
Rectal columns, 150
Rectum, 150, 151
Red line of lip, 106
Red pulp of spleen, 98, 99
Reissner's (vestibular) membrane, 240, 241

Renal corpuscle, 172, 174
—papilla, 172, 173, 176, 177
—pyramid, 172, 173
Reticular cell of bone marrow, 54, 55
— —of lymph node, 92–95
—fibers of liver, 158, 159
— —of lymph node, 92, 93
Reticuloendothelium of liver, 156, 157
—of spleen, 98
Retina, 237–239
—blind, 236, 237
—ciliary, 236, 237
—iridial, 236
—optic, 236, 237
Retzius, lines of, 112, 113
Riolan, ciliary muscle of, 236, 237
Rods of retina, 238, 239
Root canal of tooth, 112, 113

S

Salivary glands, 116–121
Sarcolemma, 58, 60
Sarcoplasm, 58, 60, 61
Satellite cells, 72, 73
Scala tympani, 240, 241
—vestibuli, 240, 241
Schmidt-Lantermann clefts, 68, 69
Schreger, bands of, 112, 113
Schwann's sheath (neurolemma), 70–73
Sclera, 236–239
Sebaceous gland of eyelid, 232, 233
— —of integument, 100–103
— —of lip, 106, 107
— —of penis, 202, 203
Seminal vesicle, 198, 199
Seminiferous tubule, 192–195
Serosa of gall bladder, 160, 161
—of large intestine, 146, 147
—of small intestine, 140–143
—of stomach, 130, 131
Serous demilunes, 118–121
Sertoli cell, 194, 195
Sinusoids of bone marrow, 44, 45, 48, 49, 54, 55
—of liver, 154–159
—of lymph node, 90–95
—of spleen, 98, 99
Skin, Cajal's trichromic stain of, 100, 101
—of palm, 100, 101
—of scalp, 102, 103
Small intestine, 140–145

Spermatid, 194, 195
Spermatocyte, primary, 194, 195
—secondary, 194, 195
Spermatogonium, 194, 195
Spermatozoa, 194, 195
Sphincter, anal, 152, 153
—pyloric, 138, 139
Spinal cord, 74–77
—cervical region, 74, 75
—thoracic region, 76, 77
Spiral ganglion (of Corti), 240, 241
—lamina, osseous, 240, 241
—limbus, 240, 241
—sulcus, external, 240, 241
— —internal, 240, 241
Spleen, 98, 99
Splenic cords (of Billroth), 98, 99
Spongiocytes, 190, 191
Stain, acid fuchsin, mitochondria, 158, 159
—Altmann's, mitochondria in liver cells, 158, 159
—aniline blue, bone, 40, 41
— — —nerve, 70, 71
—azan, hypophysis, 184, 185
—Best's carmine, glycogen in liver, 158, 159
—Cajal's silver, cerebellum, 78, 79
— — —spinal cord, 74, 75
— — —nitrate, cerebral cortex, 80, 81
— —trichromic, skin, 100, 101
—cresyl blue, reticulocytes, 52, 53
—del Rio Hortega's, reticular fibers, 158, 159
—Fontana's silver, argentaffin cells, 142, 143
—hematoxylin-orcein, elastic cartilage, 38, 39
—iodine, glycogen in vaginal epithelium, 224, 225
—Janus green, mitochondria in leukocytes, 52, 53
—Mallory-azan, nerve fibers, 70, 71
— —Purkinje fibers, 88, 89
—May-Grünwald-Giemsa, peripheral blood, 52, 53
— — —bone marrow, 56, 57
—neutral red, leukocytes, 52, 53
— — —loose connective tissue, 28, 29
—orcein, aorta, 84, 85
—osmic acid, fat, 158, 159
— — —bile canaliculi, 156, 157
—Protargol, nerve fibers, 70, 71
—Van Gieson's, esophagus, 126, 127

—Verhoeff's, elastic fibers, 34, 35
Stellate cell of cerebellum, 78, 79
— —of liver (Küpffer cell), 156, 157
Stereocilia, 196–198
Stomach, chief cells of, 130–135
—foveolae of, 130–135
—fundus or body of, 130–135
—gastric pits of, 130–135
—gastric glands of, 130–135
—mucosa of fundus or body, 134, 135
—parietal cells of, 130–135
—pyloric mucosa of, 136, 137
—zymogenic cells of, 130–135
Stratum corneum, 100–103
—germinativum, 100–103
—granulosum, of skin, 100, 101
— —of ovary, 204–209
—lucidum, 100, 101
Striated border of epithelium, 16, 17, 142–145
Striated duct, 116–121
Striations in muscle, 58–61
Stroma, corneal, 234, 235
—ovarian, 204–209
Subcapsular sinus (marginal sinus) of node, 90–95
Subendothelium of artery, 82, 83
Sublingual gland, 120, 121
Submandibular gland, 118, 119
Submucosa, of appendix, 148, 149
—of esophagus, 122, 123, 126, 127
—of rectum, 150–153
—of small intestine, 140–145
—of stomach, 130, 131, 138, 139
Substantia propria of cornea, 234, 235
Sulcus, posterior median, of spinal cord, 74–77
Suprachoroid layer of eye, 238, 239
Sudoriferous gland, 100–103
Sweat gland, 100–103
Sympathetic ganglion, 72, 73, 84, 85
— —cells, 72, 73
—lateral nucleus, of spinal cord, 76, 77
— — —cells, 76, 77

T

Tactile corpuscle (Meissner's), 100, 101
Tarsal gland, 232, 233
Tarsal muscle, 232, 233
Tarsus, 232, 233
Taste buds, 110, 111
Tectorial membrane, 240, 241

Teeth, 112–115
—development of, 114, 115
Tendon, 32, 33
Testis, 192–195
Theca externa, 206, 207
—follicular, 204, 205
—interna, 206, 207
—lutein cell, 208–211
Thymus gland, 96, 97
Thyroarytenoid muscle, 164, 165
Thyroid gland, 186, 187
Tissue, adipose, 34, 35
—bone, 40–43
—cardiac, 60, 61
—cartilage, 36–39
—connective, 28–35
— —dense, 30–33
— —embryonic, 34, 35
— —loose, 28–31
—epithelial, 14–27
—fibrous connective, 28–33
—muscular, 58–61
—nervous, 62–73
—skeletal muscle, 58–61
—smooth muscle, 58–61
Tomes, fibers of, 114, 115
—granular layer of, 112–115
—layer of, 112–115
—processes of, 114, 115
Tongue, 108–111
—longitudinal section of, 108, 109
—transverse section of, 110, 111
Tonsil, laryngeal, 164, 165
—palatine, 94, 95
Tooth germ, permanent, 114, 115
Trabecula, of bone, 42, 43
—of lymph node, 90–93
—of penis, 202, 203
—of spleen, 98, 99
Trachea, 166, 167
—cartilage of, 36, 37
—glands of, 36, 37
Tracheal cartilage, 166, 167
—muscle, 166, 167
Tubules, collecting, of kidney, 174–177
—distal convoluted, 174, 175
—proximal convoluted, 174, 175
—seminiferous, 192–195
Tunica adventitia of an artery, 82–85
—albuginea, of ovary, 204–207
— —of penis, 202, 203
— —of testis, 192, 193
—intima, 82–85
—media, 82–85

U

Ureter, 178, 179
Urethra, cavernous, 202, 203
—prostatic, 200, 201
Urinary bladder, 180, 181
Uterine glands, 214–219
Uterine tube, 212, 213
Uterus, follicular phase of, 214, 215
—menstrual phase of, 218, 219
—progravid phase of, 216, 217
Uvea, 236, 237

V

Vagina, 224, 225
—exfoliate cytology (smears), 236, 237
—glycogen in cells of, 224, 225
Vas deferens (ductus deferens), 198, 199
Vasa vasorum, 82–85
Vein, central, of liver, 154–159
—interlobular, of kidney, 172–175
—intralobular (central) of liver, 154–157
—portal, 82, 83
— —of liver, 154–159
—renal, 172, 173
—transverse section of, 82–85
—tunica adventitia of, 82–85
— —intima of, 82
— —media of, 82–85
Ventral (anterior) median fissure, 74–77
Ventricle, of heart, 86–89
—of larynx, 164, 165
Vermiform appendis (appendix), 148, 149
Vestibular (Reissner's) membrane, 240, 241
Villus, of intestine, 16, 17, 138–145
—of placenta, 220, 221
Visceral pleura of lung, 168, 169
Vitreous chamber of eye, 236, 237
—humor, 236, 237
Vocal cord (vocal ligament), 164, 165
—folds, false, 164, 165
— —true, 164, 165

W

White matter of spinal cord, 74–77
—of eye, 236
—pulp of spleen, 98, 99

Z

ZEISS, glands of, 232, 233
Zinn, zonule of, 232
Zona glomerulosa of adrenals, 190, 191
—fasciculata of adrenals, 190, 191
—pellucida of ovum, 206, 207
—reticularis of adrenals, 190, 191
Zymogenic cells of stomach, 132-135
— —of pancreas, 162, 163
— —of small intestine (Paneth cells), 142, 143